THE *REAL* TRUTH

ABOUT

AGING

A SURVIVAL GUIDE FOR
Older Adults and Caregivers

NEIL SHULMAN, MD
MICHAEL A. SILVERMAN, MD, MPH
ADAM G. GOLDEN, MD, MBA

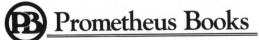

Prometheus Books

59 John Glenn Drive
Amherst, New York 14228–2119

Published 2009 by Prometheus Books

Inquiries should be addressed to
Prometheus Books
59 John Glenn Drive
Amherst, New York 14228–2119
VOICE: 716–691–0133, ext. 210
FAX: 716–691–0137
WWW.PROMETHEUSBOOKS.COM

13 12 11 10 09   5 4 3 2 1

Library of Congress Cataloging-in-Publication Data

Shulman, Neil.
    The real truth about aging : a survival guide for older adults and caregivers / by Neil Shulman, Michael A. Silverman, and Adam G. Golden.
        Includes bibliographical references and index.
        ISBN: 978–1–59102–719–5 (pbk. : alk. paper)
        1. Aging. 2. Aging—Physiological aspects. I. Title.
QP86 .S527 2009
612.6/7 22   2009005802

Printed in the United States of America on acid-free paper

THE *REAL* TRUTH

ABOUT

AGING

DISCLAIMER

The information in this book is intended for general information. The information does not imply an endorsement of any drugs or medical procedures. This book is not a substitute for medical advice from a doctor. Always consult a physician about all issues relating to your health.

CONTENTS

Why we age has been a question that has confused humankind throughout history. We simplify many of the complicated concepts regarding the molecular mechanisms associated with aging.

Many changes to the different organ systems occur with aging. These age-related changes often play a role in the development of many health issues that develop in a person's later years.

What steps can you take to lead a healthier life? We describe the major preventive tests that are currently available. Some tests are simple and may lead to interventions that allow you to live longer and healthier. Other tests may be expensive, involve potential complications, and/or have no proven benefit. We will tell you which ones are appropriate for both the healthy and the frail older adult.

Many products claim to reverse aging and improve one's memory, strength, and sex drive. We will give you the tools you need to analyze these claims for yourself.

We review the latest research regarding the effectiveness and potential side effects of "anti-aging" hormones (growth hormone, testosterone, and DHEA).

Millions of seniors take vitamins, herbs, and other supplements for the prevention of specific diseases and to improve their overall health. What does the research say about the benefits of these products? You may be surprised by what you find.

It is well known that exercise is good for the mind as well as the body. However, knowing which exercises are safe and effective for older adults is not so simple. An exercise routine designed for young adults may lead to injuries for seniors. This chapter will review the precautions that elderly patients need to be aware of before starting an exercise program.

Seniors account for about 12.5 percent of the population but they consume over 30 percent of all prescription medications. This chapter will provide an explanation of:

- *why many seniors are prescribed too many drugs*
- *why seniors are at an increased risk of medication side effects*
- *which drugs are considered dangerous for seniors to use*
- *the potential problems with the Medicare Part D prescription benefit*

PART 2. THE TWENTY-FIRST-CENTURY HEALTHCARE SYSTEM

As people live longer, there will be more people who are unable to take care of themselves. Many seniors will need to be moved to assisted living facilities or to nursing homes. Today's hospitals and nursing homes are far different from those of yesteryear. These facilities are now taking care of patients who are older, frailer, and sicker than ever. This chapter discusses the major changes in our healthcare system and its impact on the frail elderly. We also discuss other options for long-term care besides nursing homes.

Today's doctors are expected to see more patients in less time. Elderly patients with multiple health problems may be uncomfortable with this fast-paced setting. This chapter will provide you with valuable tips to help you maximize the limited time you have to see your doctor.

Many different healthcare professionals are involved in the care of the elderly. This chapter defines the level of training and the responsibilities for each of the following professions and how they can help your elderly parent:

- *nursing assistants*
- *nurses*
- *physicians*
- *dieticians*
- *home health services*
- *pharmacists*
- *physical/occupational/speech therapists*
- *social workers*
- *case managers*

Many older adults fear being placed in a nursing home more than they fear death. The perception by many in the public is that nursing homes are dirty places where residents are abused, neglected, and left to die. This chapter explores the reasons why so many negative stereotypes exist. Many resources that discuss how to choose a nursing home provide inaccurate and misleading information. We provide the reader with a realistic list of issues to consider when choosing a nursing home.

While hospitals provide lifesaving care for millions of Americans each year, these medical centers are often dangerous places for frail elderly patients. The modern hospital is an unfamiliar environment that can be especially frightening for those with dementia or poor vision. The hospitalized senior is at high risk for becoming delirious, falling, developing bedsores, and acquiring antibiotic-resistant infections. Knowing whom to turn to for help or for answers to your questions can often be difficult to figure out. This chapter will walk you through the modern hospital system and provide you with insights about what to expect.

PART 3. CARING FOR THE FRAIL SENIOR

Falls are common and may lead to a variety of injuries, including head injuries and hip fractures. Falls usually do not have one single cause but rather are the result of a complicated process involving a variety of age-related body changes, environmental factors, and medical conditions. This chapter will discuss the things you can do to lower your risk of falling.

Osteoporosis weakens your bones. In many cases it can lead to fractures of the bones in the hip, spine, and wrist. This chapter explains how osteoporosis is diagnosed and what you can do to slow down the effects of this disease.

Many seniors are sent to nursing homes for rehabilitation. Others may receive therapy at home or at an outpatient center. Their progress will often determine to what extent they will be able to take care of themselves once they recover. This chapter will discuss:

- *the basic structure of a rehabilitation program*
- *the special issues involved with rehabilitation following hip or knee surgery*
- *the prevention of contractures*

Family and caregivers need to know how to safely help frail older adults with the basic activities of daily living. We will also discuss the proper use of mobility aids (walkers, canes, and wheelchairs).

The elderly are not only at higher risk for developing infections, but they are also more likely to die from infection. This chapter will discuss causes and treatments of the four most common infections in the senior population:

- *skin infections*
- *pneumonia*
- *urinary tract infections*
- *infectious diarrhea*

Malnutrition *and* starvation *are terms that may elicit strong emotions and suspicion of abuse or neglect. Such suspicions usually do not reflect the truth regarding malnutrition in the frail elderly. Malnutrition is often the result of multiple poorly understood age-related organ changes, medical illnesses, and psychological issues. This chapter will discuss the difficulties in evaluating this problem. It will also provide an overview of current treatments.*

Feeding tubes were initially developed for use in children and in patients with cancer of the throat and esophagus. Today, they are often used to provide nutrition to elderly patients with end-stage dementia. There are many misconceptions on the part of families and even many healthcare professionals regarding the benefit of this "medical intervention." Feeding tubes can lead to a variety of medical complications.

About half of frail older adults cannot control their urine. We cover the causes and treatment options for this discouraging problem.

Depression is often difficult to diagnose in the elderly. Older adult patients may only exhibit signs of anxiety or physical symptoms, such as weakness, fatigue, or pains in the abdomen, chest, or back. Patients with dementia may not have any complaints but manifest their depression in the form of a variety of abnormal behaviors. This chapter will discuss the difficulties in diagnosing depression in this population, as well as the importance of treating this disease. An explanation of the common medications used to treat depression will be reviewed. Misconceptions regarding electroconvulsive therapy will also be discussed.

By the age of eighty-five, 40 percent of people will have a diagnosis of dementia. While Alzheimer's disease is the most common cause of dementia, other forms do exist. In this chapter we discuss the major categories of dementia. We also discuss current therapies for the prevention and treatment of dementia.

Most patients with dementia will eventually exhibit one or more abnormal behaviors. In fact, for many families it is the behavioral problems rather than the loss of memory that is most troublesome. This chapter will give you the insights you need to address the following behavioral problems:

- *agitation*
- *anxiety*
- *depression*
- *hallucinations/delusions*
- *sleep disturbances*
- *wandering*

This chapter will explain why so many seniors have trouble sleeping. A variety of age-related body changes, medical illnesses, and medications play a role in this common problem. Sleep problems can often be addressed without the use of medications. If you do need medication, be careful! Many sleep medications have harmful side effects.

Bedsores, also known as decubitus ulcers *or* pressure ulcers, *frequently occur in the nursing home or hospital setting. Many people are appalled when they hear that these bedsores were "allowed to happen." Many books will tell you that bedsores are usually the result of poor care. This chapter will explain the real reasons why some frail elderly develop bedsores. We will explain why they are not only difficult to prevent but also difficult to treat.*

Too often, pain is not addressed because it's thought to be a normal part of the aging process. The failure to address pain can have serious psychological and health consequences. We discuss:

* *the benefits and potential side effects of commonly used pain medications, as well as nondrug options*

PART 4. PLANNING AHEAD BEFORE IT'S TOO LATE

The longer you live, the more money you will need for your retirement. The financial collapse of 2007–2009 did not help seniors. Money carefully set aside to last twenty years may not last for ten years. Investment uncertainties and increasing healthcare costs are two of the many factors that make financial planning difficult. Most people are not ready. This chapter will tell you what to expect and how to prepare for this financial challenge.

The factors that place some older drivers at risk for auto accidents are often quite subtle and may be difficult to recognize. This chapter will provide tips for recognizing if there is a problem and will also give advice on what to do once a problem is recognized.

Following retirement, many older adults have more free time to visit family and to travel. Whether they will be spending several months in another city with family or vacationing in exotic locations, they need to consider important health issues.

With millions of seniors living in Florida, the Carolinas, and the Gulf Coast, the threat of hurricanes is something that we can no longer ignore. The affected regions usually have several days to prepare. Other disasters, such as earthquakes and terrorism, occur without any warning. Having a disaster plan may mean the difference between life and death. This chapter will give the information that seniors need to survive.

Advanced directives allow patients an opportunity to express their healthcare wishes before they are no longer able to make those decisions for themselves. Advanced directives can take many forms, such as a living will or a healthcare surrogate. This chapter will review the important issues regarding the different types of advanced directives. We will also discuss how patients are assessed for their decision-making capabilities.

Death is a reality we all must eventually face. The last days can be quite frightening for family members to watch. For many, this can be a difficult time that is full of fear and guilt. This chapter will discuss how hospice can help both the patient and the family. It also reviews what to expect and what can be done to try to make the patient more comfortable.

INTRODUCTION

"Be careful about reading health books. You may die of a misprint."

Mark Twain (1835–1910)

As life expectancy continues to increase, millions of seniors are living well into their eighties and nineties. In fact, people eighty-five years and older represent the fastest-growing segment of the population. Many suffer from multiple medical illnesses, and others are already at the stage where they are losing the ability to take care of themselves.

To avoid becoming sick and disabled before they reach old age, people want to know what they can do to stay healthy. Many of these same people are already caregivers for an elderly spouse or parent.

Dr. Neil Shulman, a former nursing home director, and geriatric experts Dr. Michael Silverman and Dr. Adam Golden have written *The Real Truth about Aging* to be a survival guide for this difficult and inevitable phase of life. This book provides REAL answers in clear, easy-to-understand language that will help seniors and their families prepare for the challenging road ahead.

As doctors of geriatric medicine, we have extensive experience caring for seniors. Over the years, we have spoken to thousands of patients and their families. They come to us with many questions, such as "Do anti-aging therapies work?" or "When should grandpa stop driving?" Unfortunately, the answers to these questions are complicated and there are often no simple cures or fountains of youth. In many cases good clinical research does not exist to answer these questions.

Finding a doctor to discuss these issues is not easy. Physicians who specialize in geriatric medicine are hard to find. Most other physicians will either be too busy or may not even know the answers themselves. We have discovered that many topics regarding aging are never taught to doctors during their medical school or residency training, and much of what is taught is actually wrong. We suspect that if you read this book, you will probably know more about geriatric medicine than your doctor.

WHAT IS GERIATRIC MEDICINE?

Geriatric medicine is the branch of medicine that specializes in the clinical care of the elderly patient. It is a field of medicine that focuses on the needs of the entire patient. For example, as geriatricians we understand that older adults are usually suffering from multiple chronic illnesses, take a high number of medications, and remain at high risk for dementia, falls, depression, malnutrition, and bedsores.

WHAT IS THE DIFFERENCE BETWEEN GERIATRICS AND GERONTOLOGY?

We get asked this question a lot. *Geriatrics*, or geriatric medicine, is the medical subspecialty that focuses on the assessment and treatment of illnesses in the elderly. *Gerontology* is a term that refers to the study of a variety of non-medical, aging-related fields. For example, gerontology encompasses animal research looking for genes that increase longevity, as well as the social science (social work, psychology) and economic issues of the older adult population.

HOW IS THIS BOOK DIFFERENT FROM ALL THE OTHER BOOKS ON AGING?

Numerous books and Web sites focus on the issues of aging. Most resources either focus on healthy aging or on caregiving issues. In the first category are the resources that offer the "secrets" to a long and healthy life. These books concentrate on the benefits of healthy diets, nutritional supplements, and anti-aging therapies. The second category tries to address the concerns of families caring for frail older adults.

Most books present oversimplified and inaccurate explanations of very complicated healthcare issues. Every problem seems to have a simple cause and a simple solution. The reader walks away with a false sense of personal empowerment. We believe that personal empowerment comes from *both* knowing what you can do to stay healthy and a realistic awareness of what to expect as you grow old.

The idea for the format of this book came about through a discussion that Dr. Shulman had with his cousin Dr. Michael Silverman, who was on active duty with the United States Army. Dr. Silverman mentioned that he had reviewed many survival guides used to prepare soldiers for what they would encounter in new and often strange environments. As a geriatrician, he realized that there were no senior health resources that he felt comfortable recommending to patients and families to prepare them for what was often a new and strange environment—the uncharted territory of aging. The two doctors then enlisted the assistance of geriatric expert Dr. Adam Golden and began to write a survival guide for seniors and caregivers.

This book draws on our extensive geriatric experience as well as an exhaustive analysis of the current medical literature. We do not sugarcoat any issues. If people are faced with making life-and-death decisions, they need to know the straight facts. This is the first book to call a spade a spade. We will expose many geriatric myths and explain why, for example:

- Anti-aging hormone therapies could shorten your life
- Most antioxidant vitamin studies have shown no benefits in humans
- Older adults need to be very careful when starting a yoga regimen
- Many seniors are overmedicated and others are not getting enough medication
- Many primary care doctors don't want new Medicare patients
- Many people are afraid of ending up in a nursing home
- Lots of bedsores are not preventable
- Some Medicare Part D providers put price over drug safety
- Many seniors would rather take the risk of dying than being shipped off to a hurricane shelter
- The drugs used to treat Alzheimer's disease often do not work
- Social Security will place a huge financial burden on tomorrow's workforce
- Living wills are often outdated and so vague that they may be useless

This book has four parts. The first eight chapters focus on the aging process and what seniors can do to stay healthy. The second part helps seniors and their families understand the modern and often confusing healthcare system. The third part of this book provides information about the common problems affecting frail older adults. The final part highlights what seniors and families need to do to plan ahead. While this book is written for patients and their families, we recognize that healthcare professionals will also find this information helpful.

If you learn anything from reading this book, let it be that for many of the medical problems that seniors face there are no simple answers. The issues are often complicated and the truth is that even with many years of experience, geriatric physicians do not know all the reasons that elderly people become frail. In many cases, good clinical research is lacking.

You may be asking yourself, "If the experts in geriatric medicine don't have the answers, what are seniors and their families supposed to do?" Although we do not have all the answers, we will give you the straight facts we do have so that you and your family can prepare for the challenges ahead and avoid being exploited by so-called experts who claim to have all the answers.

We apologize if some of this information seems discouraging; it may seem like we are presenting an overwhelmingly negative body of facts. We don't want people to lose sight of the positives that come with aging, such as having free time to pursue one's interests, and let's not forget senior discounts.

However, this book is not about the lighter side of aging. Our aim is to give you the real nuts and bolts of what you are likely to experience as you age. You already know the positives. We'd like to enlighten you to what you may not know already, namely, the complex physical reality of aging.

Part 1

FIGHTING THE AGING CLOCK

Chapter 1

WHAT DOES IT MEAN
TO GROW OLD?

*"Age is not a particularly interesting subject. Anyone can
get old. All you have to do is live long enough."*
Groucho Marx (1890–1977)

While Groucho's humor is timeless, we believe that this statement is
partially incorrect. The study of aging is an exciting field of science that incorporates the latest research in molecular genetics, medicine, and
nutrition.

In order to make sense of the information in this book, we first need to
give you a foundation about what aging means and its effects on the different
organs of the body.

WHAT IS AGING?

When we look at a person who is elderly, we see many characteristics that tell
us the person is old. It may be the white hair, the wrinkles, or the stooped posture that conveys to us we are looking at an old person.

Although *Merriam-Webster's Dictionary* defines aging as "to become old,"
this definition does not really help us understand what it is.[1] We prefer to use
a more scientific approach that defines several characteristics of aging:

- Increased risk of dying
- Increased risk of disease
- Changes in tissues and organs
- Decreased ability of the body to respond to environmental stresses, such as changes in the temperature, diet, and infectious organisms[2]

In the past we distinguished between the changes of "normal aging" and the changes that result from chronic illnesses, such as diabetes and hypertension. In reality, this distinction is quite blurry. The changes that occur with normal aging may increase the risk of developing chronic illnesses. Changes to the heart and blood vessels, for instance, will increase the risk of developing high blood pressure and suffering a heart attack. On the flip side, many chronic illnesses often speed up or exacerbate the aging process of a particular organ or tissue. Diabetes, for example, can speed up age-related changes to the heart and other organs.

IS THERE AN AGING CLOCK?

The notion that the length of a person's life is predetermined is an idea that people have thought about throughout history. In recent years scientists have shown that our DNA provides genetic signals that tell individual cells to stop dividing or die. From the day we are born we are getting older. No one has figured out how to stop cells from aging. Even the cells of the healthiest person will eventually die.

Is there anything we can do to prevent our cells from killing themselves? There is one scenario where these programs are turned off. It is called cancer. But of course cancer brings its own threats to our longevity. Some scientists believe that cancer cells arise when a cell no longer has the normal mechanisms to eventually stop dividing and die.[3] This is important because many books on aging will tell you that you must try to stop or reverse the aging process. Not only are these goals unobtainable, but they could also cost you a lot of money and endanger your health. Instead, our focus is going to be on healthy aging.

ARE THERE SPECIFIC GENES THAT DETERMINE HOW LONG WE LIVE?

There is no easy answer to this commonly asked question. We know that genes play some role. People whose parents lived to be one hundred are more likely to live longer than those whose parents died at earlier ages.

Scientists have discovered more than a dozen genes in yeast and fruit flies that are involved in aging. Whether these genes have any role in human longevity at all remains unknown.

Unfortunately, just because a gene plays a role in the longevity of a fruit fly does not mean that it will play a similar role in humans. Part of the problem is that the genetics involved with a human are infinitely more complicated. The environment a human lives in is also more complicated and variable than that of a yeast cell living in a Petri dish in a research laboratory.

So has anyone discovered the gene responsible for aging in humans? The answer is a definite NO! There is no single aging gene, per se. Rather, our best guess is that many genes are responsible for our growing old. How these many genes work together remains a complete mystery.

DOES EVOLUTION PLAY A ROLE IN AGING?[4]

When we think about Darwin's concept of evolution, we also need to remember that this theory relates to the ability of an animal to reproduce. Darwin's theory is based on survival of the fittest—individual organisms that are able to survive and thrive will pass their genes on to the next generation. Darwin showed those traits that allow an organism to reproduce more effectively will be "selected for." However, the theory of evolution may not be related to longevity. Natural selection enables the strongest organisms to survive through their reproductive years. It does not necessarily work to improve how long the animal will live once it stops reproducing. For example, the traits that allow a silverback gorilla to be more muscular will improve his chances of mating, but they will not make him live longer. The point is that there is no evolutionary selection pressure that would allow organisms to live beyond their reproductive years. Therefore, the genetic factors that allow a fruit fly to live longer do not have to be the same as in other animals or in humans.

WHAT IS THE *FREE RADICAL THEORY OF AGING?*

Like a car engine, our bodies require fuel in order to work. Where does this fuel for the body come from? It comes from the food we eat. In the process of breaking down food into fuel, our cells make a bunch of molecules known as *oxidants*, or *free radicals*. Free radicals are used by the cell to carry out many of its normal functions. However, if the levels of these molecules get too high, the cell's DNA, proteins, and membranes can get damaged. Fortunately, the cells in your body make a variety of enzymes that work to neutralize these oxidants and to keep the amount of damage to a minimum.

In order for these enzymes to work well, they need to partner with a *cofactor*. Cofactors include the vitamins A, C, E, beta-carotene, and the vitamin B family. (We discuss these vitamins at length in chapter 6.)

The *free radical*, or *oxidative stress theory* on aging holds that the greater the amount of exposure to toxic substances, the greater the free radical damage to the cell. At a certain point, this damage will make it harder for cells to multiply or even survive. The theory holds that the better these "clean-up" enzymes work, the less free radical damage will occur and the longer a life the organism will live.

While free radicals are damaging, don't forget that the over the years your body takes a beating. Like a set of tires that have been driven for eighty thousand miles, you will certainly see signs of wear and tear regardless of how carefully you've driven. With a decreased ability to repair damage and make new cells, your tissue and organs will accumulate the wear and tear of aging.

DOES THE FREE RADICAL THEORY CORRECTLY EXPLAIN WHY PEOPLE AGE?

The free radical theory of aging makes a lot of sense and has much research to support it.[5] Fruit flies and mice with genetic mutations that increase the ability of the enzymes to remove free radicals often live longer than those without these mutations. Most books on aging will highlight this exciting experimental data in an attempt to explain why you need to be eating specific antioxidant foods and taking specific antioxidant vitamins. A number of authors suggest that the research perfectly supports this theory.

The **real truth** is that many good research studies do not show a relationship between free radical damage and aging.[6] Other studies do not show a correlation between the amount of food metabolized and the amount of oxidative damage that results.[7] We mention these contradictory studies not to suggest that the free radical theory is without some merit but to show that the molecular mechanisms responsible for aging are infinitely complex. We should therefore not be surprised that human research studies involving people using antioxidant vitamins have failed to show that they live longer.[8]

ARE THERE ANY OTHER THEORIES ON AGING?

While science has given us some insights, no one theory can neatly and completely explain how and why people age. Scientists have noted for years that many proteins in the body become damaged, causing them to work less efficiently. In addition, scientists believe that the weakening of the immune system also plays a role in the aging process. As the immune system weakens, the body becomes more susceptible to a variety of cancers and illnesses.

Many scientists have noted dramatic changes in the levels of certain hormones with aging. Do these changes play a role in the aging process? (We discuss this at length in chapter 5.)

Ultimately, the aging process is complex and we have much to learn. Beware of anyone who claims to have the simple answer.

REALIZE YOU CAN'T STOP THE BODY FROM AGING!

We have no way to escape the natural process of aging. While you may be able to slow down the rate a bit, all cells must eventually die or stop dividing. As the cells die, all tissues and organs in the body will get weaker. At a certain point, even the youthful Dick Clark stopped looking like America's oldest teenager and started looking his age.

The important point here is that no matter how successful you are at slowing down the aging process, it is inevitable that at some point in the future you will look in the mirror and notice that you are staring at an old person.

AT WHAT AGE IS SOMEONE CONSIDERED A GERIATRIC PATIENT?

This is a question that we are often asked. From a medical standpoint, there is no specific age, per se. In the United States, the age of sixty-five seems to be a landmark age. This is the age when you qualify for Medicare. Many people also begin collecting their Social Security at this age. This is also the age when many companies force their employees to retire.

WHAT IS SO SPECIAL ABOUT THE AGE OF SIXTY-FIVE?

From a medical standpoint, the answer is actually nothing. There is no specific change that occurs in your body on your sixty-fifth birthday. The real reason the United States began using sixty-five as the age for retirement and paying out Social Security is that we were copying the Germans.[9] In 1889 Germany passed the Old Age and Disability Insurance Bill. This piece of legislation provided a pension for workers who reached the age of seventy. In 1916 it was lowered to sixty-five. If you think that the Germans were being generous, consider that the average life expectancy at that time was only forty-five. So if you lived twenty years past the average life expectancy, the government threw you a bone.

THE ELDERLY ARE NOT ALL ALIKE

The term *senior citizen* is often used for all people over sixty-five years of age. Other terms that may apply to this large segment of the population include *elderly*, *geriatrics*, and *older adults*. Because we are all aging at a different rate, one must be careful about labeling all people sixty-five and over. A sixty-seven-year-old man who still works and plays golf is quite different from a ninety-two-year-old woman who lives in a nursing home and is unable to take care of herself. While we are going to discuss normal aging, we need to always remember that the frail older adults who live in nursing homes are often a whole generation older than the healthy elderly people we see playing golf or tennis daily.

One of our aims is to highlight the differences between these two segments of the senior citizen population. The medical literature refers to the former group by using the adjectives *community-dwelling* or *healthy*, while referring to the latter as *frail*.

WHAT DOES IT MEAN TO BE FRAIL?

We will be using the term *frail* often in this book. The word represents a concept that, like pornography, is best defined as *you will know it when you see it*. We all have a picture in our mind of what a frail person looks like. Although every reader may have a different image of what that means, as geriatricians we think of a frail person as someone who is very far along in the aging process.

A college football player has strong bones that can withstand the impact of getting tackled hundreds of times. The last time we checked we did not see any ninety-five-year-old men playing football for the University of Miami Hurricanes. A ninety-five-year-old's bones may be so thinned out by osteoporosis that they will break if the person merely slips in the locker room.

Marathon runners have lungs and a heart that are strong enough for them to run the 26.2 mile distance. In contrast, our ninety-five-year-old will likely get short of breath walking up several flights of stairs.

Frailty should not be thought of as an all-or-nothing phenomenon. It is not like being pregnant. A woman is either pregnant or not pregnant. There is no in between. In contrast, elderly people can be a little frail or very frail. Some ninety-year-old men may need a little help fixing their ties and tuxedos while others are sequestered day and night in bed at a nursing home. People don't just wake up one day and become frail. This is usually a gradual process.

WHY IS IT IMPORTANT TO KNOW ABOUT THESE CHANGES?

This concept of frailty is important in understanding many of the problems that arise in geriatrics. Many times a family member will say something like "My mother was doing so well until she came into the nursing home," or "My father was doing so well until he got sick and came to the hospital." "Doing well" may not be the best term to use in these situations. "Barely getting by," in many cases, is the more accurate description. The person whose body is gradually deteriorating may not notice any difference until it goes below some threshold level.[10] For the person who is "just getting by," the stress on the body from an acute illness may be too much.

Chapter 2

WHAT HAPPENS TO
OUR BODIES AS WE AGE?

"Every day you get older—that's a law."
Butch Cassidy and the Sundance Kid

To a certain extent we all fear getting old. With aging, we may fear that our looks will fade or that we will not be able to do the things we once enjoyed. The focus of this chapter is to discuss the major changes to the different organ systems that occur with aging. It is only through an understanding of these changes that we can begin to discuss our fears about growing old and the reality of what frail elderly people will face.

While it is true that we do get older each day, the age-related changes that we will describe in the following pages proceed at different rates in each person. It is also important to realize that in any specific individual the changes occurring in each organ system may be proceeding at different rates. In other words, in one person, the kidneys may be aging faster than the lung tissue, whereas the opposite may be true in another person.

To make matters even more complicated, many of the age-related changes discussed below were discovered by comparing young people to older individuals.[1] Since the younger patients grew up in a different era, some of the differences that we see may not be due to age alone. Changes in diet, the environment, and modern medical care may also play a role.

DOES MY BRAIN STILL WORK?

The size of the brain decreases to a certain extent with aging. This shrinkage, which can be viewed on MRI and CT scans, is referred to by the terms *cerebral atrophy* or *brain atrophy*. This shrinkage is due to a decrease in the size and the number of nerve cells.

Balance and reflexes change with aging. The ability of the nerves to sense hot and cold objects with our hands and feet also decreases with age. So be careful in the kitchen!

There is also some slowing of our thought processes. As you get older, there is a decrease in your ability to learn new things and remember information. This natural slowing of our mental abilities and reflexes should not be mistaken for Alzheimer's disease. Alzheimer's disease and other forms of dementia are not part of normal aging.

WILL I STILL BE ABLE TO BREATHE?

The chest wall consists of the rib cage and the muscles of the chest and back. When we take a breath, our chest rises and our diaphragm (the wall of muscle that separates the chest from the abdominal cavity) lowers. This expansion of the chest wall allows the lungs to expand.

As we age, the ability of the chest wall to expand decreases. Part of the problem is a result of the osteoarthritis that can form in the small joints between the ribs and the sternum (breastbone).

Other factors also play a part. The muscles between the ribs shrink in size as we get older. These muscles are needed to pull on the ribs in order to expand the chest wall. If that wasn't bad enough, many elderly people have humps in their backs from osteoporosis. The abnormal hump is due to curvature of the spine, which in turn prevents the lungs from fully expanding. Try hunching over and taking a deep breath. Now stand up straight and take a deep breath. Notice the difference?

Even if the chest wall were to expand normally, the lung tissue itself undergoes changes. There is loss of *elastin*. Elastin forms microscopic rubberlike fibers in the lungs that allow them to expand and then recoil spontaneously. The springlike action of the lung tissue relaxes. With the loss of elastin, the smaller airways in the lung have a harder time staying open, making it more difficult for air to flow through. This can lead to

- a gradual loss of the ability of the lung tissue to extract oxygen from the inhaled air
- air being trapped in the lungs that can cause a buildup of pressure, which will impede the flow of blood to certain parts of the lung

What we've just discussed are the normal changes to the lungs that occur with aging. If the person was a smoker or continues to smoke, this loss of lung function with aging may be much greater. Many older patients will say they had a relative who smoked until he was in his eighties with no problems. We like to respond by saying he might have had "no problems" into his nineties if he hadn't smoked.

THE HEART

It's Not Pumping Like It Used To!

There is a loss of muscle cells in the heart with aging. There is also an increase in the number of *collagen fibers* and cells called *fibroblasts*, which together can be thought of as the mortar that keeps the heart muscle together. With a decrease in muscle cells and an increase in this mortar material, the heart becomes thicker and stiffer. The heart, therefore, will pump blood less efficiently.

It Doesn't Relax Like It Used To!

As blood flows from the veins to the heart, the heart muscle needs to relax and expand. The expanding (stretching) heart muscle allows the heart to accept more blood in its chambers. In some sense, a heart muscle filling with blood is like a balloon filling with water. As water comes into the balloon, the balloon expands. The balloon can expand because balloons are made of a flexible material.

The increased stiffness of the aging heart makes it more difficult for the heart muscle to relax and expand when blood flows into it. So instead of acting like a water balloon and expanding, the aging heart acts more like a plastic bottle that can only handle a fixed amount of water. Long-standing high blood pressure can make this stiffness even worse.

In fact, about a third of older adults with a diagnosis of congestive heart failure will suffer from symptoms caused by the inability of the heart to relax. We normally think of heart failure as being associated with a heart that cannot pump the blood out well. What we are discussing here is a stiff heart that cannot expand well when blood is trying to flow into it. The pressure can build up in the blood vessels of the lungs and can cause severe shortness of breath. We refer to this form of heart failure as *diastolic heart failure*, or *diastolic dysfunction*. Literally, the heart is unable to relax during the diastolic (relaxed) phase.

The Arteries Sure Are a Lot Harder!

The arteries that receive the blood from the heart also become thicker and stiffer due to a variety of complicated factors. This means that the heart will have to work even harder to pump blood into these stiffer vessels. The stiffness of the arteries is a major contributor to the increase of the systolic blood pressure (the top number of the blood pressure reading) with age.[2]

It Sure Doesn't Beat as Fast as It Used To!

The resting heart rate in general does not change as a person ages. However, with aging, the heart rate does not increase as much in response to such stresses as exercise, fever, and dehydration as it does in a young person. Part of this effect may be due to the decrease in the number of pacemaker cells that stimulate the heart to beat.

The older heart is therefore stiffer and less able to speed up its rate. So what can the older heart do to increase its rate in response to exercise or stress? The heart tries to compensate over time by dilating the size of its chambers. This increase in size increases the stress on the wall of the heart, much like the tension on a balloon increases as you blow it up. This increase in wall tension also increases the need for oxygen. However, the blood vessels supplying the heart are likely to be clogged to a certain extent. It is not a surprise that advanced age is a significant risk factor for a heart attack.

WHERE DID ALL MY MUSCLES GO?

As we age, the size of our muscles gradually decreases. Between the ages of thirty and eighty there is a 30–40 percent decrease in muscle mass. If you think about it, you have never seen an eighty-year-old man playing football in the NFL or competing in the Mr. Olympia bodybuilding tournament. Today, Arnold Schwarzenegger is playing the role of a politician and not that of Conan the Barbarian.

Why do the muscles shrink? No one really knows for sure.[3] We have determined that muscle shrinkage is due more to a decrease in the size of the muscle cells rather than from a loss in number of muscle cells. This decrease in the size of the cells is caused by a variety of changes that includes:

- shrinkage (atrophy) resulting from decreased activity
- decreased activity in the enzymes involved in the production of energy inside the muscle cells
- decreases in the stimulation of muscle cells by nerve cells
- increased protein breakdown due to a variety of medical illnesses (see chapter 19)

This decline of the muscles is one of the many factors that leads to increased weakness and falls in the elderly. It also can affect how the body deals with many common drugs. We discuss what you can do to minimize the muscle wasting caused by aging in chapters 5, 6, and 7.

While there is a loss of muscle mass, the total body weight may not drop that much. We cannot begin to tell you how many times seniors have proudly told us that they weigh the same as they did when they were twenty years old. They may weigh the same, but they certainly do not look the same. In all cases, they have less muscle but more body fat.

WHAT'S GOING ON WITH MY TENDONS, LIGAMENTS, AND CARTILAGE?

Just as important as the changes to the muscles are the changes to the tendons, ligaments, and cartilage. Tendons attach muscles to bone, while ligaments connect bones together. Both tend to become stiffer as people age and as the water content of these tissues decreases. As a result, most people become less flexible. Both tendons and ligaments tend to tear more easily, and when they tear, they heal more slowly.

Cartilage is the area of padding between bones that absorbs impact and acts as a lubricant. Think of the cartilage as a moist sponge. The water content of this sponge decreases with normal aging. The cartilage gradually thins and its ability to act as a shock absorber decreases. The moist sponge has now become a thinned, crunchy, dried-out sponge. This can be a big problem in certain areas, such as the knees and spine, that need to absorb a lot of impact.

On a microscopic level, small breaks in the structure of the cartilage can be seen in the elderly. If the cartilage thins too much, the bones in the joints will begin to rub against each other. This can cause stiffness and pain in the joints that people associate with osteoarthritis.

The majority of seniors have one or more joints with osteoarthritis. Repeated injury, the lifelong use of joints, and obesity will speed up the damage to the cartilage and often lead to osteoarthritis. Arthritic joints may cause pain as the joint surfaces no longer easily glide over each other. An understanding of these changes is essential to an appreciation of how difficult it is to structure an exercise program for an elderly person (chapter 7). Bone changes that predispose the frail elderly to osteoporosis will be discussed in chapter 15.

DOES THE BODY STILL MAKE HORMONES?

Insulin

In the older adult population about 40 percent will have either diabetes or what we call *impaired glucose intolerance*, or *prediabetes*.[4] Most adult-onset diabetes is due not to a lack of insulin but rather to an inability of the tissues to react to the body's own insulin. You may hear the term *insulin resistance* used to describe this problem. Be aware that many common medications, such as prednisone and hydrochlorothiazide, can make this problem of insulin resistance even worse.[5]

Estrogen

With menopause comes a gradual loss of estrogen. This leads to a variety of changes in the body. The density of bone decreases. This estrogen loss also leads to changes in the vaginal tissue.[6] There is a decrease in the quantity and acidity of vaginal secretions. Because of this change in acidity, there are fewer normal bacteria, known as *Lactobacilli*. Instead, bacteria from other parts of the body may colonize the area. This is an important risk factor for developing urinary tract infections. The lack of estrogen also leads to shrinkage (atrophy) of the pelvic muscles. This weakening of the pelvic muscles can cause many older women to leak urine when they cough, sneeze, or laugh (chapter 21).

Growth Hormone and Testosterone

There is a gradual decrease in the amount of the growth hormone and testosterone with aging. Many doctors claim that the declining level of these hormones is responsible for many of the changes that occur with aging. These changes include muscle weakness, decreased virility, decreased concentration, and increased fatigue. Most of us have seen ads or infomercials showing elderly men who took either testosterone or growth hormone and appear to be active, virile, and muscular.

These hormones have been studied in the relatively "healthy" elderly. They have not been well studied in the older and sicker nursing home population. We discuss the potential benefits and side effects of hormone therapy in greater detail in chapter 5.

DHEA

DHEA (another hormone that is largely produced by the adrenal gland) decreases by five- to tenfold by the age of eighty. No one is quite sure what this hormone does, but many people are touting it as a fountain of youth. Some people also think it may help in the treatment of depression. Simply giving this to the frail elderly may be dangerous as it can be converted by the body into either testosterone or estrogen. (We will discuss this topic in further detail in chapter 5.)

DOES MY IMMUNE SYSTEM NEED A BOOST?

When studying the changes that occur in the immune system, scientists often have trouble determining which changes are truly related to getting older and which are the result of one or more illnesses. That being said, with aging comes a decreased ability of the immune system to attack the bacteria, viruses, and fungi that cause disease. More recent studies have suggested that the weakening of the immune system may be partially responsible for the increased risk of cancer that we see in the elderly.[7]

Normally the immune system activates white blood cells known as *T cells* and *B cells* (the ones that produce antibodies) during an infection. The ability of these cells to function properly is impaired with aging. Studies have shown that older adults produce fewer antibodies when they receive flu and pneumonia vaccines. A decrease in some of the chemicals of the immune system (called *cytokines*) also impairs the ability of the T cells and the B cells to function properly.

On the other hand, other cytokine levels may actually increase when you get sick. These cytokines are associated with a variety of serious problems, including an increased risk of postoperative complications, malnutrition, bedsores, and hormonal imbalances.

WHAT ABOUT THE BLOOD?[8]

Although the bone marrow may not produce as many blood cells as when you were young, aging by itself is unlikely to cause *anemia,* a deficiency of red blood cells. Anemia should therefore always be investigated as a problem of its own.

AM I THE ONLY ONE WHO CANNOT SEE?

Poor vision is another major problem in the elderly. Twenty to thirty percent of people age seventy-five and over have impaired vision.[9] Poor vision is associated with an increased risk of falls, accidents, and increased confusion on hospitalization. *Presbyopia* is a common problem in older adults that prevents seniors from focusing on objects that are close. In addition to difficulty focusing on objects, the ability of the eyes to adapt to a dark room can be delayed severalfold. Older adults also have a harder time discriminating between different surfaces. These difficulties place the older adult at further risk for falls. Dry, irritated eyes are another common problem, as there is decreased tear production.

Age-Related Eye Disorders

Millions of Americans have *age-related macular degeneration* (ARMD). It is the most common cause of blindness in the developed world.[10] ARMD leads to the loss of straight-ahead vision. This type of vision is needed to read or to recognize faces. Patients with this type of vision loss often benefit from the use of magnifying devices and other aids, such as large-print books.

Fifty percent of seniors age seventy-five and over will have a cataract.[11] Cataracts are so common that we almost consider them to be a normal part of the aging process. Cataracts occur when the protein molecules in the lens of the eye begin to clump up. This leads to the lens of the eye becoming cloudy.

When you see an older person with a white, milky-looking eye, this is a cataract. Cataracts develop at a different rate and reach a different level of severity for each person. They may even form at different rates in the two eyes of the same person. Cataracts often cause blurry vision, increased sensitivity to glare, and the appearance of halos around lights. The risk factors for cataracts include diabetes, use of steroids (prednisone), smoking, and long-term unprotected exposure to sunlight.

Cataracts are often removed surgically with a procedure that is relatively quick and has minimal risk of injury. With modern cataract surgery, the cataract is removed through a tiny opening in the cornea (clear part of the eye). A new lens is slipped through the same tiny opening.

Another eye problem that can be fixed surgically is an *ectropion*. This is a sagging lower eyelid that can produce constant dryness in the eye and happens with the loss of tissue holding the lower eyelid in place.

DID YOU SAY SOMETHING?

Hearing loss is very common in the frail elderly: it is estimated that 80 percent of people eighty-five years of age and older are affected.[12] Much of this hearing loss is a result of excessive noise exposure over the course of a person's life. So turn down the loud music before it's too late and don't get lazy about wearing ear plugs if you work at a job with a lot of noise exposure.

Recognizing and treating hearing loss is important. Hearing loss is associated with major psychological impairments, including social withdrawal, loneliness, depression, and irritability.[13] Hearing is also an important factor when assessing someone's memory. It may be even more important than vision. The person who can't see will tell you, but patients who can't hear may just nod their heads and make up an answer for an unheard question.

We had a couple of patients who had been labeled as demented. On closer evaluation, it turns out that they were both severely hearing impaired. When they were given hearing aids, their "dementia" miraculously improved.

As it turns out, the high-frequency (high-pitch) sounds and those involving certain consonants (*f*, *s*, *t*) often give seniors the most difficulty. This leads to the older adult perceiving that people are mumbling. Speaking louder will not help. Therefore, if your family member is having trouble hearing you, raising your voice often does not help. Other older patients may have trouble hearing when there is a lot of background noise, such as at a dinner party or sporting event.[14]

How Can I Tell If My Loved One Has a Hearing Problem?

Many older persons are unaware of their hearing loss. If you notice that your loved one turns up the TV loud or is cupping his ears when he is talking to you, there may be a hearing problem present.

Many studies have shown that simply asking a senior one of these simple questions can help you tell whether he or she has a hearing problem:

- Would you say that you have any difficulty hearing?
- Do you have trouble hearing?
- Do you feel you have a hearing loss?
- Do you think you have a hearing problem?[15]

The elderly patient who cannot hear a whispered voice from six inches away from her left or right ear is over six times more likely to have a hearing problem.[16]

When speaking to seniors with hearing problems, make a point to do the following:

- Make sure they wear their glasses and/or hearing aids
- Maintain good eye contact so they can see your facial expressions and read your lips
- Use appropriate gestures
- Make sure there is good lighting for facial gestures
- Eliminate background noise
- Lower the tone of your voice
- Speak at a slightly slower pace
- Repeat important segments of what you are trying to say: ask them to repeat what they heard
- Avoid complex sentences
- Do not shout!!!!!!!

Hearing Aids Are Not Always the Answer!

Only 16 percent of older adults with a hearing problem have a hearing aid or assistive device, and only 8 percent use the device. Hearing aids are expensive, and they are not covered under Medicare. Many seniors will spend a lot of money only to discover that they cannot figure out how to put the hearing aids inside the ear or how to adjust the settings. Others forget to use them or find them too uncomfortable.

Some seniors forget to change the batteries. Wearing a hearing aid with a bad battery will only make the problem worse because the person will have the underlying hearing problem and will also have the hearing aid acting like a plug. It seems as though some seniors find them hard to use, but easy to lose. The point is that hearing aids are not for everyone.

CHANGES IN THE DIGESTIVE SYSTEM

A decrease in both taste and smell occurs with the normal aging process, causing a 50 percent decrease in the ability to taste food by age eighty. The loss of bitter and sour tastes is greater than the loss of sweet tastes. It is therefore not surprising that many frail seniors have a craving for sweets and carbohydrates. For some patients, the loss of smell and taste can become significant risk factors for malnutrition. In the mouth there is a general thinning of the lining of the cheeks and gums. The saliva produced is generally much thicker. The mouth of the frail older adult is marked by receding gums, tooth decay, and wear. These factors will have a direct impact on the frail older adult's ability to chew and can also be a source of pain. Poor dentition may also increase the risk of pneumonia and possibly even cardiovascular disease.

Normally when we eat, the food stimulates a reflex that causes the stomach to expand to accommodate more food. In the elderly, this reflex is impaired. When food enters the stomach, acid is released to help digest food. The stomach produces the same amount of acid.

Many changes take place in the colon (large intestine). Normally, digestive waste products are gently pushed through this large tube-shaped organ through a coordinated contraction of muscle that starts at one end of the colon and moves down to the rectum at the other end. With aging, the movement of stool through the colon becomes slower, especially as the muscle contractions of the colon become less coordinated. Also important, for some unknown reason, the number of receptors for opiates increases. This makes the colon of an older individual more susceptible to the side effect of constipation from narcotic pain medications, such as morphine, codeine, and oxycodone.

In addition, the liver shrinks in size and receives less blood flow. The number of liver cells declines and the cells that do remain increase in size. Despite these changes there is no change in the ability of the liver to carry out its normal functions.

WHAT IS SO IMPORTANT ABOUT THE KIDNEYS?

Urine production may not be the most appealing thing to talk about, but the responsible organ, the kidney, is very important. It controls the elimination of water, minerals, and waste products from the blood. By controlling the elimination of these products, the kidney regulates how much fluid is in our body, and how much acid and waste products are in our blood. Approximately 25–30 percent of kidney mass is lost between the ages of thirty and eighty. There is a 7.5–10 percent decline per decade in the ability of the kidney to filter the blood. It also loses some of its ability to regulate sodium and potassium levels in the blood. The ability of the kidneys to hold onto water when the body is dehydrated also decreases.

Seniors take a lot of medications. Many of these drugs are excreted by the kidney. As the kidney function declines, drug levels in the blood may increase. Many common drugs are also more likely to cause kidney damage in seniors. These are some major reasons why seniors are at a higher risk of having side effects from medications (see chapter 8).

MAINTAINING THE RIGHT AMOUNT OF WATER IN THE BODY

The elderly have multiple risk factors for becoming dehydrated. Muscle tissue has far more water in it than fat tissue. As noted earlier, you lose muscle mass as you get older. This loss of muscle mass means that the total amount of water stored in the body is also decreased. The body's sense of thirst is impaired with aging as well. Therefore, seniors will be less thirsty when they become dehydrated. The ability of the kidney to hold on to water during periods of dehydration is also impaired.

CHANGES TO THE SKIN

The skin is the largest organ in the body. If you examine the skin of many seniors you will notice that it feels like paper. There are a variety of changes that occur to both the outer layer (*epidermis*) and the inner layer (*dermis*) with normal aging. The epidermis loses about 30 percent of its thickness. The rate of cell regeneration in the epidermis is slower. The outermost portion of the epidermis works as a barrier to protect the skin and to keep water from leaving the skin. As this layer thins the skin is more likely to dry out. The border between the epidermis and the dermis normally has ridges that keep these two layers fastened together. With aging these ridges flatten making the epidermis more vulnerable, so it is more likely that the skin can tear off (something that we call, appropriately, a *skin tear*).

The number of immune cells, known as *Langerhan's cells*, also decreases. The loss of these cells may play a role in the emergence of skin cancer, since the remaining immune system cells will have a harder time trying to find and destroy the abnormal cells.

The inner layer (the dermis) thins, providing less support and protection to the underlying structures, such as muscle and tendons. This thinning is due to the fact that there are fewer cells, known as *fibroblasts*, that constitute the main structure of this tissue. There are also fewer immune cells known as *mast cells*. There are also fewer small blood vessels, and the ones that are present are more disorganized in their structure. Moreover, there are also fewer sweat glands. These changes are part of the reason that the frail elderly can get severe bruising with just minimal trauma.

IT'S NOT SO EASY TO BE 98.6!

Your body is a very efficient machine that has numerous parts that must all work together. For the cells and organs to function, body temperature must be maintained at a point near 98.6°F. If the temperature is cold outside, the body has some built-in mechanisms to prevent body temperature from dropping. In very warm weather, the body will sweat in order to cool down.

In the winter time, older adults are at risk for becoming ill from their body temperatures dropping, a problem known as *hypothermia* (*hypo* means low). There are several reasons to explain this potentially lethal problem. As we stated earlier, older adults have less muscle. With less muscle, there is less shivering. Because of this, they produce less heat per pound of body weight. Normally, when the temperature drops, the small vessels that supply the skin with blood contract. By decreasing the amount of blood flowing to the surface of the skin, less body heat is lost. This constriction of these specific blood vessels is called *vasoconstriction*. Older adults have less vasoconstriction when they are exposed to the cold.

On the other hand, older adults may also have the problem of getting overheated during the summertime. This failure of the body to lower its body temperature in response to heat leads to *hyperthermia*. Older adults have decreased sweat production, and a higher body temperature is needed to initiate sweating. To make matters worse, the elderly patients have a decreased sense of thirst and are more likely to become dehydrated.

As a result of the changes described in this chapter, the organs of the older adult have a decreased capacity to handle the stresses that occur to the body from a variety of illnesses.

Chapter 3

THE REAL TRUTH ABOUT PREVENTIVE MEDICINE

"If I knew I was going to live so long, I would have taken better care of myself."
                    Henny Youngman, "King of One Liners"
                                        (1906–1998)

In the thirteenth century, the philosopher Roger Bacon (c. 1214–1294) wrote down his secrets for a long and healthy life. To live to the age of eighty in the thirteenth century was quite impressive. There was poor sanitation, no antibiotics, and no medical care. Roger Bacon believed that the secret to a long life was strict adherence to the following:

- exercise
- good hygiene
- inhaling the breath of a young virgin
- moderation in lifestyle
- proper rest
- a sensible diet

Jumping ahead to the year 2004, a large study was published in the prestigious *Journal of the American Medical Association* (*JAMA*) that showed healthy seventy- to ninety-year-olds who adhered to a Mediterranean diet, moderate alcohol use, physical activity, and a nonsmoking lifestyle had a 50 percent decrease in the rate of death.[1] These research findings do not seem too far off from what Roger Bacon described over seven hundred years earlier with the exception, of course, of inhaling the breath of a young virgin.

Modern medical research has also identified other factors that appear to increase your chances of living a long life. These include:

- Good genetics: People whose parents lived to be very old have a higher chance of living a long life as well. We really don't know much more than that. The specific genes involved in the human aging process remain unknown.
- Increased lipoprotein size and increased HDL cholesterol levels in your blood: There is some evidence that components of your cholesterol may be protective factors for heart disease and strokes. Higher levels of these proteins are more commonly seen among people who live to be one hundred.
- Being lucky! Not being in the wrong place at the wrong time. We all know of people who have been in a bad car accident or were the victim of a violent crime. Others have rare or unexplained illnesses.
- Proper preventive medical care.

WHAT IS PREVENTIVE MEDICINE?

We have all heard the saying "An ounce of prevention is worth a pound of cure." Taking the proper steps to avoid developing illnesses is important, as is diagnosing illnesses early. Prevention, therefore, can take several forms. It can involve:

- Modifying one or more risk factors that can lead to the development of a disease. Quitting smoking, for example, may help prevent a heart attack or stroke.
- Trying to identify a disease at an early stage before it leads to a serious illness or death. For example, a colonoscopy attempts to identify and remove small polyps in the colon before they turn into colon cancers.
- Keeping a close eye on people who already have an illness. Women who have had breast cancer are at much higher risk for developing further breast cancer and will need closer monitoring.

WHAT IS THE PROPER PREVENTIVE SCREENING FOR AN ELDERLY PATIENT?

The guidelines for the proper screening of an elderly person are not clear. Part of the confusion is that there is so much variability among the elderly population. Surely, you would be less likely to order a colonoscopy for a severely demented 102-year-old nursing home resident than a 66-year-old woman who still plays tennis daily.

Another part of the problem is that many of the medical specialty societies do not agree as to which tests are appropriate to order for elderly patients. For example, the American Cancer Society and the American Urological Association recommend that doctors offer men over age fifty a yearly blood test to measure the *prostate specific antigen* (PSA) along with a digital rectal exam.[2] The PSA is elevated in many patients with prostate cancer. Other medical organizations, such as the United States Preventative Health Task Force, believe that there is not enough evidence to recommend that doctors order PSA blood tests for their male patients.[3]

WHAT ABOUT A YEARLY PHYSICAL EXAM?

We have all grown up thinking that a yearly physical is an essential factor in making sure we remain healthy. While we all have different ideas of what this exam should encompass, most believe that it should involve a full discussion of all healthcare issues, a full head-to-toe examination, and lab work. The **real truth** is that this standard format has not been shown to be of any benefit for detecting new, potentially life-threatening diseases.[4] It is, however, an opportunity to discuss exercises and to make sure the patient is up to date on his or her immunizations and cancer screening.

Research has shown that tests often ordered yearly in otherwise *healthy* seniors are not beneficial. These tests include:

- chest x-ray
- complete blood cell (CBC) count
- blood chemistry panel
- electrocardiogram (EKG)

On the surface, it would seem that these tests would be useful. But as it turns out, ordering these tests routinely each year will rarely identify any new diseases.

SEVEN THINGS YOU CAN DO TO PREVENT DISEASES

1. Stay out of the sun!

In chapter 2 we discussed many of the skin changes that occur with normal aging. Excess sun exposure leads to a variety of additional skin changes that we refer to by the term *photoaging*. Sun damage will make you look older. This damage occurs both at the skin's outer layer (epidermis) and at the inner layer (dermis). Photoaging can make people in their forties and fifties look twenty years older.

You will also get blotchy spots, or *liver spots*. In the dermis, there is damage to the collagen and elastic tissue that leads to wrinkles. You may also see areas reddened with tiny blood vessels. These vessels are known as *telangectasias*.

To lessen the damage to the skin, we recommend:

- Wearing a hat that covers the top of the ears and the back of the neck. A baseball cap is not good enough.
- Stay out of the sun during peak hours. Do your outdoor activities in the early morning or late afternoon.
- Use sunscreen. Check the label on the bottle. You want to use one with an SPF of at least 15 that protects against both UV A and UV B rays.
- In addition to staying out of the sun, stop smoking! Smoking increases the changes in the skin.

Taking these steps has been shown to decrease the rate of skin aging and lowers the risk of some skin cancers. We find it quite ironic that some people will spend so much money on makeup and hair products but will refuse to take the simple steps listed above to prevent the sun from damaging their faces.

What about a moisturizer?

Many products come with claims that they will "restore" or "rejuvenate" the skin. If you really want to slow down the aging of your skin, you don't need any expensive creams or lotions. A simple moisturizer will do. Expensive products may not be any better than the cheaper ones you can get at a convenience store. Look for a moisturizer and/or exfoliant that contains hydroxyl acid. But beware! If you use a product with hydroxyl acids on your skin, it will actually increase the ability of ultraviolet B (UV B) rays to penetrate your skin. So once again, stay out of the sun!

2. It is never too late to quit smoking!

We often hear comments like "I've smoked my entire life and I feel fine! I don't feel sick." We answer by saying that "you don't feel sick *yet*!" We have all seen the public service announcements talking about the strong link between smoking and lung cancer. In reality, lung cancer is only the tip of the iceberg. Smoking is a major risk factor in the development of:

- cancers of the mouth and throat
- chronic obstructive pulmonary disease (COPD)/emphysema
- heart disease
- pneumonia
- poor circulation
- poor wound healing
- osteoporosis
- sinusitis
- strokes

If that's not enough to convince you, it will also make your skin wrinkle faster too! So watch out, smoking will make you look older.

3. Put down the bottle!

Studies have shown that a "small amount of alcohol per day may have important benefits." For seniors, a small amount means no more than one drink per day and no more than two on any special occasion.[5] By "one drink" we mean either 5 ounces of wine, 12 ounces of beer, or 1.5 ounces of spirits.

The problem is that many seniors have a problem with alcohol abuse or alcoholism. Drinking too much over long periods of time is bad for your liver. It can cause your liver to turn into shrunken scar tissue, which we call *cirrhosis*. Alcohol can also interfere with many common medications, such as benzodiazepines (chapter 8). Drinking too much also increases your risk of car crashes (chapter 29) and fall-related injuries (chapter 8).

4. Get your blood pressure checked!

As we discussed in chapter 2, the systolic blood pressure (the top number) gradually increases with age. Many studies have shown that a high systolic blood pressure over time will increase your risk of strokes and heart attacks.

At what age can we stop checking the blood pressure? The answer is NEVER. Controlling blood pressure is so significant that it is recommended by all medical organizations even for patients who are very old and frail.

A Few Words about High Blood Pressure

You hear so much about the dangers of high blood pressure that many patients become worried when they are told that their blood pressure is high. If you have high blood pressure it is important that you take your blood pressure medication as directed, plus there are other things that you need to aware of:

- Your blood pressure will vary from moment to moment depending on what you are doing.
- For most people, there is no real danger if your blood pressure is a little elevated for a few hours or a few days.
- Caffeine and nonsteroidal anti-inflammatory drugs (such as ibuprofen and naproxen) can increase your blood pressure.
- If you check your blood pressure at home, record the results to show your doctor.
- Bring your blood pressure cuff with you to the doctor's office. By comparing it to the one in your doctor's office, you will be able to tell if it is accurate.

5. Check your cholesterol.

Patients with a history of coronary artery disease, peripheral vascular disease, diabetes, or strokes should continue to get their cholesterol checked regularly as they get older. Lowering the cholesterol (specifically the LDL, or "bad cholesterol") can prevent atherosclerosis from clogging up your arteries and lower your risk of dying from a heart attack or stroke.

What about patients in their eighties or nineties who have never had a heart attack or stroke and do not have diabetes? Here is where it gets controversial. Some doctors will say that there is no evidence that treating these patients for high cholesterol will help. If they haven't had a problem so far, then the high cholesterol is not likely a risk factor in this patient.

In the last few years, some doctors have become more aggressive in treating elevated cholesterol levels in the elderly. There is now data suggesting that lowering cholesterol may also slow down the progression of dementia and macular degeneration. It may also lead to the shrinkage of plaques in arteries that can later cause strokes and heart attacks.

6. Stay up to date with your vaccinations.

All elderly patients should receive the influenza vaccine (flu shot) every year. The flu strikes as a wave in which many people become sick at the same time. In the nursing home both residents and staff will get sick. Most of the people who die from influenza each year are seniors. It is also important that health-care workers get vaccinated.

We have heard many excuses for not getting vaccinated, such as "I don't get sick," "Vaccines can cause you to get the flu," or "I have never needed to get one before." We explain to elderly patients that not getting a flu shot every year is a dangerous and foolhardy decision. You need to get it annually because the infectious strain changes each year.

Contrary to popular belief, you can't get the flu from getting the flu shot. The shot may stimulate your immune system so that you may have some temporary flulike symptoms, but it is impossible to get the flu from the vaccine.

Other people will say that they got the flu even though they received the vaccine. The vaccine covers only one of many strains of the influenza virus. Also, there are many other viruses other than influenza that can cause respiratory symptoms, fever, body aches, and so on.

It is recommended that all elderly patients receive the vaccine for pneumonia once every five to eight years. However, receiving this vaccine will not give total protection from getting pneumonia, as it only protects against a small fraction of the many types of bacteria that can cause pneumonia (chapter 17).[6]

Don't forget your tetanus booster every ten years. Tetanus is now a very rare disease with fewer than one hundred cases per year in the United States, but about half of all cases occur in older adults.

7. Check for cancer?

Ordering medical tests to look for cancer may seem pretty straightforward. Many tests exist that can be used to detect specific types of cancer. Before you run off and get a whole bunch of medical tests, there are some things to consider:

- Seniors with limited life expectancies can suffer a lot of pain and suffering from unnecessary testing and aggressive treatments, only to die of other things, such as heart attacks, pneumonia, and so on.
- Clinical guidelines for the elderly are often ambiguous and research often excludes older adult patients.

- In some cases, doctors may be too aggressive in ordering screening tests, since they fear being sued if they do not order these tests and the patient does develop cancer.
- The healthiest people with the lowest risk of disease are those most often screened. Minority patients are often underscreened.

Breast Cancer Screening

Important facts about breast cancer in the elderly:

- One out of every nine women will get breast cancer at some point in her life.
- Fifty percent of cases occur after the age of sixty-five.
- Breast cancer takes several years to grow from the first cell to a lump that can be felt in the breast.
- Most research studies have focused on patients younger than seventy.

Do I Need a Mammogram?

A mammogram is one of the best ways to screen and identify breast cancer before it gets too large and spreads. Screening for breast cancer is improved when the mammogram is combined with a regularly scheduled examination of the breasts by a physician. There is no evidence that self-examination of the breasts improves your chances of discovering breast cancer before it is too late.[7] That being said, we do not recommend that you stop checking your breasts. If you note any new lumps on your breasts or in your armpits, you need to bring it to the attention of your doctor.

So When Can I Stop Getting Mammograms?

There is no clear point at which you can say that mammograms are no longer needed. Recommendations for seniors vary among different organizations. Part of the confusion is due to the fact that all of the studies looking at the benefit of mammograms excluded patients over the age of seventy-four.[8] Nevertheless, Medicare will cover yearly mammograms regardless of age.

As both an oncologist (cancer doctor) and a geriatrician, Dr. Silverman strongly believes that there is no age limit per se. He recommends that women continue to get them as long as they are healthy enough to be able to tolerate surgical mastectomy (removal of the breast) and radiation therapy, should a tumor be found. It makes no sense to screen for an illness if the patient is too frail to tolerate the potential treatments.

What about a Breast MRI?

You may have heard on the news that an MRI of the breast is better than a mammogram for detecting breast cancers. There have been several studies that have shown that this is, in fact, the case for young and middle-aged females.[9] Whether an MRI is better for elderly women is unknown at this time. Before you dial up your doctor's office demanding an MRI, realize that these studies are so new that Medicare does not cover the cost of MRIs as a routine screening procedure for breast cancer.

Cervical Cancer Screening

The Pap smear is an important screening test for cervical cancer. Forty percent of cervical cancers occur in women over the age of sixty-five. Just because you had a hysterectomy does not mean you are out of the woods. Sometimes, the cervix is left behind. Women over seventy years of age with an intact cervix may choose to stop having Pap smears if they have:

- three or more documented, consecutive, normal/negative Pap smears
- no abnormal/positive Pap smears within a ten-year period before the age of seventy
- no new sexual partners

Doing a pelvic exam on a frail older woman can be distressing and uncomfortable. For some older women a Pap smear may be associated with some potential harms. In some cases she will get a positive Pap smear but the woman does not have cervical cancer. We call this a "false-positive" result. The patient will be under great emotional stress and will need more invasive tests. Therefore, the potential harm may exceed benefits among older women who have had normal results previously and who are not otherwise at high risk.

What about Ovarian Cancer?

In the United States, ovarian cancer is the fifth leading cause of cancer-related death among women. There are two screening tests for ovarian cancer. One is the transvaginal ultrasound. This test involves inserting the ultrasound device into the vagina in order to visualize the ovaries. The other test is a measurement of the blood levels of a protein known as *CA-125*. Patients with ovarian cancer often have increased levels of this protein.

Unless you have one or more first-degree relatives who have had ovarian cancer, most health experts recommend against routine screening with a transvaginal ultrasound and CA-125. One problem is that most of the time when one of these tests is positive, the woman will end up not having ovarian cancer. Before we can tell her that she does not have cancer, she will be under much distress and will need further invasive testing. In some cases women will undergo needless surgery. In other cases, we may find the cancer sooner, but the person does not end up living any longer.

PROSTATE CANCER SCREENING IN THE ELDERLY

How Common Is Prostate Cancer?

Six and a half million men in the United States over seventy-five years of age will have cancer cells in their prostate. Prostate cancer cells can be found in the prostates of 40 percent of men over the age of eighty-five. In most cases the prostate cancer grows very slowly. Most elderly men die *with* prostate cancer, not *because of* the prostate cancer.[10] There are many treatments available.

How Do You Screen for Prostate Cancer?

- Digital rectal exam—this involves having the patient bend over while the doctor inserts a finger to feel if there are any hard nodules on the prostate.
- Prostate Specific Antigen (PSA)—this blood test checks for a protein that comes from the prostate. The level of PSA is increased with prostate cancer and when the prostate is enlarged (benign prostatic hyperplasia, or BPH for short).

If the doctor feels a hard lump in your prostate, you may have prostate cancer. A PSA test value of four or higher indicates a possible problem with the prostate. In either case, your doctor will likely refer you to a urologist for a prostate biopsy. This involves sticking an instrument into your rectum and taking six small tissue samples from your prostate. Many men find this painful.

Should I Be Checked for Prostate Cancer?

While Medicare covers the cost of a yearly PSA exam, there is currently tremendous debate over whether to do a PSA test or a rectal exam on a yearly basis. The American Cancer Society urges men over fifty to have both tests done each year in order to catch prostate cancers early. The US Preventive Services Task Force does not think that there is enough evidence to recommend the digital rectal exam or the PSA as effective screening tests for prostate cancer. In fact, this organization recommends against screening men over the age of seventy-five.[11] Some of the problems with these tests are:

- The PSA and digital rectal exam (DRE) identify about two-thirds of prostate cancers, so many men with prostate cancer will have a negative test. Thus, the cancers will often be missed.
- Only one in four men with a PSA between four and ten has prostate cancer. Many men will have elevated PSAs but do not have prostate cancer. Imagine the needless psychological turmoil that these men must go through when they are initially told they might have cancer. These men will all need to go through the painful process of having their prostate biopsied.
- Many men will be diagnosed with prostate cancer and will be treated either with surgery or with hormonal treatment. Common side effects from surgery include impotence and incontinence. Studies have shown that most elderly men have a cancer that is not highly aggressive. For seniors with a life expectancy of less than a ten years, they are more likely to die from other illnesses than from their prostate cancer.[12]

PREVENTING COLON CANCER

Colon cancer is the third most common lethal form of cancer, behind breast cancer and lung cancer. Screening for colon cancer is essential because identifying and removing suspicious polyps can prevent most cases.

Although a variety of procedures exist, colonoscopy remains the best way to look for colon cancer. It is the only test that allows the physician to see the inside walls of the entire colon and to take biopsies of any suspicious areas. Medicare will pay for a screening colonoscopy once every ten years. The key word here is "screening." This means that all older adults with Medicare can get checked for colon cancer with this gold-standard test. Medicare will also cover for a colonoscopy sooner if the patient has one or more of the following signs/symptoms:

- anemia (low red blood cell count)
- black, tarry stools
- change in bowel habits
- rectal bleeding

At What Age Should Seniors Stop Getting Colonoscopies?

There is no simple answer to this commonly asked question. Without sounding like politicians, we like to say it is when the benefit of having the test outweighs the potential risks. It has been our experience that many frail elderly patients have difficulty getting ready for a colonoscopy. Your doctor will order one of several liquid laxative products available for you to drink the day before the colonoscopy in order to clean out the colon. The colon needs to be cleaned out entirely in order for the doctor to be able to see the walls of the colon as she passes the camera through this long tubular organ. If the waste is not completely clear then your colon is not clean enough for the test. As the colon empties, the patient will need to go to the bathroom many times. For patients with mobility problems this can be quite difficult. Patients also need to avoid eating and drinking after midnight on the evening prior to the test.

While colonoscopy is the gold-standard test, the situation for the elderly is not so simple. The elderly are less likely to be able to clean out their colons properly. They are also at a higher risk for complications.[13] Elderly patients are several times more likely to have their colon walls punctured or have heavy bleeding if a biopsy is done during the procedure. Sedation and longer recovery time may be required.

We generally recommend to our patients that they do not take any of their diuretics ("water pills") the day before and the day of the colonoscopy. The laxatives, along with not eating, place the frail elder at an increased risk of becoming dehydrated. Because the doctor may biopsy an area that looks suspicious for a cancer, you need to stop taking aspirin and other blood thinners, such as clopidogrel (Plavix) and aspirin/extended-release dipyridamole (Aggrenox), for at least one week prior to the procedure. If you are on warfarin (Coumadin), talk to your doctor about what you need to do before you have this test.

Can't I Just Get a Virtual Colonoscopy Instead?

You may hear a lot of people talking about the virtual colonoscopy as the new alternative to the standard colonoscopy. Instead of shoving a long tube with a camera through your colon, the virtual colonoscopy uses a computed tomography (CT) of the abdomen and pelvis to view the walls of the colon. This test does not require sedation. This test not only looks for masses in the colon, it can also see if the cancer has spread to the lymph nodes and liver.

Before you get excited, however, you need to realize that the virtual colonoscopy is not a simple test. You still have to drink all the nasty fluid the day before to clean out your colon. As with a regular colonoscopy, air will need to be pumped into the colon in order to separate the collapsible walls of the colon.

Analyzing the films produced during these virtual colonoscopies can be difficult for even a skilled radiologist to interpret. If any suspicious areas are seen on the films, then the person will need to have a traditional colonoscopy. With the traditional colonoscopy you have the advantage that biopsies of suspicious areas can be obtained at the same time.

Because of these difficulties, the use of this procedure is not recommended by the American College of Physicians, the American Cancer Society, or the US Preventive Services Task Force. Also, the cost of this procedure is not covered by Medicare.

SCREENING FOR LUNG CANCER

There are no recommendations at this time for any screening tests for lung cancer.[14] We have known for many years that getting a chest x-ray yearly in general is a bad way to screen for lung cancer. In most cases, this test will not help you find a lung cancer at an early enough stage that it can be treated. There is some evidence that spiral CT scanning may be able to detect small lung cancers in patients at high risk for cancer (namely, smokers).[15] Just be aware that Medicare will not pay for this type of screening.

WHY NOT GET A YEARLY WHOLE-BODY CT SCAN?

In theory, the idea of getting a CT scan of the entire body makes sense. By getting a detailed picture of the inside of the body, doctors may be able to catch a disease, such as cancer, before it is too late. But the **real truth** is that these tests may lead to many problems.[16]

Whole-body CTs do not involve the use of IV contrast. While this makes the procedure safer, it also makes it much more difficult for the doctor to really see what is going on inside. The doctor will therefore have trouble making a definitive diagnosis if he sees any abnormalities.

Most of the findings on these CTs will turn out to be nothing serious. The problem is that in order to find out if everything is OK, you may have to undergo additional testing that may involve the use of IV contrast. In other cases you may have to undergo procedures involving needles or even surgery. Some experts believe that the risk of getting injured during the follow-up is greater than the chances of finding something serious on a whole-body CT.

The idea of getting yearly CT scans to screen for cancer comes with a bit of irony, since the radiation exposure from a CT scan is about fifty times greater than what you would receive from a chest x-ray. Many scientists now believe that the radiation from multiple CT scans may increase your risk of developing cancer.[17]

DO PREVENTIVE BODY SCANS PREVENT HEART ATTACKS?

This is a tough question to answer. The idea behind using the new special CT scanners is to identify patients who do not have any symptoms yet may have significant blockages in their coronary arteries.

In the last few years special CT machines have been developed that look at the amount of calcium in the coronary arteries. Traditional CT machines were unable to visualize the small coronary arteries due to the motion of the heart when it beats.

What are the coronary arteries? They are the small arteries that supply the heart muscle tissue with blood. The heart's function is to pump blood to the body. But the heart itself needs blood in order to work. If one of its arteries becomes blocked, then the blood flow to the muscle supplied by this artery is cut off and the tissue dies. We call this a *myocardial infarction, MI,* or *heart attack.*

Since calcium is often found in the atherosclerotic plaques in the coronary arteries, the rationale behind preventive body scans is that arteries with more calcium are more likely to be atherosclerotic and at higher risk for becoming blocked. Some studies have shown that patients with a low calcium score have an extremely low chance of having significant blockage in their arteries.

Other scientists have expressed concerns that a calcium score is not a precise measure of atherosclerosis. Many cardiologists are concerned that this test may give misleading results, as calcium is only one of several components that may block your coronary arteries. Cholesterol deposits, blood platelets, and cellular debris cannot be seen by the CT machine, but may also contribute to the blockage of arteries.

In most cases, Medicare will not pay for this CT scan. Before you go and spend money on this test, talk to your primary care doctor or to a cardiologist.

ARE THERE OTHER TESTS TO LOOK FOR HEART DISEASE?

Narrowing of the coronary arteries can be seen on a cardiac catheterization. This invasive test involves threading a long thin tube from your right groin all the way up to your heart. Special dye is then injected into the coronary arteries. This test is done in many centers on thousands of patients every day. It is very safe, but whenever needles are stuck into arteries, there is a risk of bleeding and infection.

Another test that can be done is a thallium stress test. In this test, the heart is "stressed" by having the patient exercise or by injecting Persantine into a vein. Both act to stress the heart by increasing the amount of work that the heart muscle has to do. The thallium is then measured to see if it is absorbed by the different parts of the heart muscle. The results will show if there are areas of heart muscle that receive no blood flow (prior heart attack) or receive poor blood flow due to blockages in the coronary arteries.

We hope that the information in this chapter gives you a better understanding of the tests that will allow you to live longer and healthier.

Chapter 4

THE FACTS ABOUT
ANTI-AGING THERAPIES

*"Whatever poet, orator, or sage may say of it, old age is
still old age."*
Henry Wadsworth Longfellow

In 1513 Ponce de Leon began searching along the Florida coast for the fountain of youth. He was told that anyone who drank from this fountain would be cured of all diseases and would remain youthful. With a sketchy map of the eastern Caribbean and tales from Indian legends, Ponce de Leon embarked on this doomed campaign. Almost five hundred years later, many Floridians and people around the world continue the search. While Ponce de Leon searched through swamps and forests, today's explorers search the Internet and bookstores for a secret that will allow them to remain healthy and active into an extremely old age.

Although science has given us important insights into the molecular mechanisms of aging, no one has unraveled the mystery of how to stop the aging process. In a sense, we know as little about the aging process as Ponce de Leon knew about the land of North America.

ANTI-AGING MEDICINE?

In the previous chapter we discussed the things that you can do to try to slow the rate of age-related changes to your body. Anti-aging products often go one step further by claiming a treatment that can reverse the decline in organ and tissue function. Advertisements often focus on a product's ability to do one or more of the following:

- improve the immune system
- increase energy and strength
- increase lean muscle mass
- improve sexual performance
- reduce body fat

Before we proceed any further, let us be perfectly clear: there is no such thing as an anti-aging therapy or an anti-aging medicine. You may see testimonials or hear about people living in remote villages where everyone is active and happy into their nineties. When you hear such claims, big flashing warning lights should go off in your head.

It is beyond the scope of this book to discuss each of the thousands of claims individually. Instead, we will give you the insights that will help you analyze the facts behind these claims yourself. In chapter 5 we will focus on the most popular anti-aging hormone and skin therapies. Chapter 6 will discuss the use of vitamins, herbs, and other nutritional supplements.

MOST PRODUCTS FOCUS ON ONE OF SEVERAL AGING THEORIES

The people who market anti-aging treatments usually try to link their product to one or more of the aging theories that we discussed in chapter 1. Many treatments are based on the free radical or oxidative stress theory of aging. Free radicals are small chemicals formed when your body is exposed to toxic substances. Free radicals are also produced as waste products by our bodies when we convert food into the energy we need to live. The more free radicals there are in your body, the greater the chances of damage that will occur in the DNA, protein, and walls of your cells.

According to the free radical theory, longevity is based on how well the body neutralizes the harmful effects of these chemicals. Many anti-aging products claim that changing the diet or taking a supplement can decrease the number of free radicals formed or even increase the rate at which these toxins are removed from the body.

The **real truth**, however, is that the science behind the free radical theory of aging is extremely exciting but not definitive. There are many studies that have thrown a monkey wrench into this theory.

The free radical theory is not the only game in town. Other products focus on different theories of aging, such as:

- the immune system becomes weaker with aging, which leads to the development of a variety of medical illnesses
- there is a loss of certain hormones that leads to the changes associated with aging

Beware! Research has shown that no one theory or combination of theories can adequately explain all the complicated changes that occur with aging. Let us not forget that we are working with an extremely primitive map of the molecular pathways involved with aging, so products that are devised to deal with the above issues cannot realistically be expected to slow down or halt the aging process.

THE FDA DOES NOT REGULATE NATURAL ANTI-AGING PRODUCTS

Many anti-aging products are marketed aggressively as "natural" treatments for common medical and age-related problems. Yet, these products are registered as food supplements, not as drugs. By doing so, the manufacturers avoid the scrutiny of the Food and Drug Administration (FDA) that would ordinarily apply to a drug. The FDA has strict regulations and oversight of drugs. The agency reviews the following:

- effectiveness
- purity
- manufacturing, packaging, and distribution
- side effects

The key point is that these regulations apply only to the companies producing drugs. Because many anti-aging products are registered as food supplements, they are completely exempt from this oversight.

LET'S CLEAR THE AIR BEFORE WE DISCUSS THE SPECIFIC PRODUCTS

Most claims touting the benefits of anti-aging treatments are often not supported by good, quality evidence.[1] This is a significant point that cannot be overemphasized. What separates modern medicine from superstition and snake oil remedies is the reliance on scientific research.

There are many rules and procedures to follow when conducting clinical research using medications. These rules were not created by close-minded scientists to discriminate against alternative medicines. Instead, the medical community has learned that these rules need to be followed in order to protect the public from bogus and potentially dangerous treatments. At the core of these rules is the notion that medical research should be done in a manner that others can follow and potentially reproduce. If the results can't be duplicated, you cannot say the treatment works.

Any new products should also be monitored for potential side effects. The people trying to sell you anti-aging products often do not report this information. Instead, the snake oil salesman will present many people who can testify that they are "cured." Where are the people who did not get cured or who got sick when they tried this treatment?

HOW DO YOU RESEARCH WHICH PRODUCTS ARE WORTH TAKING?

We hear many nonmedical people say that they have "researched" a particular product. We know that they are not working in a lab or doing actual research. They usually mean that they have read about a product on one or more Web sites or in books.

If you want to learn more about a product, how can you tell that your reading material has merit? The ability to analyze the quality of medical research is another topic that goes well beyond the scope of this book. We can, however, give you some useful pointers that can help you investigate the benefits and risks of anti-aging therapies.

I FEEL SO MUCH BETTER AFTER USING AN ANTI-AGING PRODUCT!

Anybody can make such claims in a book or in an infomercial. To borrow a line from a 1980s Wendy's commercial, you should be asking yourself: "WHERE'S THE BEEF?" In other words, what kind of evidence do they have to prove that their products work? The makers of most anti-aging products do not have research studies in humans to back up their claims. Instead, they will rely on testimonials and before/after pictures. Therefore, you need to ask yourself:

- Are these people really product users or are they actors?
- Where are all the patients who did not respond to this treatment? If many thousands of people feel better, then these companies really have no excuse for not publishing their medical data.
- How do you know it was the product and not other factors, such as better nutrition, more exercise, giving up alcohol, and so on? Many people start using products at a time when they are making other changes in their lifestyle.
- Could these testimonials be explained by the *placebo effect?*

A *placebo* is a pill, solution, or lotion that contains no real medicine. The patient, however, thinks that he is taking a real medicine. This is really important. You would be surprised at the number of people who feel better when they take a placebo. Thirty to forty percent of the people taking a placebo for depression, pain, arthritis, and enlarged prostates will feel better. What this means is that many people will feel better if they believe that they are taking a medicine, even if they are receiving no medicine at all.

BUT THE AD SAYS, "RESEARCH STUDIES" SHOW THAT THE ANTI-AGING FORMULA WORKS

1. Look for research from peer-reviewed medical journals. These are journals that have independent editorial boards. Before an article can be published in one of these medical journals, the research must be reviewed for its quality by an expert or experts in the field. The article can be published only if the experts believe that the study was done correctly and the article is written in an unbiased manner.

2. Look for studies involving humans. Many research studies involving aging use either fruit flies or mice. These organisms are used for many reasons. Their lives are much shorter than those of humans. Thus, experiments can be done in a relatively short period of time. Flies and mice breed in large numbers, making it easy to do large experiments also in a relatively short period of time. Because of extensive past research we know a tremendous amount about how their bodies work. This makes it easy to continue to use these animals. While there has been much interesting research that has come from flies and mice, we must always remember that they are not people. What works in a mouse may not necessarily work in a human.

The last point to make is that if there are studies involving humans, you then want to see how similar the study patients are to you. If you are an eighty-year-old African American woman, a study using men in the Chinese army may not be relevant to you.

3. Look for studies that compare the use of the anti-aging therapy against a placebo group. Ideally, you would like to see a *randomized double-blind placebo-controlled study*. The term *randomized* means that neither the scientist nor the patient can choose who will receive a drug or who will receive a placebo.

The term *blind* means that neither the scientist nor the patient knows who is getting the treatment and who is getting the placebo. One group will get the drug and the other group will get an injection or pill that looks exactly the same but lacks any active ingredients. A *single-blind* study means that the patient does not know if she is receiving the treatment or the placebo. The investigator, however, knows what the patient is receiving. In order to minimize the potential bias of the investigator treating the patients differently, we always prefer the *double-blind* placebo-controlled study. In the double-blind design, neither the investigator nor the patient knows who is receiving the drug and who is getting the placebo.

Randomized double-blind placebo controlled studies are very labor intensive and expensive to conduct. However, if done correctly, they provide powerful evidence that any differences between the treatment group and the control group are due to the effect of the drug.

4. Look to see whether or not the researchers conducting the study have a financial interest in the marketing of a particular product. The people who own the company are less likely to report data that show their product did not help or was harmful. An impartial scientist with no financial interest in the product is more likely to report his or her findings regardless of the result.

WHERE CAN I FIND OUT IF RESEARCH STUDIES HAVE BEEN DONE?

Now that you have an idea about what to look for, you need to know where to look. A great Web site to use is PubMed, found at www.pubmed.gov.[2] This free site is a database of all the articles that have been published in most of the peer-reviewed medical journals. You can type in the name of a drug or treatment and PubMed will list all the articles that have ever been published on this topic. Not only will it give you the title, author, and journal, it also gives you the abstract, which is a summary of how the study was designed and what results were obtained.

In many cases, simply typing in the term that you want to look up will give you a list that may contain hundreds or even thousands of articles. In order to focus this list to the articles that you need, click on the tab in the upper left corner that says "Limits." Now you can add the parameters that will allow you to focus your search. For people without a medical background, we suggest that you:

- click on "Human"
- click on "Review Articles," "Meta-Analysis," and "Randomized Control Studies"
- limit your search to the last five years

If you want to see if there are studies specifically in the elderly, you can click on "Age 65+ years" under the tab "Ages."

A FRIEND OR FAMILY MEMBER SWEARS BY A PRODUCT

- Once again do not underestimate the power of the placebo effect.
- How do you know it was the product and not other changes in his or her lifestyle, such as better nutrition, more exercise, or giving up cigarettes?

DO NOT FALL FOR THE CONSPIRACY ARGUMENT

We are often told about a hidden extract or ancient formula that is so good that the medical community and the big drug companies are trying their best to keep the information from getting out. Reading between the lines, this means that there is no good research to show that their product works. Rather than assume that there is a conspiracy to hide an unproven product from the public, the **real truth** is that over the years, we have seen thousands of products give false hope to desperate patients.

HOW CAN MY DOCTOR ADVISE ME ABOUT THIS TREATMENT IF HE IS NOT "FAMILIAR WITH IT"?

You cannot expect your doctor to know about every product that is on the market. This does not mean that your doctor is ignorant or close-minded. He or she may be, but do not assume this to be the case. There are numerous products out there and many have very little data to support their use. The burden of proof is on the maker of the product to prove that it works. It should not be the charge of the medical community to prove that it does not work.

In fact in some cases you could argue that it is unethical to recommend these treatments. As doctors we take the Hippocratic oath to "first do no harm" to our patients. To prescribe treatments based on poorly designed, biased research that can have serious side effects violates this important ethical principle.

SUMMARY OF IMPORTANT POINTS TO CONSIDER
BEFORE USING ANY ANTI-AGING PRODUCTS

- Do not rely only on testimonials!
- Has the product been tested in studies involving humans?
- Has the product been tested in randomized trials comparing it to a placebo?
- Has the product been tested in a double-blind test?
- Has the product been specifically tested in older patients similar to you?
- Have you been warned of any potential side effects?

As doctors, we know that patients are vulnerable to false claims. We don't like to see people spending their hard-earned money on unproven and potentially harmful products. Remember, many who make these conspiracy claims also make a lot of money by promoting these products. In the most tragic cases, patients use these bogus products in place of medically beneficial procedures and remedies.

Chapter 5

DO I NEED HORMONE REPLACEMENT THERAPY?

Late in his life, Hollywood legend Cary Grant was approached by a fan who commented, "You don't look like Cary Grant." He replied, "No one does, ma'am."

There is much talk in the media about the use of growth hormone, DHEA, and testosterone to make elderly men more active, virile, and muscular. Many books have also been written about this topic.

We have all seen advertisements showing an older man who now has big muscles after starting hormone therapy. If you buy into the notion that a picture says a thousand words, then these photos can be quite convincing. After reading this book you should be able to appreciate the fact that nothing that deals with the elderly is simple and straightforward. Every issue has a variety of complicating factors. When you encounter these promotional pictures ask yourself:

- Are the people actually stronger or do they just have bigger muscles? Some people who take growth hormone may get bigger muscles, but when you measure their strength, it is unchanged.
- Is it the hormone that is responsible for these changes? Some scientists believe that the increased muscle is due to the changes in diet and exercise that go along with the hormone treatment. The only way to tell if the effects are due to the hormone is to do a double-blind placebo-controlled trial, where half the subjects involved in the study will receive

the hormone while the other half receive a placebo (chapter 4). Neither the patient nor the scientist know who is getting the placebo. It is uncommon to see an anti-aging product spend the money and resources to do studies with a double-blind placebo.

- Have these hormones been studied mostly in the relatively "healthy" elderly who live at home? It is less likely that they have been studied in the older and sicker homebound and nursing home populations.
- Might they have serious side effects? While they are promoted as health elixirs, they really should be thought of as poorly understood and potentially dangerous medical treatments.

WHAT ABOUT GROWTH HORMONE?

Growth hormone is a hormone secreted by the pituitary gland in the brain. Growth hormone stimulates the production of another hormone called *insulin-like growth factor-1* (IGF-1). Don't get confused, IGF-1 is not insulin. IGF-1 got its name because the molecule is similar in structure to insulin. Growth hormone through IGF-1 is responsible for a variety of functions in the body. It helps prevent protein breakdown and increases the breakdown of fat cells. Growth hormone levels gradually decrease through adulthood, especially in women after menopause. This age-related decrease may lead to:

- decreased energy
- decreased muscle mass
- decreased sex drive
- increased blood pressure
- poor sleep

THE DIAGNOSIS OF GROWTH HORMONE DEFICIENCY

Growth hormone deficiency is usually diagnosed by measuring IGF-1 levels in the blood. Growth hormone is not cheap. You're looking at spending anywhere from five hundred to a thousand dollars per month, and don't expect your insurance company to help pay for it. It is not going to be covered. In addition, you will need to have blood drawn several times a year to check the levels of IGF-1. The monitoring of IGF-1 levels is necessary to make sure you are not being given too little or too much. Again, your insurance will not cover you for this blood work or for the office visits to see the doctor prescribing this medication.

Many *endocrinologists* (doctors who specialize in the treatment of hormonal diseases) say that measuring IGF-1 levels is not the appropriate way to even gauge growth hormone deficiency. Technically, the FDA does not even consider the use of growth hormone as an anti-aging treatment for older adults to be a legal use of this steroid.[1]

What are the legitimate medical uses of growth hormone? Human growth hormone was developed to help boost the growth rates in children with low growth hormone levels to help them develop properly. It has since been shown to also be of benefit to young adults who have low growth hormone levels due to AIDS or injuries to the pituitary gland.[2]

Much of the regulation of growth hormone has come about because of reports of athletes and bodybuilders using it as a performance enhancer. The athletes are trying to get their IGF-1 levels in the super-high range.

Are older adults breaking the law by taking growth hormone as an anti-aging therapy? We personally think that this falls into a gray zone, but there are many endocrinologists who would say that the use of growth hormone for this purpose may be unethical and possibly harmful.

FIRST, THE GOOD NEWS ABOUT GROWTH HORMONE

Since the early 1990s, small studies have shown that healthy elderly men with low IGF-1 levels benefited from growth hormone injections.[3] The men who received the hormone had less body fat and more muscle mass than those who received the placebo. The men also reported that they had more energy and more interest in sex. It is important to remember that these studies were done in healthy seniors. There is currently no evidence to show any benefit when growth hormone is used to treat frail elderly patients.

NOW FOR THE BAD NEWS ABOUT GROWTH HORMONE

The question that we often hear is "Isn't it worth paying all this money to improve your health?" This question assumes that growth hormone has a proven health benefit. The actual data are not so clear-cut. Yes, those who take these hormones may have bigger muscles, but clinically significant improvements in strength, exercise endurance, memory, and sex drive have not been proven with the use of growth hormone or any of its precursors or derivatives.

In a randomized double-blind placebo-controlled study of healthy seniors, leg swelling was seen in 39 percent of the people taking growth hormone and none of the people receiving the placebo pills.[4] Carpal tunnel syndrome (a swelling of the tissues of the wrist causing much pain and weakness in the hands) was seen in 32 percent of those taking growth hormone and none of the placebo patients.[5] Painful joints and diabetes or glucose intolerance were also seen more commonly in those taking growth hormone. The advertisements for these products largely ignore these serious side effects.

NOW FOR THE REALLY BAD NEWS

Even if you believe all the beneficial claims about growth hormone, there is no evidence showing that growth hormone can prolong a person's life. In fact, there is evidence that the opposite is true. There is some scientific evidence in both animals and humans suggesting that high levels of growth hormone are associated with a shorter life span. Another way to think about this is that lower growth hormone levels may be associated with living longer.

SOME OF THE DATA INVOLVING HUMANS

- One study of 864 middle-aged policemen in Paris showed that men with increased growth hormone levels had a higher mortality.[6]
- Another study showed that low levels of IGF-1 in the blood are more common among people who are very old.[7]
- Defects in the ability of the cells to sense IGF-1 were more commonly seen in people who live to the age of one hundred years.[8]
- A large study looked at the effect of growth hormone on malnourished patients in an intensive care unit. The patients were randomized to receive either growth hormone or a placebo. The study had to be stopped early because the patients who received the growth hormone were discovered to have a much higher chance of dying.[9]

SOME FINAL THOUGHTS ABOUT GROWTH HORMONE

At present, there is no definite evidence that seniors really benefit from restoring growth hormone and IGF-1 levels to that of a young adult. You may be asking yourself, Why do many athletes want to take it if it is so ineffective? There is a difference. Athletes are young and already have normal growth hormone levels. By taking growth hormone, athletes hope to raise these levels way above normal. In the case of anti-aging, the idea is to raise someone with below normal levels to those of a "normal" young adult.

We find it quite surprising and unfortunate that medications touted as anti-aging treatments may actually decrease your life expectancy.

IS A LOW TESTOSTERONE LEVEL A PROBLEM?

Low testosterone levels are found in 20 percent of men in their sixties and 50 percent of men who are eighty years of age or older. Low testosterone may be associated with a decrease in muscle strength, bone density, sex drive, and memory.[10] It is also associated with increases in body fat, complaints of insomnia, and symptoms of depression. This constellation of problems in a patient with low blood levels of testosterone is referred to by some doctors as *andropause*, the male equivalent of menopause.

HOW WILL I KNOW IF MY TESTOSTERONE LEVELS ARE LOW?

- Blood levels of testosterone need to be drawn. The *free testosterone level* is the most significant. The free testosterone level is the amount of testosterone that is floating in the blood unattached to specific plasma proteins. Blood drawn in the early morning is the most accurate.
- The testosterone levels need to be measured on at least two separate occasions prior to diagnosis. Don't make a treatment plan based on only one measurement.

DOES TESTOSTERONE REPLACEMENT WORK?

Testosterone can be taken in the form of pills, patches, or injections. Most studies on the use of testosterone therapy focus on middle-aged men and not the elderly. In 2006 a double-blind placebo study involving elderly men with low testosterone levels showed that giving testosterone did not improve their strength or quality of life.[11]

However, the carefully monitored use of low-dose testosterone seems to be pretty safe. As with any medical treatment, you need to discuss it with your physician and you should know the potential side effects. These include:

- fluid retention
- *gynecomastia* (the growth of breast tissue in a male)
- *polycythemia* (abnormal increase in the amount of red blood cells in the bloodstream)
- sleep apnea
- possible increased risk of prostate cancer and/or benign prostatic hyperplasia (enlargement of the prostate). A digital rectal exam and a PSA blood test (chapter 3) need to be done prior to starting hormone therapy.

Make sure you see your doctor every three months for the first year and then every year thereafter.

WHAT ABOUT DEHYDROEPIANDROSTERONE (DHEA)?

DHEA is sold as a food supplement at health food stores. No one is quite sure what this hormone does, but many people have touted this product as a fountain of youth. DHEA is a steroid hormone that is secreted in short bursts by the adrenal gland. Normally, these bursts are larger and occur with increasing frequency at night.

Trying to interpret whether the impact of lower DHEA levels on the aging process is complicated. Most books say that DHEA levels decrease with aging. However, in one large study one out of three patients actually had an increase in their DHEA levels over the eight-year study period.[12]

DOES DHEA WORK?

If the person already has normal levels of DHEA, taking extra DHEA is a waste of time and money. A double-blind placebo-controlled study looking at elderly women and men with low levels of DHEA found that taking it as a supplement had no effect on body weight, muscle size, or percentage of body fat.[13] It also had no effect on aerobic endurance, muscle strength, or insulin sensitivity. Another recent double-blind placebo-controlled trial showed that older adults who took DHEA had no improvement in their cognitive performance or in their sense of well-being compared to those who received the placebo.[14]

If you still believe that taking DHEA will have some benefit, a variety of questions remain unanswered in the medical literature:

- What is the correct dose to take?
- How long should you take this product?
- What is the best time of the day to take it?

IS DHEA SAFE?

If you have low DHEA levels, it is probably safe to take this supplement. Of course you should consult your doctor first. Some doctors remain concerned that the DHEA can get converted to testosterone in men or estrogen in women. This is a concern because higher testosterone levels may affect the prostate. In women, increased estrogen levels may increase a postmenopausal woman's risk of breast cancer, uterine cancer, heart attacks, or strokes.

Chapter 6

WHICH VITAMINS AND HERBAL SUPPLEMENTS SHOULD SENIORS TAKE?

"Wisdom doesn't automatically come with old age. Nothing does—except wrinkles. It's true, some wines improve with age. But only if the grapes were good in the first place."

Abigail Van Buren (Dear Abby) (1918–)

In January 2007 the American Association of Retired Persons, better known as the AARP, and the National Center for Complementary and Alternative Medicine published a survey of 1,559 people age fifty and older regarding their use of complementary and alternative medicine. The majority reported using one or more therapies. Vitamin and herbal supplements are the most popular types of complementary and alternative medicine treatments.

WARNING—DON'T FORGET TO TELL YOUR DOCTOR!

The majority of seniors who use vitamin and herbal products do not tell their doctors about it. We can't stress enough the point that if you plan to use any of the products discussed in this chapter, you need to tell your doctor and ask him for his opinion about it.

WHY WON'T MY DOCTOR GIVE ME A STRAIGHT ANSWER ABOUT VITAMINS?[1]

Part of the difficulty with interpreting studies involving the health benefits of vitamins is that many of the foods we eat in the United States are already fortified with vitamins and minerals. Also, most vitamin studies involve either middle-aged or healthy elderly subjects.

This issue is further complicated by the research that has shown that patients who take vitamins eat a more nutritious diet and lead a healthier lifestyle than those who do not. Therefore, how do you know whether it is the vitamins or the diet that is benefiting the patient? The answer is that we don't know without a double-blind placebo-controlled study. Don't forget that there is no uniformity between brands of a specific vitamin. Also, batches may even vary within a brand. Thus, you and your doctor cannot be 100 percent sure as to the dose and quantity of the vitamins you are taking .

VITAMINS

What about a Multivitamin?

It is probably a good idea for older adults to take a daily multivitamin. We generally recommend a vitamin that has a complete balance of many vitamins and minerals. You don't need to buy the expensive brands at the health food store. Some of the cheaper brands from a convenience store may work just as well. For patients with a poor appetite who are not eating well, the multivitamin may be the only way that they are going to meet the daily requirement of vitamins and minerals.

It is important to realize that the multivitamin is not a magic bullet. The use of a multivitamin has not been shown to decrease the risk of cancer or heart disease.[2] It has not been shown to reduce the risk of dying or lower the risk of infections.

What about Antioxidants?

In chapter 1 we discussed how the excess production of *free radical molecules* can cause a lot of damage to the cells and especially to the DNA itself. In order to protect against this damage, the body has a variety of enzymes that work to remove the buildup of these toxic molecules.

Simply put, antioxidant vitamins don't actually remove the oxidants themselves. Instead, the vitamins bind to the neutralizing enzymes to make them work better. In theory, the better these enzymes work, the more efficiently the bad free radicals will be removed. The more oxidant molecules are removed, the less damage there will be to the cells and the slower the aging process.

Many health books on aging claim that taking these antioxidant vitamins will make you live longer since you will be slowing down the production of free radicals. Before you run out and buy a vitamin product you just saw in an infomercial or in a magazine advertisement, you need to be careful.

The **real truth** is that to date, dozens of randomized clinical trials have been done with antioxidant vitamins. If you look at all the data from these studies, there is no evidence that antioxidant supplements will make you live longer.[3] Many scientists are concerned that the use of antioxidant vitamins by cancer patients receiving chemotherapy or radiation therapy may have an increased risk of dying compared to those who do not take vitamins. These scientists believe that the vitamins may somehow help protect the cancer cells from being killed by the chemotherapy drugs or by radiation therapy.[4]

Vitamin E

Vitamin E is an antioxidant that was touted by many doctors in the 1990s to be effective in preventing heart disease, cancer, and Alzheimer's disease. More recent studies have not shown any of these benefits to be the case. It may even increase your risk of death. Vitamin E can also increase your risk of bleeding. If you are already taking blood-thinning medication, such as warfarin (Coumadin), aspirin, or clopidogrel (Plavix), you need to talk to your doctor before you start taking vitamin E.

Beta-Carotene

Initial studies suggested that beta-carotene intake might serve to protect against the development of some types of cancer. These studies observed that populations with a higher intake of beta-carotene in their diet had a lower risk of getting certain cancers. When randomized double-blind placebo-controlled studies were done, the patients who took beta-carotene had, in fact, a higher risk of getting cancer.[5]

Folate

Many people take folate in order to prevent heart disease. Others take it to prevent memory loss. There is much research now showing that high levels of the amino acid homocysteine is associated with an increased risk of heart attacks and strokes. It is also associated with an increased risk of developing Alzheimer's disease. The treatment for an elevated homocysteine level is to take a folate tablet daily.

Does it work? No one really knows. The use of supplements containing folic acid has been shown to decrease homocysteine levels in the blood. However, research studies have not been able to show that taking folate will decrease the risk of heart attack, stroke, Alzheimer's disease, or death.[6] Part of the difficulty is that in the United States all cereal-grain flour products are now fortified with this vitamin. So if everyone is already getting a large amount of folate from their diet, it becomes very hard to tell whether folate pills will help. Even though we can't tell you if it works, we do know that it is very safe to take and has minimal side effects and drug interactions.

Vitamin B12

Vitamin B12 is commonly taken by older adults for a variety of ailments. A vitamin B12 deficiency is sometimes associated with anemia as well as a variety of neurologic and psychiatric problems. Measuring vitamin B12 levels in the blood is not the definitive test for B12 deficiency. It is only a screening test. If there is a strong suspicion for a vitamin B12 deficiency, then your doctor may want to check methylmalonic acid and homocysteine levels in the blood.

If it turns out that you have vitamin B12 deficiency, injections of vitamin B12 usually correct the neuropsychiatric abnormalities. You can also take a vitamin B12 tablet daily. The dose needed is 1 mg per day. We strongly recommend that you talk to your doctor about this. She may use a prescription brand rather than an over-the-counter preparation. This dose is much larger than the amount found in most over-the-counter B-complex vitamin preparations. When you buy over-the-counter products, there is no guarantee that the dose on the label is the actual dose of the pills.

Vitamin B12 injections in patients who do not have vitamin B12 deficiency do not improve their energy level. If someone tells you that in his or her experience it does, we think it is most likely the placebo effect (chapter 4). Medicare will not cover B12 injections unless there is a blood test confirming a low B12 level or a high homocysteine level.

Vitamin A

There have been several studies suggesting that taking high levels of vitamin A may make the bones weaker and increase the risk of fractures.[7] A recent analysis of the randomized studies involving vitamin A reveals a small increased risk of dying.

Coenzyme Q10

The food that we eat gets converted into energy units (adenosine triphosphate, or ATP for short) and water. This process occurs primarily in the *mitochondria* of the cells. The mitochondria can be thought of as the power plants of the cells. Coenzyme Q10 helps in this conversion process as well as in neutralizing the free radicals produced.

Placebo studies have shown that the use of coenzyme Q10 supplements may benefit patients with congestive heart failure[8] and Parkinson's disease.[9] There is some research suggesting that taking the cholesterol medications referred to as *statins* (Lipitor, Zocor, Crestor) may lower your coenzyme Q10 levels. While taking coenzyme Q10 with the statin may restore coenzyme Q10 levels, it is unclear if this leads to a benefit in the patient's health.[10]

Selenium

In 1996 a large study was published showing that people who took supplements containing selenium had a lower risk of developing cancer of the lung, colon, and prostate.[11] Further analysis, however, showed that these same were also at a higher risk for developing diabetes than those who took the placebo.[12] Further studies have failed to show that selenium supplements help prevent cancer.[13]

What's All the Buzz about Vitamin D?[14]

We have known for a long time that vitamin D, along with calcium, is important in order to maintain strong bones. We will discuss the effect of calcium and vitamin D on the bones later in this chapter.

What you may not be aware of is that humans get vitamin D both from their diet and from sunlight. The majority of frail older adults are at risk for vitamin D deficiency because they do not get enough sunlight and have poor diets.

In the last several years there have been many studies showing that patients who took vitamin D had a slightly lower risk of dying.[15] There are also many studies showing that patients who took vitamin D supplements had a 20 percent lower risk of falls. We think that vitamin D may actually play a role in maintaining muscle strength. Recent evidence also suggests that vitamin D supplements may help lower the risk of colon cancer.

So how much vitamin D should you take? Previous recommendations of 400–600 IU per day are probably inadequate. Most researchers now recommend between 800–1000 IU per day.[16]

Just a word of caution: studies have shown an increase in kidney stones in postmenopausal women taking this supplement. Patients with high calcium levels in their blood should avoid taking this supplement. Make sure your doctor knows you are taking calcium and/or vitamin D.

Do Vitamins Help Prevent Macular Degeneration?

Macular degeneration is the most common form of blindness in the elderly (chapter 2). If you watch TV, listen to the radio, or surf the Internet, it is not hard to find advertisements for vitamin products that will protect your eyes. The US government conducted a large randomized placebo-controlled trial to study the effect of the use of vitamins to slow down the progression of macular degeneration.[17] The formula they used contained 500 mg of vitamin C, 400 IU of vitamin E, 15 mg of beta carotene, 80 mg of zinc in the form of zinc oxide, and 2 mg of copper as cupric oxide.

The results of this study showed that there was no benefit for people with mild disease, but there was a 30 percent reduction among people with more advanced age-related macular degeneration.

Before you rush out to buy these products, be careful! Not all vitamins are the same. Read the label on the bottle. Many do not contain the recommended doses used in the study described above. Some may have the vitamin E and beta carotene removed for the reasons we discussed earlier. If you have any concerns, talk to your doctor.

HERBAL THERAPIES

All herbal products are regulated as food supplements, not as medications. Because of this lack of rigorous oversight, the quality and quantity of herbal product can vary considerably among different brands and even among different batches from the same manufacturer.

What about Garlic?

This herb has been used for its medicinal properties for thousands of years. Many people use garlic as a natural treatment for atherosclerosis. By inhibiting platelets from clumping together, garlic, in theory, can help lower the risk of heart attacks and strokes. Garlic is also marketed as a natural way to lower your cholesterol. Clinical studies measuring the ability of garlic supplements to lower cholesterol have not been encouraging. Neither has its effectiveness at lowering blood pressure been so easy to demonstrate.

Stop using garlic at least seven days before any surgery or invasive medical procedures. If you are already taking aspirin, clopidogrel (Plavix), aspirin, or warfarin (Coumadin), talk to your doctor before beginning a garlic regimen.

Does Echinacea Help Treat or Prevent Infections?

Echinacea is an herb that many people claim will boost the immune system. Many people take this in an attempt to prevent and shorten the course of respiratory and viral infections. Several studies suggested that this herb could stimulate the immune system. However, other studies have shown that the product is no better than a placebo at treating or preventing an infection.[18] Studies specifically with elderly patients are lacking.

Does Saw Palmetto Help Men with Enlarged Prostates?

Saw Palmetto is an herbal product that is used by many men with enlarged prostate conditions. There have been many studies looking at the effectiveness of this product to decrease the urinary symptoms that are associated with enlarged prostates. While this herb has been shown to be very safe, its medical benefit is unclear. There are studies showing some improvement in symptoms, while others show no benefit at all.

What about Ginkgo Biloba?

Ginkgo biloba is a popular herbal product that is marketed as an alterative therapy treatment for people with memory loss to help improve their memory. Studies have been done to see if this herb has any effect on memory. Some studies show a benefit while more carefully designed ones show that it is no better than a placebo.[19] Ginkgo is generally very safe to use.

In theory, ginkgo may have some effect on the ability of the platelets in your blood to effectively form clots. Most research, however, has shown that this effect is not clinically important.[20] Despite the lack of evidence for an increased risk of bleeding, ginkgo should still be used with caution in patients who are already on blood thinners, such as aspirin, heparin, warfarin (Coumadin), and clopidogrel (Plavix).

What about Valerian?

Valerian is an herbal supplement that has been shown to help people fall asleep. The doses used in studies ranged from 400 to 900 mg. Before you rush out and buy this product, you may want to keep a few things in mind. This medication has not been studied in the frail senior. Therefore, we do not know whether this medication is effective or whether the dose needs to be lowered in frail patients or in those who take many medications.

What about Green Tea?

For years, researchers have thought that green tea contains a chemical that may have strong antioxidant properties. Many studies have suggested that drinking green tea may lower the risk of cancer, heart disease, and diabetes.[21] In 2006 the medical journal *JAMA* published a large study from Japan showing that people who drank five or more cups of green tea per day had a lower risk of dying than those who drank less than one cup per day.[22] More recent studies suggest that green tea may contain substances that can lower cholesterol, improve diabetes, and protect the body against cancer. On rare occasions, there have been reports of people damaging their liver from using green tea products.

OTHER SUPPLEMENTS

What about Omega-3 Fatty Acids?

The fat in fish oil is high in omega-3 fatty acids. Scientific research has shown that the omega-3 fatty acids found in fish are metabolized to produce the anti-inflammatory molecules PGE3 and LTB5.

Not all omega-3 fatty acid supplements are the same. Some are rich in alpha-linolenic acid (ALA), which can be found in flaxseed and walnuts. Others contain the longer molecules eicosapentaenoic acid (EPA) and decosahexanic acid (DHA), which are found in fish oils. Alpha-linolenic acid is a precursor of EPA and DHA. However, for some unknown reason, this conversion of flaxseed oil into EPA and DHA is not an efficient process in males, and most of the ALA will not get converted into EPA and DHA. This is important because it is the EPA and DHA that have the anti-inflammatory effect.

Can Omega-3 Fatty Acids Prevent Heart Disease?

The American Heart Association has recently endorsed the use of omega-3 fatty acids for the prevention of heart attacks in patients who already have heart disease.[23] This is the first time that this prestigious organization has ever recommended a nutritional product for patients with heart disease.

How much fish oil should you consume?[24] If you have heart disease you should take 1 g a day of DHA and EPA. Read labels carefully because most fish oil pills are only 30 percent DHA and EPA. If you do not have heart disease, the recommended dose is only 500 mg per day.

Final Thoughts on Fish Oil

Fish oil is commonly used in the treatment of arthritis pain (chapter 27). Fish oil may have some anti-inflammatory properties when taken in high doses. Taking an NSAID (on the same days you are taking omega-3 fatty acids) may decrease the anti-inflammatory properties of the fish oil since it may lead to the blockage of the conversion of omega-3 fatty acids to PGE3. If you are taking this supplement for your arthritis, do not expect it to work immediately. It may take up to four weeks for you to notice an effect.

We regard fish oil as one of the good guys. There are good data supporting its benefits and it is very safe. It is also very cheap. Fish oil supplements do not contain mercury. While fish oil probably won't increase your risk of bleeding, you should still talk to your doctor if you are already on a blood-thinning drug (Coumadin, Plavix, aspirin).

What about Glucosamine?

Glucosamine is a compound that is found in many arthritis nutritional supplements. While many nutritional products have not been studied, glucosamine is a different story. While the initial studies seemed promising, more recent studies show no benefit to using this supplement.[25]

Chondroitin sulfate is another nutritional compound that you may see being promoted for patients with arthritis. The research does not show any benefit by itself or in combination with glucosamine.[26] Chondroitin is often combined with glucosamine. Fortunately, both of these products are reported to be very safe.

Should I Also Take Calcium?

All patients at risk for osteoporosis should be taking calcium (chapter 15). In every study involving the medications for osteoporosis, every patient was also on calcium. If you buy calcium supplements, look for ones that have vitamin D included. The vitamin D helps the calcium absorb better. We recommend calcium citrate over calcium carbonate tablets. We have found that calcium citrate tablets are more easily digested.

So How Much Calcium Do I Need per Day?

According to the National Osteoporosis Foundation, if you are over the age of fifty, you should take 1,200 mg of calcium daily.[27]

WHAT TYPE OF DIET IS THE BEST?

Many people believe that a diet low in saturated fats and high in fiber is ideal. These low-fat diets are recommended by many doctors and nutritionists. Two recent research studies have compared a low-fat diet to a Mediterranean diet (that is, a diet rich in olive oil and nuts).[28] Patients on the Mediterranean diet also had a few glasses of wine per day. In both studies, those on the Mediterranean diet had lower blood glucose levels, lower blood pressures, and lower cholesterol levels.

Will a Calorie Restriction Diet Make You Live Longer?

You may have seen news stories about research showing that reducing the number of calories you eat may increase your life span. This theory is referred to as *calorie restriction.*

Studies have shown that calorie restriction can increase the life span of fruit flies and rodents. Many studies in mice have shown that even a small decrease in the amount of calories eaten can lead to a big increase in longevity. In fact, calorie restriction is science's most effective intervention for increasing longevity in mice and fruit flies.

How does it work? No one is really sure.[29] To use the explanation that fewer calories means less free radical formation appears to be too simplistic. An emerging theory is that decreasing caloric intake somehow signals the cell's mitochondria (where nutrients are converted into energy) to increase in number and work more effectively.[30] At the present time, we do not know what these signals are, but we suspect that a family of genes (SIRT1, SIRT3, SIRT4, and SIRT5) may be involved.

To get a better understanding of whether calorie restriction is beneficial, studies have been conducted looking at the effect of calorie restriction in monkeys. By cutting the calorie intake by 30 percent, the researchers noted that there was a decrease in LDL (the bad cholesterol), blood pressure, insulin levels, and oxidative damage to muscle tissue.[31] There was also an increase in the number of times the fibroblasts could duplicate before they stop dividing. This is important because, as we discussed in chapter 1, cells in the body can undergo only a certain number of genetically programmed divisions. Calorie restriction may somehow delay the normal genetic mechanisms that tell a cell to either stop dividing or die.

Have There Been Any Studies Looking at Calorie Restriction in Humans?

Conducting these studies in humans is quite difficult since humans age much slower than mice. The scientists would most likely die before the study was finished. There have been several short-term studies with humans showing that calorie restriction may have a variety of beneficial effects.[32]

What about Resveratrol?

In a country where obesity is such a problem, getting people to eat less than normal could be a challenge. Trying to find a substance that can mimic the effects of calorie restriction is an area of research for many scientists.

One compound that has received a lot of attention is resveratrol. Originally isolated from the roots of the white hellbore and the Japanese knotweed, this substance has also been found in red wine.

Studies in yeast cells and fruit flies strongly suggest that resveratrol may have anti-inflammatory and anticancer properties. It even appears to extend the life span in these organisms by a mechanism similar to that of calorie restriction,[33] possibly involving the SIRT family of genes. Recent studies in mice show a similar benefit.[34]

So why can't you just drink a glass or two of red wine? Found primarily in the skin of the grape, the concentration of resveratrol can vary over twenty-fold depending on the brand of wine. At this time, no studies have been done in humans to see if resveratrol works. One reason that there are no studies in humans is because no one really knows how much resveratrol humans would need in order to see these beneficial effects. We assume that you would have to drink many gallons of wine per day. Part of the reason a person would need a large quantity of resveratrol is that our bodies break it down in minutes.

Currently, there are resveratrol tablets on the market. These tablets are sold as food supplements and not as a drug (see chapter 4). The dose in these pills is probably not going to be enough to have any effect. Therefore, the race is on in the pharmaceutical industry to develop a pill form that can deliver high doses of resveratrol in a manner that is not so quickly broken down by the body and would have no side effects.

As we discussed in the previous two chapters, always talk to your doctor before you start taking any nutritional supplements or alternative therapies. Your doctor may be able to give you some good advice that can save you some money and help you avoid potentially harmful side effects.

Chapter 7

THE REAL TRUTH ABOUT EXERCISE

"I get my exercise acting as a pallbearer to my friends who exercise."
Senator Chauncey Depew (1834–1928)

HOW IMPORTANT IS REGULAR EXERCISE?

Exercise is vital for any older adult who wants to remain healthy. Studies have shown that older adults who exercise regularly have:

- better balance and a lower risk for falls
- better control of their blood sugar levels
- better flexibility
- better quality sleep
- fewer symptoms of depression
- improved muscle strength
- less arthritis pain of their hips and knees

We have all read many books and articles encouraging people to exercise. Understanding that exercise is a good thing is the easy part. Figuring out the ideal exercise program is often very difficult. Patients all have different body shapes, different medical issues, and different musculoskeletal problems. We are therefore very reluctant to recommend any exercise regimen that is not adjusted to meet the specific needs of the individual older adult.

As doctors, we do tell our patients that they need to exercise more. Some may join a gym and get a personal trainer. However, just because a trainer has big muscles does not mean that he knows what he is talking about. Many athletic trainers who work at gyms and health clubs are not trained to understand all the potential risks and dangers involved with training the elderly.

The elderly person needs someone who understands the subtle issues that come with aging muscles and ligaments. In addition, many seniors have arthritis and osteoporosis, which changes the normal body alignment during exercise. Others may have degenerative changes in the spine. If your trainer does not pay attention to these details, you could get hurt. You have to train a seventy-eight-year-old woman differently than an eighteen-year-old football player.

So be very careful!

AEROBIC EXERCISE

Endurance exercise helps to strengthen both the heart and the lungs. It will also give you more stamina. Before you get started, beware: many older adults have much *atherosclerosis* (plaque) in their coronary arteries. This places older adults at a higher risk for heart attacks. An older adult who has not exercised for years should talk to his doctor before starting an aerobic exercise routine. The doctor may determine that the patient's heart would be unable to tolerate the increased exertion associated with exercise.

You may have heard the recommendation that people should try to exercise for thirty minutes at 75–80 percent of their maximum target heart rate. The maximum heart rate is calculated using the simple formula *220 minus your age in years.*

This formula does not work well for many seniors. For the older adult who has been inactive for years and now wants to start exercising, we generally recommend a goal of 60–65 percent rather than 75–80 percent. For those who cannot exercise for a full thirty minutes, two fifteen-minute periods or three ten-minute periods may suffice.

Before you run off to buy one of those heart rate meters, you need to be careful. Many older adults may be on heart medications called *beta-blockers*, which can slow down their heart rate.

Commonly used beta-blockers in the United States include:

- atenolol (Tenormin)
- carvedilol (Coreg)
- labetalol (Normodyne, Trandate)
- metoprolol (Lopressor, Toprol-XL)
- propranolol (Inderal)

Diltiazem and verapamil are two other popular heart medications that may slow the heart rate down. Many pacemakers regulate how fast the heart can beat. If you have an irregular heart rhythm problem called *atrial fibrillation,* you need to be careful as well. So how hard should elderly patients exert themselves? We suggest that they should be able to talk comfortably while exercising.

STRETCHING

Our advice with regard to stretching is to be careful! Many seniors have not stretched in decades. During that time their tendons (which attach muscles to bone) and ligaments (which attach bones together) have undergone a variety of degenerative changes and the water content decreases. The water content of cartilage also decreases. Consequently, most people become less flexible as they age. Tendons and ligaments tend to tear more easily, and when they tear, they heal more slowly.

The National Institute on Aging offers some helpful hints on stretching:

- Stretching exercises should be done only after your muscles are warmed up. You can warm up by walking or by doing some gentle bicycle riding. This is especially important during the winter when it is cold outside. The cold weather will make your joints and ligaments stiffer.
- Stretching should cause some minor discomfort, but it should not be painful. If you are experiencing pain with stretching, you need to lessen the tension or stop.
- Move slowly into a stretching position. Quick jerking motions can lead to injury.
- Hold the position for at least twenty to thirty seconds. If you can't hold the stretch that long, then you are overstretching and need to do it more gently.
- We believe that all frail elderly patients should consult with their physician or a physical therapist before starting a stretching regimen. Don't

just do stretching exercises that you saw someone perform on TV or at the gym. Even a yoga or Pilates class that is not specifically designed for the untrained older adult can lead to injuries.[1]

WHAT ABOUT WEIGHT TRAINING?

There is some truth to the saying "use it or lose it!" The **real truth** is that many elderly patients do not have much more that they can afford to lose. This brings up the concept of *functional reserve* that we alluded to in chapters 1 and 2. Functional reserve refers to the amount of extra work that can be done by an organ or muscle when needed. By the time some seniors reach their eighties and nineties, they have such a small functional reserve in their muscles that they can barely get out of bed or walk.

Many seniors take up exercise programs that involve lifting weights. By lifting weights their muscles will grow in size and become stronger. Weight training would appear on the surface to make sense. Increasing muscle size and strength could help many seniors who have lost some of their size and strength over the years.

The **real truth** is that older adults need to be careful before beginning a weight-lifting program. Proper instruction with the correct weight and form is critical. We cannot overemphasize the danger that a poorly designed weight-training regimen poses to the joints, tendons, and ligaments of seniors. Studies have shown that a carefully designed regimen may make seniors' muscles a little bigger and stronger. Any benefits gained have usually been lost once the study is over. Researchers have not been able to show that weight-training exercises by themselves can decrease the level of disability among frail seniors.[2]

SOME RECOMMENDATIONS FOR THOSE OF YOU WHO HAVE NOT EXERCISED IN DECADES

1. *Walking*—it is so simple yet so effective. Even fifteen minutes twice a day can help improve one's lung function and lower the blood sugar levels in patients with diabetes. For people who are out of shape, this is a nice way to exercise without putting a lot of stress on your joints.
2. *Pool exercises*—you don't have to do laps in the pool. Walking in the pool or simply moving your arms and legs as you stand in the shallow end of the pool is an excellent way to exercise. Buoyancy provides support to

joints during movement and even some resistance. Muhammad Ali used to do pool exercises to help him train for many of his fights. It works very well for patients with arthritis of the hips and knees as a way to exercise arthritic joints without putting much weight-bearing stress on the joints.

3. *Stationary bicycle*—when done at low speeds and low resistance this exercise can be of great benefit to patients with arthritic knees.

4. *Tai chi*—we like this Chinese martial art because it promotes balance and strengthening without putting much stress on the joints and ligaments. You commonly see videos of elderly people in China doing their slow tai chi exercises in the morning. Although it does not involve punching or kicking, it is still considered a martial art. It has also been shown in several studies to improve balance and decrease the risk of falls in older adults.[3]

5. *Yoga*—many older adults enroll in yoga classes in order to enjoy its many health benefits. These benefits include increased flexibility, improved balance, and an improved sense of well-being. However, we have found that older adults need to be very careful. There are yoga classes that cater to clients who have medical challenges as well as older clients. Look for a yoga instructor with experience in adapting poses for individual needs.

6. *Custom exercises*—for patients who can no longer walk, there are even exercises that a physical therapist can design to be done in bed or in a chair.

7. *Power Plate*—is a new exercise device that involves a flat rubber-matted circle that vibrates at very fast speeds. By standing on the plate in a variety of different positions, seniors can potentially receive an effective workout, even if they are unable to walk. We strongly recommend that seniors use this device only under the supervision of a trained professional.

We recommend to our patients that they should always start to exercise slowly. Once started, some patients get quite motivated and excited about their new exercise regimen. The improvement in how they feel and in their exercise performance serves to motivate them further. As the amount of exercise increases, we often see that many of them succumb to joint and ligament injuries. The point is that even if you think or know you can do more, we advise you not to do so.

QUESTIONS TO ASK YOUR DOCTOR

1. Is it safe for me to exercise?
2. What type of exercise should I be doing?
3. Are there exercises I should avoid doing?

The main point we want to leave you with is to proceed with caution when starting an exercise program. Start easy and work your way up slowly.

Chapter 8

AVOIDING THE COMMON DANGERS OF MEDICATIONS

"Doctors are men who prescribe medicines of which they know little, to cure diseases of which they know less in human beings of whom they know nothing."
Voltaire (1694–1778)

We cannot overstate the benefits that modern medications have had on our society. They allow tens of millions of Americans to lead longer and more productive lives. They form the cornerstone of modern therapy for congestive heart failure, diabetes, hypertension, COPD, and infectious diseases. Simply stated, without these drugs, many older adults would be in the hospital or dead.

Despite these advancements, it is hard to watch the news or read the newspaper without seeing stories that focus on the dangerous side effects of prescription drugs and their exorbitant prices. The media inundate us with so much information that many older adults are afraid to take them. We have cared for many patients who refuse to take medications after reading an article in a magazine or newspaper or even after reading the warning on the package insert.

WHAT DOES THE FDA DO?

In order for a drug to be sold in the United States, it must first be approved by the Food and Drug Administration. The FDA will review in great detail all research studies involving the medication. It will assess how beneficial the medication is in treating one or more illnesses. It will also determine whether there are potentially dangerous side effects.

Each drug is approved for one or more specific illnesses. Once the drug is available to the public, doctors may then use this medication to treat additional illnesses that were not studied in the initial approval process. We call this the *off-label use* of the medication. Just because a medication is being used off-label does not mean that it is being used recklessly or incorrectly. In many cases, the off-label use is supported by excellent research studies and good clinical judgment.

There Is No Good System for Monitoring Drugs Once They Are Approved!

The drug studies that the FDA reviews prior to approval often involve several thousand carefully selected patients. Frail elderly patients, those suffering from other severe illnesses, and those taking lots of other drugs are often excluded. These studies usually do not run longer than a few months to a year.

Once a drug is approved, it is ready to be used in the real world. This means that it will be used in the same types of patients excluded in the initial drug studies and might be used for a period of years. With potentially hundreds of thousands of people now taking the drug, new problems may start to be seen. If there is a problem with the drug, the FDA won't know unless it is voluntarily reported by doctors and the drug company.

"I'm Scared to Take the Medication after Reading the Package Insert!"

We hear this comment quite often from patients. All medications come with a package insert that is a piece of paper with very tiny print that lists the potential side effects of the drug. It also lists other medications to avoid while taking the particular drug. The FDA requires drug companies to list all the possible drug side effects. The key word here is "all." For the consumer, this can be frightening as the lists are often very long. Many of these side effects are so uncommon that to list them merely causes concern and anxiety among patients.

The **real truth** is that all medications have the potential to cause side effects. As we will shortly see, however, the frail elderly are at a very high risk for medication side effects.

So how do you know which side effects on the list you need to worry about? Ask your doctor or other healthcare professional. The important questions to ask your doctor are:

- What are the side effects thatI need to worry about?
- Is the benefit of taking the medication greater than the risk of a serious side effect?
- Do safer alternative drugs or treatments exist?

Why Do Seniors Have So Much Trouble Taking Their Medications?

Elderly patients often do not to take their medications as prescribed. There are many reasons to explain why this problem is so common:

- seniors take more medications than younger adults
- many seniors have memory problems
- many drug names sound alike, for example, Celexa is an antidepressant and Celebrex is an anti-inflammatory drug. In the last few years the FDA has recognized this problem and is now very careful about how market names are assigned to drugs.
- many seniors suffer from depression (chapter 21)
- some drugs need to be taken more than two times per day
- a poor understanding by many patients of their medical issues and the need to take the medication
- poor vision and difficulty hearing verbal instructions
- poor communication between the patient and the doctor
- lack of money to pay for the medications

If you get confused about how to take your medications, you need to talk to your doctor. It a good idea to bring all your medications with you to your doctor's office during a visit. You should also be honest and tell the doctor if you are not taking one or more of your pills. We have seen many cases where a doctor starts a patient with high blood pressure on a second, third, and fourth high blood pressure pill only to find out that the patient was never taking any of the prescribed hypertension drugs in the first place.

WHY ARE OLDER PEOPLE TAKING SO MANY MEDICATIONS?

Once again, there are no simple answers. Older adults generally have more illnesses than younger patients. All of the following, for example, are seen more commonly in older adults:

- arthritis
- chronic obstructive pulmonary disease (COPD)/emphysema
- congestive heart failure
- coronary artery disease
- diabetes
- hypertension
- strokes

It is also not uncommon to see older adults with a combination of several of these illnesses. Because they have more medical illnesses, it is not surprising that they take more medications. A ninety-two-year-old with hypertension, heart failure, and diabetes should be on more medications than a twenty-five-year-old suffering from only hypertension.

Older adults also see more doctors for their medical illnesses. Because it is so tricky to take care of seniors with multiple medical problems, doctors are usually very hesitant to stop the medications that one of their colleagues has prescribed. Patients also commonly use a wide variety of "as needed" medications for ailments, such as pain, constipation, and anxiety.

SO WHAT NUMBER OF PILLS IS CONSIDERED TOO MANY?

There really is no straight answer to this question. Many HMOs and healthcare systems have set different cut-offs for the number of medications that an older person should be prescribed. We have seen the number vary from as few as five to as many as fourteen. The **real truth** probably varies and lies somewhere between the two. For example, a diabetic patient with congestive heart failure should be on an ACE-I, digoxin, spironolactone, a beta-blocker, a cholesterol medication, and one or more diabetic medications. If the doctor does not have the patient on all these medications, these same organizations will tell her that she is not providing quality care. At the other extreme, if the person is taking fourteen or more medications, you have to wonder if there is any room in the stomach for food.

DON'T JUMP TO ANY CONCLUSIONS!

There is a tendency by many who teach geriatrics to doctors to oversimplify the issue and say that the elderly take too many drugs. Unfortunately, such statements ignore the fact that many medications are actually underused in this population. For example, many postmenopausal women are not on any medications to prevent or treat osteoporosis. Similarly, the majority of older adults with depression do not receive an antidepressant medication.

WHY DO DRUGS COST SO MUCH IN THE UNITED STATES?

It is distressing for consumers to see how much these drugs can cost. It currently costs hundreds of millions of dollars to develop, test, and bring a new drug to the market. What people forget is that for every product that makes it to the market, there are many trial compounds that will fail. The further along in this process the drug is before it fails, the more money that the company will have to write off. The other thing to remember is that not every drug is a blockbuster moneymaker for the company. Like automobile models, some medications never get a good market share and become money losers. The drugs that do *make it* have to make up for all these losses. Without a profit incentive, the companies will not invest the billions of dollars needed to develop new drugs.

This explains why the companies need to charge so much, but it does not explain why drugs are so much cheaper in other countries. Many countries impose price controls on the drug companies. In other cases, the medications are cheaper overseas because certain countries do not respect US patent rights. In these countries the drugs can be made with cheaper labor and less attention to issues of quality control. Because of this, the American consumer is in a sense subsidizing the cost of drug research and development for the rest of the world.

ARE THE DRUG COMPANIES CONSPIRING TO PUSH DRUGS?

Let's not be naive; the pharmaceutical industry wants to make a profit. The reason there are so many commercials for medications on TV and in magazines is that the companies want to motivate people to ask their doctors for them.

WHAT IS THE MEDICARE PART D DRUG PROGRAM?

In January 2006 Medicare began offering insurance coverage for prescription drugs. The idea behind this program was to help seniors afford the medications they need. These plans are run by profit-driven private companies that are approved by Medicare. The prescription drug benefit provided by these companies is not free. The basic plan requires that you pay:

- a monthly premium
- a yearly deductible
- a percentage of the cost of each prescription (a copayment)
- when the amount paid by you and the drug plan for the year exceeds $2,510, you pay the next $3,216 of the costs (this is referred to as the "donut hole")
- 5 percent of the costs after the drug cost exceeds $5,726 for the year[1]

Patients with a low income can qualify for reduced payments. Seniors who were on Medicaid or have an individual income of less than $15,600 ($21,000 for a married couple living together) can sign up for special plans with no premiums, deductibles, or donut holes.[2] The copayments are only several dollars per prescription. The rest of the senior population can pay a higher premium in order to lower the amount of the donut hole.

Seem kind of confusing? It has been our experience that the seniors with the most medical illnesses (the ones taking the most medications) often do not know the names or the dosages of the drugs they are taking. Many are unable to even follow the directions on a pill bottle. To expect all of them to understand this complicated system is absurd. A recent study in *JAMA* showed that 60 percent of seniors enrolled in Medicare Part D, which provided "patient education," did not even know they were responsible for a large percentage of their drug costs.[3]

We have also seen many patients who stop taking their medications during this donut hole period. The patients who can't afford to pay for their drugs during this period will still have to pay their monthly premiums to the drug plan. They must also purchase all their drugs from their Part D provider. If they do not, they will not get credit toward the donut hole.

Are your drugs covered? Just because your specific medications are listed as covered by a plan does not necessarily mean that the medication will be covered for *you*. In many cases, the company imposes hoops and hurdles for you to jump through before they pay for these medications. These games usually go under the term *prior authorizations*. Your doctor will have to submit paperwork stating that you have tried other medications that failed or that your specific disease requires the medication. In other cases your doctor or her staff will have to call these companies and answer questionnaires.

It gets worse.... You will have a choice of plans. On the surface, having a choice sounds great. We have grown up in a culture in which choice is thought to be a good thing. In making your decision you can look at the cost and medications provided. Once you pick a plan you cannot switch plans for at least a year. (Unfortunately, the plans can change the specific medications that are covered ... after you have signed up.) How's that for a confusing system?

Over time the problems with the Part D programs will only get worse. These companies want to maximize their profits. An obvious way to do this is to charge more and to institute more stringent regulations on how they will pay for medications. Many of these companies have had a lot of success in developing rules to limit the use of specific drugs. Unfortunately, their experience has been with employee health and retiree plans. Now they are applying this model to people who in many cases are demented or have hearing and vision problems. How is this population group possibly going to navigate the increasing hurdles that the pharmacy benefit companies are putting in front of them?

There will also be pressure from Medicare to cut benefits. Since its inception, Medicare Part D has led to increased profits for pharmaceutical companies. Seniors can now get the drugs that in the past they could not afford. The companies handling the Medicare Part D benefit are also making a great deal of money. With companies making tons of money off this program, the cost of the Part D benefit to the government will increase from $49.5 billion in 2007 to $141.8 billion in 2017.[4] Over time, the government will become more aggressive in its attempts to keep expenses down.

We believe that in the years to come, the drug plans will therefore become more strict in what they will actually pay for. Many companies will make patients use generics before they will pay for a brand-name drug. Premiums, deductibles, copayments, and the donut hole will all likely increase. We believe that such stringent policies defeat the whole purpose of a drug plan in the first place. If seniors are going, in many cases, to be forced to use generics that cost only four dollars per month at Wal-Mart and pay higher copayments, does it really benefit to have a drug plan in the first place?

SHOULD I BE WORRIED ABOUT MEDICATION SIDE EFFECTS?

The frail elderly are at a very high risk for drug-related side effects. The three main reasons seniors are at such a high risk include:

- decreased functional reserve
- age-related changes in the way medications are absorbed and broken down by the body
- the use of higher numbers of medications that can increase the risk that the drugs will interact poorly with each other

What Is Meant by *Decreased Functional Reserve*?

As we discussed in chapter 2, this population lacks the *functional reserve* to handle the stress of some medications. A drug that causes a younger patient to get a little drowsy, for instance, may cause the elderly patient with a decreased brain reserve to become delirious.

Seniors also have multiple medical illnesses. Therefore, the drug used to treat one illness may have a side effect that makes another illness worse. For example, Lopressor or Toprol-XL may be needed to treat hypertension or congestive heart failure, but these drugs have the potential to makes diabetes or COPD worse.

AGE-RELATED CHANGES IN THE WAY MEDICATIONS ARE ABSORBED AND BROKEN DOWN BY THE BODY

The absorption of medication through the walls of the stomach and small intestine is largely unchanged with normal aging. A variety of factors, however, may impair how drugs are absorbed in the body. The use of drugs to suppress acid production (Prilosec, Nexium, Prevacid, Aciphex, Zantac, Pepcid) may affect the absorption of certain other drugs. The presence of food in the stomach can also affect the ability of the stomach and intestines to absorb certain drugs.

The movement of a drug throughout the body may also be different. There is often a decrease in the proteins in the blood that drugs bind to. There is also a gradual decrease in the amount of water and muscle tissue. At the same time there is a gradual increase in the amount of fat tissue. These changes in water, muscle, fat, and blood protein levels all have a major impact on how long drugs stay in the body. The ability of the kidney and the liver to eliminate drugs and toxins generally decreases with the normal aging process.

WHAT DOES IT MEAN TO SAY THAT TWO DRUGS MAY "INTERACT" WITH EACH OTHER?

You may read that the more drugs a person takes, the higher the risk that two or more drugs may "interact." But what does this mean? You may have a vision of a chemistry experiment in which you mix two chemicals to form a super-dangerous new compound. That is not what we mean by this term. Usually what we mean is that drug A will block the absorption of drug B, so less of drug B will get into your body. It may also mean that drug A may increase or decrease the body's ability to break down or excrete drug B.

Not surprisingly, studies have shown that the more medications an elderly patient is taking, the higher the risk of an adverse side effect.

How Common Are These Side Effects?

No one really knows for sure. Some experts have estimated that there may be more than 2 million cases of serious adverse drug reactions among hospitalized patients and another 350,000 that occur in nursing homes each year.[5]

Also, it has been estimated that 5–28 percent of all hospital admissions in the elderly are due to side effects from medications. In the hospital, 25 percent of patients over eighty years of age will have a drug-related side effect.[6] These adverse side effects will increase the number of days you are stuck in the hospital, as well as your risk of death and placement in a nursing home.

When we think of drug reactions in young adults, the first thing that comes to mind is the terrible allergic rash that some get when they take the antibiotic penicillin. In the frail elderly, the side effects can occur in a variety of ways, including:

- bleeding from ulcers in the stomach or in the small intestine
- delirium
- difficulty controlling one's urination
- dizziness and low blood pressure upon standing
- falls
- imbalances in the blood levels of sodium, potassium, glucose, and calcium

- kidney failure
- severe constipation—this can occur to such an extent that the stool becomes stuck in the colon, leading to a fecal impaction

The media talk often about the dangers of medication in the elderly, and you should keep a few thoughts in the back of your mind. When drugs are being tested for their safety, they are usually given to young patients. While geriatric patients are often required to be included in the studies, it is almost always younger healthier elderly patients who are selected. Patients over the age of eighty-five or who live in a nursing home are excluded. Why would the companies do that? The main reason is that the frail elderly have so many complicating illnesses and are often on so many other medications that to include them would only complicate the analysis of the research. The irony here is that the population that is at highest risk for drug side effects are in the same category of patients who are excluded from drug safety studies.

WHO'S WATCHING OUT FOR NURSING HOME RESIDENTS?

In the late 1980s the federal government got very concerned that nursing home residents were being overmedicated with potentially dangerous medications. There was a belief that psychiatric medications were being overused in order to keep residents quiet and nonactive so that the facilities could save money by hiring fewer staff members. Congress held hearings on this topic and passed legislation regulating the use of psychiatric drugs in the nursing home. Psychiatric medications refer primarily to antidepressants, benzodiazepines, and antipsychotics. These regulations are very important, as the majority of nursing home residents are prescribed one or more of these drugs. This legislation was also significant because it was the first time that the federal government got involved in the regulation of how medications are prescribed.

According to the regulations, in order to use a psychiatric medication in the nursing home, the facility needs to provide documentation for each one of these drugs to ensure that:

- it is being used for the appropriate psychiatric disorder
- the dose is not too high
- the patient is not having side effects

WHO'S WATCHING OUT FOR THE REST OF US?

The regulations discussed above only apply to nursing home residents. To address drug safety issues for the elderly population as a whole, in 1993 a group of national experts developed a list of medications that are inappropriate for the elderly. This list was updated in 1997 and most recently in 2003.[7] Some of these drugs are, however, commonly prescribed to elderly patients in the nursing home, hospital, and outpatient settings. The use of one or more of these medications may increase the risk of an elderly person getting sick or even needing to go the emergency room. In the last few years, many HMOs and government agencies have been using these lists as markers of the quality of care provided to seniors. In their eyes, a physician who prescribes more of these medications would not be as good as one who uses them sparingly. In the sections below, we will discuss some of the commonly used medications that made it onto this list of "inappropriate" drugs.

WHAT ARE THE "INAPPROPRIATE DRUGS"?

Benzodiazepines

Benzodiazepines are a class of drugs that are commonly used to treat symptoms of anxiety and insomnia (difficulty sleeping). Benzodiazepines are categorized as either "short-acting" or "long-acting" agents.

TABLE 8.1. COMMONLY USED BENZODIAZEPINES

Short-Acting Agents	Long-Acting Agents
alprazolam (Xanax)	clonazepam (Klonopin)
lorazepam (Ativan)	chlordiazepoxide (Librium)
oxazepam (Serax)	flurazepam (Dalmane)
temazepam (Restoril)	diazepam (Valium)
	clorazepate (Tranxene)

The use of a long-acting agent or high doses of the short-acting agents may be dangerous for seniors.[8] These medications act in the body in a manner that is very similar to alcohol. So beware! All of these medications are addicting. If the person has a history of alcohol abuse, he or she probably shouldn't be taking any of these medicines.

Benzodiazepines are also associated with many other problems, including increased confusion and increased memory impairment. Using benzodiazepines may also make the senior become more physically disabled. We have all either experienced ourselves or seen others who stagger after they have had too much to drink. Benzodiazepines work in the same way. Like alcohol, benzodiazepines can also leave you with a hangover.[9] They can affect your balance and increase the risk of falls and fall-related injuries, such as hip fractures (see chapter 14). Taking a benzodiazepine at night increases your risk of falls, especially if you have to get up from sleeping to use the bathroom or you already have balance and vision problems. It has been our experience that many patients refuse to believe that these risks exist.

The benzodiazepines are not all the same in their potential to cause these side effects. Diazepam (Valium) and chlordiazepoxide (Librium) are considered long-acting benzodiazepines because these medications act in the body for a long period of time (see the above list). If a young patient takes one of these long-acting medications, half of the medicine will get metabolized and excreted by the body in approximately twenty-four to thirty-six hours. Because of the changes in the musculoskeletal system and kidneys, it will take anywhere from one to two weeks for the same amount of medication to be metabolized by the frail older adult.[10]

Because of their quicker effect in the body, many doctors prefer to use the shorter-acting agents, such as alprazolam (Xanax), lorazepam (Ativan), and temazepam (Restoril). If a young patient takes one of the above shorter-acting benzodiazepines, half of the medicine will be metabolized by the body in six to eight hours. On the surface, this is great because patients can take this medication at night to help them go to sleep and by the morning it will largely be out of their system. Instead of working for only six to eight hours, this medication has been shown to act for up to twenty hours in older adults.[11] Therefore, if a senior takes one of these medications before she goes to sleep, the medication will still be active in her body the next day. Without an understanding of the prolonged effect of these medications, too many seniors are given these medications two or even three times a day.

BUT I'VE BEEN TAKING THIS PILL FOR YEARS!

Why on earth would people want to take these dangerous drugs? The answers we most commonly hear are "I need it for sleep" and "I need it for my nerves." What is so troubling is that no studies have ever shown the long-term use of a benzodiazepine has any clinical benefit in the chronic treatment of sleeping problems or anxiety. In fact, the memory of some older adults actually seems to improve when these medications are stopped.[12]

Using these drugs for a long period of time can cause you to become addicted and can make your memory worse. We have seen many seniors who are taking more than one brand of benzodiazepine at the same time.[13] There is no medical indication for a person to be taking two or more benzodiazepines.

These side effects may sound scary, but you must also remember: *do not stop these medications cold turkey.* The dose needs to be slowly decreased. If they are stopped suddenly you can potentially die from the withdrawal symptoms. We like to gradually lower the dose by no more than 25 percent each week. So if the person has been taking two tablets a day, we may tell him to break the tablets in half and take a half tablet three times a day for the first week. The following week he should decrease the dose to two half tablets per day. The third week he should just take one half tablet at night. By the fourth week he generally can stop the medication completely. We strongly suggest that you talk to your doctor to help you figure out the best way to cut down on the dose of this medication.

BEWARE OF THE ANTICHOLINERGIC DRUGS!

Many commonly used medications block the ability of the neurotransmitter acetylcholine to bind to nerve cells as well as muscle cells. We say that these drugs are *anticholinergic.* Table 8.2 lists some of the commonly used drugs that have anticholinergic side effects.

Many over-the-counter sinus, sleep, and cold medicines contain anticholinergic antihistamines. Many older antidepressants and antipsychotics also have significant anticholinergic effects. Below is a list of potential side effects of anticholinergic medications:

- blurry vision
- confusion, hallucinations, delirium
- constipation
- difficulty urinating (in men)
- dry mouth
- increased heart rate

The most common of these side effects is dry mouth. This is potentially a serious problem for frail seniors who are at high risk for losing weight (chapter 19). When a person can't make saliva, it makes it harder to taste and swallow food.

TABLE 8.2. COMMON ANTICHOLINERGIC MEDICATIONS[14]

Medication	Indication
amitriptyline (Elavil)	
desipramine	
doxepin	
imipramine	
nortriptyline	depression and chronic nerve pain
chlorpheniramine (Chlor-Trimeton)	
dexchlorpheniramine (Polaramine)	
diphenhydramine (Benadryl)	
hydroxyzine (Vistaril and Atarax)	
promethazine (Phenergan)	antihistamines used in cold and sinus medications
oxybutynin (Ditropan)	for patients with overactive bladder
belladonna alkaloids (Donnatal and others)	
dicyclomine (Bentyl)	
hyoscyamine (Levsin and Levsinex SR)	
propantheline (Pro-Banthine)	abdominal pain due to spasms of the colon
carisoprodol (Soma)	
chlorzoxazone (Paraflex)	
cyclobenzaprine (Flexeril)	
metaxalone (Skelaxin)	
methocarbamol (Robaxin)	muscle relaxers

Anticholinergic medications are especially dangerous in elderly patients with Alzheimer's disease. With Alzheimer's disease there is a destruction of many of the nerve cells that secrete the neurotransmitter acetylcholine. The loss of these cells is responsible for many of the symptoms of the disease. If you then prescribe a medication that blocks the rest of the acetylcholine from working, you can potentially make the Alzheimer's symptoms even worse.[15]

Men with enlarged prostates need to be very careful as well. Anticholinergic medications may make it even more difficult to urinate, a problem we refer to as *urinary retention*. People with heart disease need to be careful because anticholinergic drugs can speed up the heart rate. The last thing a patient with a bad heart needs is to take a pill that speeds up the heart rate.

Here are other medications that should be avoided in all elderly:

- meperidine (Demerol): this pain medication only works for a few hours and can lead to the buildup of toxic metabolites in patients whose kidneys are not working well.
- indomethacin (Indocin), ketorolac (Toradol): these two commonly used non-steroidal anti-inflammatory drugs (NSAIDs) have a higher risk of causing stomach ulcers when compared to ibuprofen (see table 27.2, p. 307). In addition, indomethacin can actually cause some older adults to become delirious.
- fluoxetine (Prozac): this antidepressant medication interacts with many medications that seniors often use. The metabolism of the drug is often slowed down in seniors as well.
- The daily use of the stimulant laxatives bisacodyl (Dulcolax) and cascara sagrada for the long-term treatment of constipation can make constipation worse.
- The daily use of NSAIDs at their highest recommended dose can increase the risk of stomach ulcers and maybe even heart attacks.[16]

Certain medications should be avoided in older adults with specific medical illnesses. For example:

- Seniors with stomach ulcers should not use the old NSAIDs or high-dose aspirin.
- Seniors with constipation should not be on either the blood pressure pill verapamil or tricyclic antidepressants, such as amitriptyline, doxepin, imipramine, desipramine, and nortriptyline. Narcotic pain medications need to be used carefully, as they can make constipation much worse.
- Seniors who are at a high risk of falling and/or have a history of falling should avoid any benzodiazepine or anticholinergic medication.
- Patients with gout, high blood calcium levels, or low sodium levels should avoid the use of the water pill hydrochlorothiazide (HCTZ).[17]

ARE OVER-THE-COUNTER MEDICATIONS SAFER THAN PRESCRIPTION MEDICATIONS?

This is a question that can be answered in two words: *it depends.* Many products can be bought over the counter without a prescription. These include herbal products, vitamins, and a host of pharmaceuticals. The elderly are more likely to use over-the-counter medications and herbal supplements than younger adults.[18] This makes sense when you consider that seniors have more illnesses.

As with everything in geriatrics, older adults need to be careful. All medications (including the over-the-counter variety) have the potential for side effects. Also, they may interact with various prescription medications. Always look at the ingredients before you buy anything. Here are some simple rules to follow:

- Do not take more than one NSAID at a time (table 27.2, p. 307).
- Do not take any products containing ibuprofen or aspirin if you are on blood thinners, such as warfarin (Coumadin), clopidogrel (Plavix), and enoxaparin (Lovenox).
- Do not take any cold, flu, or allergy products containing the antihistamines chlorpheniramine or diphenhydramine (table 25.1, p. 284). These antihistamines are very anticholinergic.
- Cold and allergy medicine containing pseudoephedrine can be dangerous in patients with poorly controlled hypertension and heart disease.
- Cimetidine (Tagamet) is a stomach medicine that is very similar to ranitidine (Zantac) and famotidine (Pepcid). It has a higher potential for causing confusion compared to ranitidine or famotidine.[19] For elderly men, cimetidine may also block the testosterone receptors, which will cause the remaining testosterone to work less effectively.

IF YOU ARE TAKING OVER-THE-COUNTER PRODUCTS, PLEASE TELL YOUR DOCTOR!

There was an interesting study of elderly women in Florida that showed one-third were taking one or more over-the-counter drugs or supplements that could interact with their prescription medications. What surprised the researcher was that the majority of these women did not consider these products to be "real" drugs.[20]

Studies have also shown that the majority of patients who take these over-the-counter medications or herbal supplements do not tell their physicians.[21] Because it is so important, we will remind you throughout this book to always tell your doctor if you are taking any over-the-counter products.

BEWARE OF THE WORDS *NATURAL* AND *HERBAL*!

As we discussed in chapter 6, the words *natural* and *herbal* imply that these products are safer than the drugs made by the big pharmaceutical companies. In many cases the opposite is true. The drug companies are tightly regulated by the Food and Drug Administration (FDA).

The makers of natural products do not have to provide any proof of safety, efficacy, or purity. This is because the natural products are classified as "food products," not "medications." The FDA is powerless to regulate them, unless they can prove that a specific product is harmful or unsafe.

THINGS TO REMEMBER!

- Do not take any medications, home remedies, or over-the-counter products without first consulting your doctor. What you are buying may have side effects or may interact with other drugs you are taking.
- Always ask the pharmacist about any potentially dangerous drug interactions among the different drugs you are taking.
- Keep an up-to-date list of all your medications. Make sure all your doctors see the list. We also recommend that you carry it with you in your wallet or purse in the event that you need emergency care.

QUESTIONS FOR YOUR DOCTOR

1. Are any of my medicines addictive?
2. Are any of my medications dangerous to take if I drink alcohol?
3. Will any of my medications impair my driving?
4. Will the medicine affect my memory or thinking?
5. Are all my medications really necessary?
6. Are there less expensive versions of any of my medications available that are equally effective?
7. Are there any generic drugs that will work for me?
8. Is it okay to crush this medicine and mix it with food or juice?
9. Are there any nonmedicine treatments that might help me instead or along with my medications?
10. Are there any over-the-counter medications I need to avoid?

Part 2
THE TWENTY-FIRST-CENTURY HEALTHCARE SYSTEM

Chapter 9

EMERGING TRENDS OF HEALTHCARE FOR THE ELDERLY

"Age will not be defied."

Francis Bacon (1561–1626)

TREND #1: PEOPLE ARE LIVING LONGER

Between 1900 and 1990 the average life expectancy increased from 47.3 to 75.4 years.[1] Much of this increase was due to improvements in modern medicine. Medical research has led to numerous breakthroughs that can either prevent or treat harmful illnesses. The flu shot to prevent influenza and the use of medications to lower cholesterol are just two of the many breakthroughs that we often take for granted in our modern healthcare system. Advances in the treatment of heart failure, atherosclerosis, cancer, and other diseases have allowed elderly patients to live for many years with one or more previously fatal illnesses. Because of the successes of modern medicine, living to an old age is now what most people should expect and plan for.

Between 1990 and 2005 the average life expectancy further increased from 75.4 to 77.8.[2] While the average life span continues to increase, it is interesting to note that the rate of increase appears to be slowing down. In other words, we should not expect to add an additional three years of life expectancy every fifteen years.

People sixty-five years and older currently account for 12.56 percent of the US population. This equates to 37.8 million senior citizens.[3] In the next twenty-five years the number of seniors is expected to double.[4] These statistics, however, only reveal some of the issues that our society faces.

While the number of people sixty-five and over continues to increase, the eighty-five-and-over age group is actually the fastest growing segment of the United States population. There are currently 5.5 million Americans over the age of eighty-five.[5] By the year 2015 this number is expected to increase to 7.3 million. By 2050, the expectation is that it will increase to 21 million and will account for almost 5 percent of the entire population.[6]

Why is this such an important issue? The healthcare needs of people in their late eighties and nineties is far different from those of active sixty-five-year-olds. They have more medical illnesses and are more likely to need assistance with basic activities of daily living (bathing, dressing, using the toilet, transferring from the bed to chair, eating, etc.). They are more likely to need nursing home care and have higher per capita costs for hospital and long-term care services.

THE CENTENARIANS ARE COMING!

Centenarian is a term used to describe a person who is one hundred years of age or older. In 1950 there were only 3,000 centenarians. In 2007 there were 80,771 centenarians.[7] By 2010 this number will increase to 114,000 and by 2020 this number is estimated to be 241,000.[8]

The explosion in the number of people living to an old age is a phenomenon that has never occurred before in human history. As a society, we have no cultural or historical experience to help us deal with the impact of this increase of the aging population on our social, economic, and political structure.

The difficulties brought about by a sky-rocketing elderly population are not unique to the United States. In 2001 the US Department of Commerce published a report showing that the world's elderly population is increasing at the rate of 850,000 per month.[9] China, for example, will have 336 million people over the age of sixty by the year 2030.[10] Who is going to take care of all these senior citizens? The Chinese government currently enforces a limit of one child per family. In the years to come you will see millions of young adults who will be caring for two parents and up to four grandparents. Japan's elderly population is now at 19 percent (compared with 12.4 percent for the United States).[11] What is so troubling for China and Japan is that both countries have a declining number of young people to support and care for the exploding population of elderly.

The percentage of seniors in Italy is 19.1 percent, the highest in Europe. Actually, every country in Europe has a higher percentage of seniors than the United States.[12] By 2030 all of Europe will have more seniors than working-age people.[13] Dramatic changes will occur in the developing world as well. By 2050 it is estimated that 80 percent of seniors will be living in third world countries.[14]

TREND #2: TODAY'S HOSPITAL PATIENTS ARE FRAILER AND SICKER

As we just stated above, patients with illnesses that were fatal just fifteen to twenty years ago are now able to live at home for many years. Now, patients are living for years with severe congestive heart failure, severe lung disease, cancer, and kidney failure. We are even taking care of patients who simultaneously suffer from all of these illnesses. When these patients become ill, their organs are so weak that our job as doctors becomes very difficult. The treatment for one illness, for example, may make other chronic illnesses worse.

Older adults have a 20 percent yearly risk of needing hospitalization.[15] Some healthcare professionals and social policy experts would then say, "We need to focus on providing the resources to keep them out of the hospital." We agree with this assessment. On the other hand, we should not fool ourselves. Most seniors will eventually become very sick and require hospitalization.

Medicare guidelines are now very strict about how sick a patient must be before hospitalization will be paid for. The old days of a patient being admitted to the hospital because the caregiver needed a break or the patient wanted some tests done are long gone. Many serious illnesses are now treated at home. The patients admitted today are really sick.

TREND #3: TODAY'S ELDERLY NURSING HOME POPULATION IS NOT ONLY FRAILER BUT ALSO SICKER!

Years ago, nursing homes were thought of as old-age homes that had a primarily social model in their design. Care was provided for those who required supervision because of senility. Others simply needed an environment that provided meals or assistance with housework. Residents and their families paid for the services provided. People without money were cared for in nursing homes that were often run by charity organizations.

Today's nursing homes operate on a medical model that is becoming ever more complex. Nursing homes do not house healthy people. Rather, they are given the task of providing for all of the needs of the sickest and frailest people in society. Eighty percent need assistance with mobility, 65.7 percent are incontinent, and 47.3 percent need assistance with eating.[16] The great majority have terminal diagnoses and limited life expectancies.

There are now approximately 1.4 million nursing home residents.[17] At any one given time only 4 percent of the elderly population will be living in nursing homes. Some interesting statistics to ponder:

- An elderly person has a 43 percent chance of requiring nursing home placement at some time in his or her life.
- Among people eighty-five years of age and older, 20 percent live in nursing homes.
- Fifty percent of those over the age of ninety-five live in nursing homes.
- Only 21 percent of residents remain in a nursing home for five years or longer.[18]

Part of the reason nursing home care has become so complicated stems from how Medicare pays hospitals. Medicare's payment fees are based on the concept of *diagnosis-related groups*, or DRGs. With the development of DRGs, Medicare pays the hospital a set fee when a senior is hospitalized. The fee is predetermined and it is based entirely on the patient's diagnosis at the time of discharge from the hospital. For example, if a Medicare recipient is admitted with pneumonia, the hospital will receive a flat fee for a person with a discharge diagnosis of pneumonia. The hospital will get the same fee whether the patient is in the hospital for three days or ten days. Thus, there is a strong incentive on the part of the hospital to discharge elderly patients as soon as possible. So what we have is a scenario where patients are getting sicker and hospital stays are becoming shorter.[19]

Also, where are you going to send these sick and frail patients? Sending them home is often not an option. As a result, they are showing up on the doorstep of the nursing home, frailer and sicker than before. These patients cannot take care of themselves and have skilled nursing needs, such as intravenous antibiotics, wound care, or rehabilitation.

TREND #4: NURSING HOMES HAVE BOTH
SKILLED NURSING UNITS AND LONG-TERM CARE UNITS

The system within nursing homes is quite complex and there is much confusion around the fact that most nursing homes have both skilled nursing units (for recent acute problems) and long-term care (intermediate care) units. The intermediate care unit is what people most often associate with what happens in the nursing home. However, the two kinds of units differ in the types of patients they care for, the amount of staff required, and the way they are reimbursed.

Skilled Nursing Unit

It is important to understand that frail elderly patients are often placed in a *skilled nursing* or *subacute section* of the nursing home when they are discharged from the hospital. While Medicare DRGs limit the amount that will be paid to the hospital, Medicare will pay additionally for this posthospital care. Medicare pays a daily rate that is adjusted depending on how sick the patient is. Therefore, there is a strong financial incentive both for the hospital to discharge the resident as soon as possible and for the nursing home to quickly accept the patient.

The length of stay averages two to six weeks. People who need rehabilitation following a stroke or following hip fractures are often placed into this category. Wound care for poorly healing surgical wounds or difficult to treat bedsores are other problems that require subacute care. Many other patients require prolonged IV fluids or IV antibiotics. Medicare covers a maximum of one hundred nursing home days per benefit period.

WHAT IS A BENEFIT PERIOD?

A benefit period is not the same thing as a calendar year. A benefit year starts on the day you go into a hospital or a skilled nursing facility. It ends after you go for sixty days without any hospital or skilled care.[20]

For many older adults, the skilled nursing unit allows them the time to recover from an illness and receive the wound care or therapy needed to be able to return home. Medicare will continue to pay for the skilled nursing care as long as the facility can document the potential for improvement. For the first twenty days of the benefit period, Medicare pays 100 percent of the costs. For days twenty-one through one hundred, the resident is required to pay a copayment. As of 2008 this deductible is $128 per day.[21]

It has been our experience that many patients in the hospital are terrified about going to a skilled nursing unit in a nursing home. They fear that once they enter the nursing home they will never leave. As family members you need to explain to your loved one that many people who go for subacute care do go home.

Long-Term Intermediate Care Unit

Dementia and the inability to perform the activities of daily living are the most common indications for long-term care placement. *Intermediate care facilities* (ICFs) provide what is commonly referred to as "custodial" care units. ICFs have lower minimum staffing requirements for nurses and nurses' aides than the skilled nursing units. Because the patients do not have a skilled need, the care is not reimbursed by Medicare.

Medicaid pays custodial care for people who are poor and too frail to be cared for at home. For example, in the state of Florida, Medicaid pays between $137 and $241 per day for each resident.[22] This is only a small fraction of what a hospital charges per day. As it turns out, the amount that Medicaid pays often does not cover the nursing home's actual cost of caring for the resident. Most facilities will charge patients who pay privately a little more in order to cover their losses from the low Medicaid reimbursement rate.

Scared of paying the high cost of nursing home care, many seniors may be tempted to put all their assets in a family member's name in order to qualify for Medicaid. If you are considering transferring assets, talk to an attorney first. This is not an easy process. Seniors have to show that the assets were not transferred for at least several years prior to applying for Medicaid benefits. Applying for Medicaid may also limit your options in choosing a nursing home, as some facilities have a limit on the number of beds reserved for Medicaid patients.

TREND #5: ALFS HAVE BECOME A VERY POPULAR LONG-TERM CARE OPTION

Many people who do not need around-the-clock assistance or twenty-four-hour supervision may benefit from an *assisted living facility* (ALF) rather than a nursing home. Some have living quarters designed to accommodate the special needs of frail older adults. The bathrooms, for example, should be handicapped equipped. The staff at an ALF will generally provide two to three meals per day, along with housekeeping and laundry.

Not all ALFs are the same! They can vary quite a lot with regard to size, quality, and services that they provide. Some ALFs may only have a few residents, while others may have several hundred. Some will provide assistance with medications and the activities of daily living. ALF residents can also hire a personal aide to help them.

The facilities do not provide their own skilled nursing services. If such services are needed, they will be performed by an outside home health agency. ALFs do not have a medical director. Physicians are not required to visit, although some do. Medicare and Medicaid do not pay for ALF placement.

It is important to understand these differences, because a lot of seniors become upset when told that they would be better off moving out of their homes and into an ALF. To them, an ALF is the same thing as a nursing home. There is a big difference. We remind them that they are too healthy to go to a nursing home. Think of the ALF as an apartment with someone who can help with the laundry, housekeeping, meals, and medications.

WHAT IS RESPITE CARE?

Respite care involves short-term placement in a long-term care facility in order to give the caregiver a much-needed break. The period of care is usually less than two weeks and is covered by Medicare.

Things You Can Do to Help!

- Find out what services are available at the ALF and what services are available at an extra cost.
- If your loved one needs to be admitted to a skilled nursing unit, try to avoid having him or her sent overnight or on the weekend when there are fewer staff members available and it is harder to contact your doctor should a problem arise (see chapter 13).

TREND #6: FINDING A NEW PRIMARY CARE PROVIDER IS NOT EASY

Many elderly patients and their families feel that their doctors do not spend enough time with them. It may seem as though the doctor is in and out of the room before the patient can even ask all his questions. Is the doctor being rude, or is she just trying to pay the bills? Without talking to your doctor, we can't really comment on her bedside manner. We can, however, give you some insights into the financial pressures that primary care physicians face.

The days when a doctor would spend an hour talking with a patient at each visit are over. Seniors often have more medical problems, have more complaints, and take more medications than younger patients. They also take a longer time to examine. Primary care doctors can make a lot more money seeing younger patients with private insurance. From a financial standpoint, it is almost impossible for an outpatient practice to provide primary care to a large group of primarily frail elderly patients.

Most of the Medicare dollars go to the hospital or to the specialists who perform procedures. The **real truth** is that Medicare does not pay a whole lot for primary care services. In fact, many primary care physicians will no longer see new Medicare patients.

As Medicare continues to nibble away at the reimbursements to doctors, many subspecialists are able to make up for the lower reimbursements by doing more procedures to make money. These physicians are always looking for new tests that they can do in their office or in an outpatient surgery center. In contrast, primary care physicians focus on diagnosing illnesses and referring patients for procedures when needed. As reimbursements decrease, the primary care physician is economically the most vulnerable. At the same time, the costs incurred by the physician (rent, malpractice insurance, supplies, staff salaries, utilities, etc.) remain high.

Not surprisingly, most medical students do not want to pursue a career in primary care internal medicine or family medicine. The fact that many medical student graduates have massive debt from student loans serves to further push future doctors away from a career in primary care. Even among doctors who pursue a residency in internal medicine, over 62 percent pursue subspecialty training, and many of the remaining doctors become hospitalists (doctors who focus entirely on the care of the hospitalized patient).[23]

Why Is This a Problem for You?

Many people think that physicians make enough money and therefore can afford to lose a few dollars. What's the big deal if they spend a little extra time with patients? The **real truth** is that it does affect you and your family. Surveys of physicians have shown that if Medicare further cuts its reimbursements to physicians, many more doctors will either decrease the number of new Medicare patients they accept or stop seeing new Medicare patients altogether. Imagine that you turn sixty-five and can't find a new doctor. Or maybe you are eighty years old and decide you are going to move to a new state. It may not be so easy to find a good doctor who will take new Medicare patients.

The National Institute of Aging prints a brochure for older adults on how to talk to their doctors.[24] They recommend making an appointment to "interview your doctor" before you choose her. While this sounds nice on paper, the **real truth** is that choosing a doctor is not like buying a hamburger from one of many fast-food outlets. When choosing a fast-food restaurant, the consumer has all the power to decide which place he or she will have lunch. Will it be Wendy's or Burger King? Subway or Dairy Queen? You will not have this much choice when you are looking for a good primary care doctor. Many doctors you want to see may not be on your Medicare Advantage Plan. Others do not take patients with both Medicare and Medicaid. Some do not accept Medicare patients at all.

TREND #7: THE NUMBER OF GERIATRIC MEDICAL DOCTORS (*GERIATRICIANS*) IS ACTUALLY DECREASING

At a time when the number of elderly Americans is rapidly increasing, the number of physicians wishing to pursue a career in geriatric medicine is declining. Before we go any further, we need to again ask, What is a geriatrician?

Geriatrics is a subspecialty of internal medicine and family medicine that deals with the medical needs of the older adult patient. In contrast with the medical trend for doctors to become ever-more specialized, geriatrics takes a more holistic approach. While the cardiologist focuses on the heart, the geriatrician will focus on how the heart medications impact the rest of the patient's body.

Geriatricians must complete residency training in internal medicine or family medicine and have been certified in the care of the elderly patient. Since 1994, becoming board certified in geriatric medicine requires the completion of a one-year fellowship specifically in geriatric medicine prior to taking a certification test. The doctor must recertify every ten years.

IS MY DOCTOR BOARD CERTIFIED?

You can see if your primary care physician is board certified with the American Board of Internal Medicine at www.abim.org, or the American Board of Family Practice at https://www.abfp.org/diplomate.

Is There Really a Shortage of Geriatricians?

You may see reports in the media that there are not enough doctors with geriatric training to take care of the sky-rocketing population of older adults. There is a lot of truth to those reports and things are only getting worse. The number of geriatricians is getting smaller. In 2008 there were 4,948 geriatricians certified by the American Board of Internal Medicine and the American Academy of Family Practice.[25] Fewer doctors are going into the field. What's even more disappointing is that over a third of all geriatricians are not renewing their ten-year recertification with the American Board of Internal Medicine.[26] To be frank, we see nothing on the horizon that will reverse this trend.

While everyone recognizes the need to have more doctors with geriatric training, a variety of factors limit the growth of this field:

- Geriatricians make a lot less money than other doctors.
- Geriatricians generally spend their time talking to patients rather than performing moneymaking medical procedures. A recent study that monitored the daily routine of geriatricians in the outpatient setting showed that 20 percent of their time is spent coordinating care for which they receive no pay.[27]
- Geriatricians attract some of the most challenging patients. If you are labeled as the geriatric doctor in a group of internal medicine or family medicine physicians, people are going to refer to you the complicated frail elderly patients. Because these patients require so much more time than younger patients, the geriatric doctor will end up seeing fewer patients and her billing will be less than her internal medicine or family medicine colleagues.
- Geriatricians have to do an extra year of training. After four years of college, four years of medical school, and three years of residency,

many young doctors don't see the point of "wasting" a year to pursue a field that will not increase their incomes.

TREND #8: THE EMERGENCE OF CONCIERGE (VIP) MEDICINE

Some people long for the good old days, when their doctor would spend forty-five minutes to an hour talking to them. They would also be able to see the doctor whenever they were sick and be able to call him or her anytime, day or night. Such practices are slowly starting to reemerge. You may be wondering how that can be, since we noted in trends 6 and 7 that seeing patients in the outpatient setting does not pay.

Some primary care doctors are now creating a style of practice that goes by many names: VIP medicine, concierge medicine, boutique medicine, or executive health medicine. These doctors have far fewer patients in their practice and will spend more time with each patient. How can they do this? By charging a fee that can run up to several thousand dollars per year, patients know that they will have easy access to their doctor. This may include same day office visits, the doctor's pager/cell phone number, and e-mail consultations. When the patient is ill, the doctor may do a home visit or accompany the patient to the ER.

The doctors who do practice this type of medicine find that they can actually make more money seeing fewer patients. Just as important, by focusing on fewer patients, these doctors believe that they can provide a higher level of customer care.

TREND #9: MANY PRIMARY CARE PRACTICE OFFICES ARE USING PHYSICIAN EXTENDERS

In many offices you may never actually see the doctor. Instead, you will be seen by an *advanced registered nurse practitioner* (ARNP) or by a *physician assistant* (PA). A nurse practitioner is a registered nurse who has undergone advanced training to achieve a master's degree in nursing. Some nurse practitioners may have even specialized in geriatrics. Most people who enroll in a physician's assistant program already have their bachelor's degree. Most physician assistant programs usually last about two years.

Do not confuse these people with medical assistants, who perform many of the routine tasks in the office, such as checking your blood pressure or drawing blood. Like doctors, ARNPs and PAs can diagnose and treat medical problems.

But only a physician can prescribe narcotics. Both types of physician "extenders" usually work under the supervision of a physician. The specific regulations vary by state. What this usually means is that the physician will be available if the extender needs assistance. Nurse practitioners and physician assistants often see patients in nursing homes. They will usually contact a physician only if there is a problem that they feel they cannot handle.

TREND #10: MANY PRIMARY CARE DOCTORS NO LONGER TAKE CARE OF PATIENTS WHEN THEY ARE IN THE HOSPITAL

As we will discuss in chapter 13, many primary care doctors will use hospitalist groups when their patients get sick. Hospitalists are doctors who specialize in the care of the hospitalized patient. Hospitalist physicians do not have an office and will not see the patient once they leave the hospital. Hospitalists usually work in shifts so it is quite common for a person to be cared for by multiple physicians during a hospital stay. If you do find a primary care doctor who sees patients in the hospital, make sure this physician has privileges at the hospital closest to where you live. Otherwise, you will likely be seen by the local hospital's hospitalist group.

TREND #11: GOOD NURSES ARE HARD TO FIND!

There is a national shortage of nurses. Many hospitals have had to close entire floors because they can't staff enough nurses. Others have begun actively recruiting from other countries, such as India and the Philippines. If we can't even find enough nurses to meet our present needs, how are we going to find the nurses to meet the healthcare needs of the aging baby boomers? Because there a nursing shortage, nurses can be selective about where and how they want to work. Many do not want to work in a "boring" nursing home or for a home care agency. The cost to recruit and retain nurses in long-term care facilities and home care agencies is expected to skyrocket at a time when reimbursements from Medicare and Medicaid are stagnant.

Chapter 10
MAKING THE MOST OF YOUR DOCTOR'S VISIT

"The secret to staying young is to live honestly, eat slowly, and lie about your age."
Lucille Ball (1911–1989)

We like to say that there are three stages of life. In the first stage, you follow grades so you will do well in school. In the second phase, you follow money so you can survive and take care of your family. In the third phase of life, you are following doctors so you can stay alive.

Before we start this chapter, we wanted to answer two questions that we are commonly asked:

At what age do I need to see a geriatrician?

There is no specific age. Geriatric medicine as a field generally focuses on the frail older adult patient. Oftentimes we see the patients whose cases are complicated and who have multiple medical problems. Because geriatricians are also experts in internal medicine or family medicine, they can handle the health issues of middle-aged and young adult patients as well.

Do all seniors need to see a geriatrician?

This is a point we discussed at length while writing this book. Not all geriatricians are the same. As with any profession, there are some who are better than others. Taking care of the frail older adult requires more patience than taking care of younger people. Seniors have more complaints and move slower than younger patients. However, just because someone completed his geriatric training does not necessarily mean he is a kind and compassionate doctor.

It is hard for us to make a blanket recommendation that elderly patients should have a geriatrician as their primary care physician. Geriatricians have special training managing the multiple health issues of a frail older adult. That being said, we know many internal medicine and family medicine doctors who provide excellent care to frail older adults.

Good communication makes for good medicine. Doctors are expected to see more patients and address more medical problems per patient than ever before. Given the constraints that are put on physicians in the modern outpatient clinic, your time with the doctor is going to be limited. By the same token, we don't want you to ignore medical problems just because you don't want to waste the doctor's time. To make the most out of the minutes that you do have, you need to be efficient. Below is a list of some realistic tips that may help you utilize your time most effectively:

BRING A LIST OF ALL YOUR MEDICATIONS WITH YOU

In fact, it would be even better if you bring all your medication bottles with you. If you see more than one doctor, she may not know what the others have prescribed. Don't forget to bring all over-the-counter, vitamin, or herbal products as well.

KEEP A COPY OF YOUR MEDICAL RECORDS

This is a very important point if you are seeing a new doctor. You may find yourself living in a different part of the country or enrolled in a new Medicare Advantage Plan. Are you going to remember the details of what happened to you in the hospital years ago? Which tests were run? The results? Don't rely on your old doctor to store the records. Over time, doctors move and retire.

You don't necessarily need all of your records, but a copy of operative reports, hospital discharge summaries, and radiology reports would be vital information to keep. Bring a copy of all recent blood work as well.

If you were recently in the emergency room or in a hospital, you may want to call the doctor's office before your appointment to make sure your records have been received. If your doctor has not received the records, it may be harder for you to receive the follow-up care you need.

KEEP A COPY OF YOUR BASELINE ELECTROCARDIOGRAM (EKG)

An EKG is commonly done to diagnose heart attack and a variety of other cardiac diseases. To the untrained eye it looks like a bunch of squiggly lines, but actually it reveals a lot of information about the structure and function of the heart. Many elderly patients have heart attacks with no symptoms. Other heart attack patients may complain of nausea, shortness of breath, or fatigue rather than chest pain. Patients with dementia may not be able to provide an accurate history. In some cases, an EKG may be the first clue that the patient is having a serious heart attack.

Because it is the change in the EKG that can help identify a heart attack or heart rhythm abnormality, it is useful to have a baseline EKG for comparison. We recommend that you keep a copy for you and your loved ones.

DON'T GO ALONE

Many seniors who have multiple medical problems, little education, or difficulty with hearing may find it hard to understand what the doctor is telling them. In these cases, it may be better to bring a family member or trusted friend along to help communicate with the doctor. A recent study has shown that seniors who bring a companion along are more actively involved in their own care and are more pleased with the care they receive from the doctor.[1]

LIMIT YOUR COMPLAINTS TO THE MOST IMPORTANT ONES

For many elderly patients, it is quite difficult to get to the doctor. Every time they come to see the doctor they have to make a copayment. Others have to pay for transportation or rely on family/friends who must miss work. To get their money's worth, many patients and families want as many issues addressed as possible.

It is important to realize that more is not always better. It has been our experience that in these situations, details are often lost when one tries to focus on too many issues at one time.

We believe that it is often better to focus on one or two issues in detail per visit rather than try to cram six or seven into a single office visit. If you feel that more issues need to be addressed, then you may want to schedule another office visit.

DON'T BE AFRAID TO ASK QUESTIONS

You may become frustrated when you are concerned about one thing and your doctor is more focused on something else. For example, you go to the doctor complaining of foot pain and your doctor seems to ignore your complaints. She seems to dwell on your elevated blood sugars. It is okay to ask your doctor why she is discussing your diabetes instead of your foot. If your sugars are dangerously high, then you have to trust the doctor's ability to see the big picture. If your doctor does not want to answer your question, then the two of you may have a communication problem. In such a case, you may want to consider getting a new doctor.

CHOOSING A DOCTOR IS NOT SO EASY!

The National Institute of Aging prints a brochure for older adults on how to talk to their doctors (http://www.niapublications.org/pubs/talking/Talking _with_your_Doctor.pdf).[2] It recommends making an appointment to interview your doctor before you choose him or her. Before you blindly follow this advice, be aware that fewer and fewer primary care doctors want to see new Medicare patients in their clinics. For financial reasons they would rather see young patients who have only one or two complaints.

FIND A DOCTOR NEAR YOU

Every older person will need medical care at some point in his or her life. We believe that it is important to live near a good medical facility. When looking for a doctor it is essential to check the credentials, but it is also essential to find out which hospitals the doctor is affiliated with. If you find a doctor you like who is far away from where you live, just be aware that your physician may not be able to see you in the hospital. The doctor may not even have a relationship with any of the hospitalists at the hospital near you.

Chapter 11

WHOM CAN I TURN TO
FOR HELP?

"It's no longer a question of staying healthy. It's a question of finding a sickness you like."

Jackie Mason (1931–)

W e have already discussed how the nursing home resident as well as the hospital patient of the twenty-first century is older, sicker, and more medically complicated than ever before. So who has accepted the challenge to take care of the frail elderly?

WHAT IS A NURSES' AIDE OR
CERTIFIED NURSES' ASSISTANT (CNA)?

Around 90 percent of direct patient care in the nursing home is provided by nurses' aides or nursing assistants. While these two terms can be used interchangeably, it is very important that you know the difference between a *nurses' aide/nursing assistant* and a *nurse.* To become a nurses' aide requires about only three months of training time. With so little training, you should not be surprised if the aide does not have a good understanding of the difficult geriatric issues with which you or your loved one is dealing. In some nursing homes you may hear the term *certified nursing assistant* (CNA). CNA describes those nurses' aides who have completed at least seventy-five hours of training and have passed a competency exam.[1] Other than that there is no real difference.

Nurses' aides have a very tough job. They are the ones who often perform the following difficult tasks:

- Assist patients with walking
- Assist with using the bedpan and urinal
- Bathe, groom, and dress patients
- Change bed linens
- Change diapers
- Feed patients
- Measure and record food and liquid intake
- Measure and record the patient's blood pressure, pulse, and temperature
- Measure urine output
- Observe patient's condition and report any change to the nursing or medical staff
- Turn and reposition bedridden patients

BEING A CNA IS NOT FUN!

You often hear people say, "I would not wipe someone else's butt for all the money in the world!" Well, someone has to do this, and the CNAs do it for far less than "all the money in the world." The average pay is somewhere between eight to ten dollars per hour. There is little opportunity for career advancement.

The average turnover rate for nurses' aides in nursing homes across the United States is approximately 71 percent.[2] The fact they do these tasks that even many family members refuse to do is only part of the hardship of their job. They are continuously exposed to body fluids (stool, urine, saliva, and blood) that can expose them to HIV as well as hepatitis. Because the job requires so much turning, lifting, and bending, CNAs are at a high risk for musculoskeletal injuries.

You hear stories in the news about nursing home residents being abused by the staff. The **real truth** is that for every one these incidents, there are many cases where the staff is abused by patients and families. In fact, studies have shown that nurses' aides experience the highest incidence of workplace violence of any American worker. The majority of events are unreported.[3] To make matters worse, the staff is often inappropriately blamed whenever something goes wrong.

It should be emphasized that there are a large number of loving, caring, and dedicated people who become CNAs because their top priority in life is to take care of people in need. They may have a small account of money, but their account of good deeds is overflowing. In our capitalistic society, it's difficult to attract large numbers of highly motivated people to go into a profession in which they are underpaid and treated badly. There are already 2.1 million nurses' aides in the United States. Most facilities and home health agencies do not have the resources to raise CNA salaries to any great extent. With an increasing elderly population, this number is expected to increase substantially in the years to come. We have no idea how nursing homes, hospitals, and home health agencies will find good people to fill all these positions.

WHAT KIND OF NURSES WORK IN A NURSING HOME?

Some states require at least one licensed nurse to be on the premise to provide twenty-four-hour supervision. Note that we said at least one. Nursing homes are not hospitals, so they do not have lots of nurses working twenty-four hours a day.

Nurses can give medications and other treatments. They can also monitor the patient and report any change in condition to the doctor. Unfortunately, most nurses do not receive any additional training in geriatric care.

Some nursing homes will have a nurse who specializes only in the assessment and treatment of pressure ulcers (bedsores) and other wounds. Others will contract out for these services. She will usually be the one the physician relies on for devising the treatment regimen for wound care. Pressure ulcers and bedsores are discussed in extensive detail in chapter 26.

PHYSICIANS

Most doctors who see patients in the nursing home are either specialists in internal medicine or family medicine. Some may even be specialists in geriatric medicine, known as geriatricians (chapter 1).

We need to emphasize again that nursing homes are not hospitals. Doctors will not be there every day to see you. Most doctors will only come by infrequently to write their monthly note on each resident. Patients in the skilled nursing unit will be seen about once per week.

Many primary care physicians do not follow their patients once they are admitted to a nursing home. In such cases, the nursing home will give you the names of one or more physicians who regularly see residents in the nursing home. So what happens if a problem arises on the days when the physician is not there? Well, the **real truth** is that most problems are handled through phone calls and faxes between the staff and the physician. Many doctors also use physician extenders.

WHAT DOES THE MEDICAL DIRECTOR DO?

All nursing homes are legally required to have a medical director. The medical director's job is to ensure that physician care is medically correct. He is also involved in projects to improve the quality of care in the nursing home and must review all incident reports. The medical director is required to serve on the home's infection control and drug review boards. Many of the residents will not be cared for by the medical director. Instead, they will be cared for by other physicians.

PHYSICIAN EXTENDERS

As we discussed in chapter 9, many doctors use nurse practitioners or physician assistants. Like doctors, they can diagnose and treat medical problems, but only a physician can prescribe narcotics. Both types of physician extenders work under the supervision of a physician. They will usually contact the physician only if there is a problem they feel that they cannot handle. These healthcare providers may also be on call for the physician at night or on weekends. The exact nature of this association varies from state to state.

DIETICIANS

Nursing homes and hospitals have dieticians on staff who help evaluate patients to make sure they are eating and drinking enough. The dietician will evaluate:

- Whether the patient is malnourished
- The nutritional needs of the patient (the daily amount of water, protein, and calories)
- The need for adjustments/modifications in the diet
- The need for nutritional supplements

Malnutrition will be discussed in much detail in chapter 19.

PHARMACISTS

The pharmacist is an important member of the healthcare team. Her primary job is to fill the medication orders of the physicians. She also makes sure that the medications prescribed are safe and do not interact with other drugs that the patient may be taking. Pharmacists can be found in all retail pharmacies, as well as in the hospital. Nursing homes are required to have a consultant pharmacist to review important issues relating to medications and to make sure federal guidelines are followed (chapter 8).

OTHER PEOPLE INVOLVED WITH THE CARE IN NURSING HOMES

Rehabilitation is an important part of the care that many nursing home residents and hospital patients receive. Physical therapists, occupational therapists, and speech therapists play significant roles in helping the older adult get stronger so that she can be as independent as possible. Speech therapists do much more than help people who have lost their ability to verbally communicate (such as after a stroke or other brain injury). They also are involved in the evaluation and treatment of patients who have difficulty swallowing. Many facilities contract out their rehabilitation services. Rehabilitation issues will be discussed in more detail in chapter 16.

Most nursing homes also have a recreational therapist whose job it is to find out what the residents' interests are. The recreational therapist will then try to facilitate activities programs that most closely meet each resident's interests and needs.

WHAT IS A CARE PLAN?

Most nursing home residents have a variety of medical, psychological, and social issues. The effect of one of these issues may have an impact on the development of another issue. For example, the resident who is depressed that his son will not talk to him is less likely to actively participate in his rehabilitation program or eat as much as he is supposed to. It is often hard for any given healthcare professional to identify and treat all the issues facing a nursing home resident.

The physical therapist may be aware that the resident is at risk for falling, while the social worker may know that the family is not supportive. In order to share this information, nursing homes have regular care plan meetings to discuss each of the residents. During these meetings, representatives from nursing, rehab, social work, pharmacy, and recreation therapy will identify each resident's current healthcare issues. They will also assess if the resident is at high risk for developing other problems, such as pressure ulcers, falls, and so on. Once the problems are identified, the team will set goals that they hope the resident will attain. They also have to design a plan that will achieve these goals. This care plan is mapped out and written down in great detail. Care plans are dynamic and change as the needs of the resident change.

A care plan for each resident is required by federal law. It is taken very seriously by the nursing home. When the nursing home is inspected, the care plans are carefully scrutinized.

These care plan meetings are not closed, secret meetings. It is quite the opposite. The resident and family are always encouraged to attend. For families, the care plans are a good way for you to learn about all the issues facing the resident. These meetings are also a nice way for you to meet many of the people who are providing care for your loved one. Your role does not have to be a passive one. You can ask questions and inquire about what you can do to help your loved one when you visit. If you do decide to go to one of these meetings, don't be surprised if the physician is absent. Unfortunately, physicians often are too busy to attend.

WHAT IS AN OMBUDSPERSON?

An ombudsperson is a volunteer of the state who visits the nursing home as an advocate for the residents by listening to their complaints and trying to work through the system to address them. Ombudspersons are not employees or even volunteers of the nursing home. They can often help the resident resolve issues by working with the nursing home staff and/or community agencies.

IS THE STAFFING AT AN ASSISTED LIVING FACILITY (ALF) DIFFERENT FROM A NURSING HOME?

- ALFs are not nursing homes. They are not required to have twenty-four-hour nursing. Some of the larger facilities may elect to have a nurse during the evening, but they are not required to do so.
- ALFs are not required to have a medical director on staff. Physicians do not have to come to the facility to see the patients.

- The ALF itself cannot provide skilled nursing services, nor can it provide physical or occupational therapy. If these services are needed, they must be coordinated through an outside home health agency.

THINGS YOU CAN DO TO HELP A LOVED ONE IN THE NURSING HOME (OR ALF)!

- Ask what kind of clothes, food, or special items your loved one wants you to buy for her.
- Visit often.
- Find out which hospital residents are sent to when they are ill.
- Try to attend the care plan meeting.

HELPING CARE FOR LOVED ONES WHO LIVE FAR AWAY

Millions of Americans are trying to provide or coordinate care for family members who live by themselves at distances of greater than one mile. If you find yourself in this role, there are things to look for when you visit:

- Is the house/apartment clean?
- Is there food in the kitchen?
- Are the bills being paid?
- Are you scared watching them drive?
- Do they appear well groomed?
- Do they know the names of their medications and what they are for?

Seniors who are having difficulty with any of these issues may need help.

THINGS YOU CAN DO AS A LONG-DISTANCE CAREGIVER

- Keep a list of your loved one's medications, diagnoses, significant test results, and physician contact information.
- Discuss advanced directives (chapter 32). The sooner you discuss this important topic, the better.
- When you visit, pitch in as much as possible to give the primary caregiver regular breaks.

- When visiting, do not change the daily routine too much.
- Make sure the patient signs a release form that allows the doctor(s) to discuss his or her medical issues with you.
- If there is no one close by to help, consider hiring a professional case manager.

WHAT IS A GERIATRIC CASE MANAGER?

This person is usually a nurse or social worker who is trained to assess the needs of the frail older adult patient. She can work with the healthcare providers to make sure the patient shows up for his appointments and is compliant with the treatment recommendations. She can also act as a source to facilitate communication between the family and the doctors. She can help the family coordinate resources in order to keep the person living at home. Such resources may include home health aides, meals on wheels, and so on. There are several things to be aware of before you hire a case manager. One is that her services are not covered by Medicare and they can get to be quite expensive. The second point is that the qualifications among case managers vary widely. Check their credentials first and ask for recommendations.

How Do I Find a Geriatric Case Manager?

Ask around. Try your doctor's office. You probably aren't the first one who has asked about this type of service. Someone in the office may be able to help you. You may want to contact the social work department at a local hospital or nursing home. The National Association of Professional Geriatric Case Managers (www.caremanagers.org) may have a list of local resources.

WHAT KIND OF SKILLED NURSING CARE IS AVAILABLE AT HOME?

Following discharge from the hospital, many patients will require healthcare services at home. The types of services commonly provided at home include:

- occupational therapy
- physical therapy
- skilled nursing care
- speech therapy

The physician needs to order these services. As with the skilled nursing facility, Medicare will pay only for these services as long as the healthcare professionals can document that the patient is expected to continue to improve. After the patient is no longer making any further progress or after the wound care or IV antibiotics are finished, Medicare will stop paying. It has been our experience that many families have a difficult time understanding the strict cutoffs imposed by Medicare.

As with outpatient services, there are copayments associated with these services. The copayments cost up to 20 percent of the bill. The copayments are waived if the patient is homebound.

WHAT DOES IT MEAN FOR YOUR LOVED ONE TO BE HOMEBOUND?

She leaves home infrequently.

She requires the assistance of others to leave the home (medical appointments and church do not count).

Leaving the home is very difficult for her due to a medical or psychiatric issue.

WHAT ABOUT HOME HEALTH AIDES?

These people can help with basic care, such as assistance with bathing, eating, household cleaning, laundry, and going to the bathroom. Legally they cannot perform nursing functions, such as using the feeding tube, giving insulin injections, or taking care of wounds.

Home health aide services are not covered under Medicare. Medicare covers "home health nursing care." There is a big difference between these terms. Medicare will pay only for the care of a "skilled nursing need," which we discussed in the previous section.

A home health aide can be an out-of-pocket expense or may be paid for through Medicaid. Long-term care policies often pay for a home health aide to keep you at home rather than pay the cost of a nursing home.

WHAT ABOUT THE DOCTOR WHO DOES HOUSE CALLS?

Depending on where you live, you may be able to find a doctor who will do house calls. As with everything in medicine, the quality of the doctor can vary greatly. Seeing your loved one at home gives the doctor important clues about how he is coping with his illnesses. In addition to a physical exam, blood can be drawn and sent to a laboratory for analysis, just like in a doctor's office. In many areas around the country there are even companies that send out x-rays and ultrasound equipment for house calls.

You may have heard people say that the days of a doctor making a house call are over. While this was true up until a few years ago, the trend is slowly reversing. There are a growing number of doctors who make only house calls. How did this happen? Well, Medicare has been increasing the amount of money it pays for doctors to make home visits. The compensation is now actually quite a bit more than for an office or nursing home visit. What is even better for the doctor is that he does not have to shell out all that money to run an office (rent, utilities, staff, etc.).

Remember, there is a caring team of compassionate dedicated health professionals who can help you take care of a loved one. These folks are available whether your loved one is in a nursing home, at an assisted living facility, or is living at home.

Chapter 12

WHY DO SOME PEOPLE
HATE NURSING HOMES?

*"I was always taught to respect my elders, and I've now
reached the age when I don't have anybody to respect."*
George Burns (1896–1996)

In the 1980s, nursing homes received a lot of negative publicity as places
where seniors were often abused and neglected. While sweeping legislation
and public awareness have improved the quality of nursing home care, many
of the stereotypes still remain. For example, if you ask one of your friends
what she thinks about nursing homes, you may likely hear one of the following
comments.

- "Nursing homes always smell like urine!"
- "They are dirty places!"
- "They are so depressing!"
- "I would rather die than go to a nursing home!"

The Henry J. Kaiser Family Foundation actually studied the perceptions that
the public has about long-term care.[1] What researchers found was that:

- 75 percent believe that nursing homes are understaffed
- 63 percent think that nursing home staff are poorly trained
- 64 percent think that there are not enough governmental regulations

WHAT DO SENIORS THINK?

Many seniors dread the thought of "being shipped off" to a nursing home. Many older people think of a nursing home as a place one goes to die. Many may feel that once they are sent there, life will lose all purpose.

In many cases, this perception is not true. Each year hundreds of thousands of seniors go to nursing homes to receive skilled nursing services after an acute illness for a three- to twelve-week period before returning home (chapter 9). This is an important point to emphasize to seniors who are afraid of going into a nursing home.

However, some other fears may be justified. It can be difficult to adjust to life in the nursing home. Moving to a nursing home represents a loss of one's personal identity. Nursing home residents were once decision makers at home and at work. In many cases, the resident is no longer thought of as a businessperson, teacher, or mother, but rather as a ninety-four-year-old with Alzheimer's disease and congestive heart failure.

Although nursing homes do try to provide as much autonomy as possible, the environment is not set up like one's home and the resident will often encounter numerous new rules. Invariably, someone will decide when they can eat, when they go to bed, or when they can urinate. There are also constraints on how the resident may decorate her room. Pets are not allowed, although pet therapy allows residents to spend some time with animals.

Seniors may also fear being further isolated from their remaining family and friends. Depending on the location of the facility, they may be right. As you reach an advanced age, many of your friends will have either moved away or died. It's not so easy to make new friends, especially when the majority of people living in the facility are either demented or can't get out of bed. Residents are also limited in the types of activities in which they can participate. They may not even be able to play cards or bingo with the other residents at night. Many people are embarrassed socially, due to speech problems or urinary incontinence.

The loss of identity and independence as well as the onset of loneliness may lead to feelings of anger, abandonment, and depression for many residents. To make matters worse, some do not get the opportunity to choose the facility where they will reside.

WHAT DO THE REGULATORS THINK?

Nursing homes are entrusted to monitor and care for people who are unable to care for themselves. Nursing homes are evaluated by comparing quality indicators that measure the frequency of falls, dehydration, weight loss, decreased mobility, bedsores, and other resident health problems. On the one hand, these indicators have led to the development of standards of care for nursing homes across the country. Facilities that routinely neglect the special needs of residents are now easier to identify, as their numbers will not look as good as those of other facilities.

Some healthcare professionals, however, misinterpret these quality of care indicators to mean that a facility should in most cases be able to rehabilitate, or restore function, among their residents. Today's nursing home residents are so frail and have so many severe illnesses that many would, in fact, meet the criteria for having a terminal diagnosis and could qualify for hospice care (chapter 26). The modern nursing home is therefore caught in a predicament of being forced to provide comprehensive and aggressive care to a population that oftentimes would be better served by focusing on end-of-life care. In many cases the residents will get worse even if aggressive care is provided.

In August 2006 *Consumer Reports* published a report on nursing homes that stated, "Bad care persists, and good homes are hard to find."[2] The magazine reported that bad care is allowed to persist because:

- The nursing home industry has a powerful lobby in many state legislatures.
- Fines against nursing homes are not severe enough.
- Lawsuits against nursing homes are hard to initiate.

ARE NURSING HOMES UNDERSTAFFED?

It depends on how you ask the question. If you were to ask the people working there if they could use more help, the answer would be yes. If you were a bed-bound resident waiting to have your soiled diaper changed, you would likely say yes as well.

Research studies have shown that nursing homes with more staff often seem to have better-quality care.[3] In response, most states have enacted laws setting minimum nursing and nurses' aide staffing standards. For example, Florida requires a minimum of 2.6 hours of contact time per day with a nurses' aide and 1 hour of contact time with a nurse. What about the other

20.4 hours a day? The **real truth** is something that we don't really ever talk about. Nursing homes do not have the staff to watch the residents every minute of the day. The staff may not realistically have several hours to feed the resident or to turn every patient precisely every two hours.

If the nursing home had more staff would the problems be solved? In some cases, they obviously would and in other cases they may not. As we will discuss in this book, blaming the nursing home every time the person falls, gets a bedsore, or loses weight may be overly simplistic. The problems that affect patients at the end of life are often the result of a complicated mixture of age-related organ changes and multiple diseases.

WHAT IS THE FAMILY'S PERCEPTION?

Dealing with Neglect?

Many families become quite frustrated when they go to visit a loved one in a nursing home. They may smell urine or hear residents screaming. They may notice that their loved one isn't being turned exactly every two hours as ordered. They may walk in the room and find that the resident is sitting in a bed full of urine or feces. They may get phone calls from the staff saying that their loved one has had a fall. In their eyes, if the resident is not kept clean or kept from falling, how can the care be any good?[4]

Families may be paying over six thousand dollars per month for care. When they are spending that much money, we can understand why they may get upset when they see that the staff is not keeping their loved one clean, getting her out of bed, or spending enough time assisting her with her meals. And where is the doctor?

Dealing with Guilt?

Families often wrestle with feelings of guilt over placing their loved one in a long-term care facility. Realizing that they were either too busy, physically unable, or unwilling to provide the care themselves, they look to the nursing home as the option of last resort. They feel terrible that their loved one has to go to a nursing home, but they rationalize it by saying to themselves that "at least there will be people to take care of their relative."

Some families have unrealistic expectations of what end of life means. They cannot understand how their loved one could have gotten pneumonia, a hip fracture, a stroke, and so on. They have been led to believe that every illness is either preventable or treatable. Part of the problem may be that we live in a society where medical science appears to have a solution for everything.

Problems such as weight loss, falls, dehydration, bedsores, incontinence, and contractures are often not preventable. In many cases these issues represent natural signs of an end-stage dementia and frailty. Many current educational resources for the public state that these events are preventable. There are very few trained geriatric specialists in the United States. So, in many cases, the healthcare professionals are unfamiliar with the science and art of caring for the very old and frail.

DOCTORS' PERCEPTIONS

Many doctors look at nursing homes as understaffed places where important clinical issues are either ignored or not treated. We have seen doctors and other healthcare professionals become upset when the nursing home does not perform to the same standard as the hospital where they work. Although the expectations have increased, nursing homes are limited in the amount of medical care that they can provide. For instance, nursing homes in Florida receive only $137–$241 per day per resident while the hospital charges thousands of dollars per day per patient.[5] They do not have the staffing or the equipment of a hospital. The danger, therefore, is that nursing homes are being held to a hospital standard without the resources to provide such a high level of care.

WHAT IS THE STAFF'S PERCEPTION?

Working in a modern nursing home is stressful. The staff are expected to deliver complicated medical care to people who no one else can or is willing to care for. It is tough work that may not always be pretty to see or pleasant to smell. The staff are sometimes physically and verbally abused by patients with dementia.

The expectations of a nursing home are high. Nursing homes are more heavily regulated than hospitals.[6] The paperwork is enormous. The turnover rate among nurses and nurses' aides is often high and recruitment of staff is a constant challenge.

HOW DO YOU PICK THE RIGHT NURSING HOME?

What Do Medicare and *Consumer Reports* Have to Say?

There are many books and Web sites that discuss this topic at length. Without ever leaving your home you can use the Medicare Web site at www .medicare.gov/nhcompare/home.asp.[7] This site provides detailed information about the past performance of every Medicare and Medicaid certified nursing home in the country. Information regarding the number of people on staff, inspection results, and quality measures is available. You can also find the *Consumer Reports* comparison of nursing homes online at www.consumerreports .org/nursinghomes.[8]

Be careful when trying to interpret the above information as you look for a nursing home. Assessing the quality of a facility is very complicated. We believe that the information in these reports is not enough to say definitively that one nursing home will provide better care to your family member than another.

In many cases, the information in *Consumer Reports* and on the Medicare Web site is a year old. During this time many things can change. What was listed as a bad home may have improved a lot. By the same token, the quality of care provided at a good home may have deteriorated. How can this be? The home may have new administrators or new owners. There may be a huge turnover among the nurses and nurses' aides. In some cases the good homes may no longer even be in business.

In addition, inspection reports do not always provide an accurate picture of the quality of care in a nursing home. A good home can potentially get a bad report. A lot has to do with the individual inspectors. Some may be tougher and more critical than others. Also, bad events can happen at a good nursing home. If something unfortunate happens at a nursing home on the day the inspectors arrive, it will be reflected in the report. If one or two families are very vocal with their complaints, it can have a negative influence on the inspection process.

Nursing homes that admit sicker patients are going to have frailer residents who will have more complications. Because the frail elderly are so complicated and different from each other, neither Medicare nor *Consumer Reports* have an accurate mechanism to really tell if the residents in one facility are as sick as the residents in another nursing home.

Save Your Time and Money!

Many books and Web sites provide information on how to choose the right nursing home. The **real truth** is that in many cases your choice may be limited by what you can afford and by which facilities have empty beds. Table 12.1 lists some helpful tips for deciding on a nursing home.

TABLE 12.1. HELPFUL TIPS FOR CHOOSING A NURSING HOME

- Find a facility that is close to family and friends. The closer the facility, the more often people will visit.
- Find a facility that is near the hospital you prefer. Remember that if 911 is called, EMS will take the patient to the closest hospital.
- Visit the place more than once at different times of the day. When you visit, take a look to see if
  - the facility appears clean
  - the residents appear well groomed
  - there is a policy on bed holding (i.e., the facility keeps the bed reserved when the resident gets admitted to the hospital)
  - the facility has a back-up plan in cases where the resident does not get along with his or her roommate
  - the facility has different levels of care
  - religious services are available.

We kept this table short on purpose. While many books will give you an extensive laundry list of items to investigate before you choose a nursing home, many of the things they list are not practical. For example, many sources will state that if the place has a strong odor of feces or urine, then the nursing home is probably a bad facility that is short staffed. These sources will also tell you to see if the resident's calls for help are being answered promptly. The **real truth** is that you cannot judge the quality of a nursing home by these variables only without making a number of visits. How do you know whether a resident happens to be demented and screams for help all day long or whether it's a rare outburst, which can happen in any facility? Were you there when the staff changed the diapers on a patient five minutes before he had his next bowel movement, which led to the foul odor? In both cases, you really won't know the full story about what is going on with the individual patients.

They also tell you to look at the results of the facility's last inspection. This report will highlight what the facility has done to address its deficiencies.

Remember that these inspection reports are to a certain degree subjective and the findings may be outdated.

Choosing a Nursing Home Is Not All Your Decision!

Some caregiving books and Web sites give you the impression that when it comes to choosing a nursing home, the consumer has all the power. Picking a nursing home is not like buying groceries, where the consumer can choose among many options.

The facility that you want may be too expensive or may not have an empty bed. You also need to be aware that while you are evaluating the facilities, the facilities in many cases are evaluating your loved one. Many nursing homes are hesitant to take residents with issues that may cause problems for the facility down the road, such as:

- extensive bedsores
- violent behavior
- sexually inappropriate behavior
- the presence of a tracheotomy (breathing tube in the neck)
- the need for dialysis
- an infection with a bacteria resistant to many antibiotics

For complicated patients with these types of problems, your choices could be quite limited. If you are relying on Medicaid to pay for nursing home care, the options will be further limited, as nursing homes place limits on the number of Medicaid patients that they will accept. These facilities will use the other beds for patients who pay privately at a higher rate.

THINGS YOU CAN DO ONCE YOUR LOVED ONE IS ADMITTED

- Visit often. Many books and Web sites say that the residents who have an involved family are less likely to be abused or neglected. This is probably true. We also think that it is important to focus on the positive emotional and spiritual benefits that families bring to their loved ones who are living in a nursing home. We believe that these benefits can have a very big impact on the quality of life of a nursing home resident.
- Attend the care plan meetings—all residents must have all of their needs discussed in a meeting involving multiple healthcare disciplines.

These meetings are required to take place every three months or sooner if there is a change in the resident's needs. These meetings do not occur in secret. Residents and family members are encouraged to attend and to be a part of the decision-making process.

Chapter 13

DANGERS ENCOUNTERED WHEN SENIORS ARE TRANSFERRED TO THE ER OR HOSPITAL

"Old age is a shipwreck."

Charles de Gaulle (1890–1970)

Years ago, there was a movie about a boy who was raised in a bubble because he had no immune system. By staying in the bubble he was protected from the dangers of the world. Most of us do not live in a bubble. We live in a world where we are exposed to a variety of dangers. Because the organ systems of frail seniors have a decreased ability to handle the stresses of additional injuries, seniors are more likely to get sick and to have a harder time recovering from a major medical illness.

To make matters more complicated, we often see frail patients who are actually suffering from two or more acute illnesses at the same time. For example, the elderly woman with a bad urinary tract infection may become weak and suffer a fall-related hip fracture while trying to walk to the toilet.

We commonly hear comments, such as "She was doing just fine at home until she came in to the hospital!" or "She used to be able to live alone before all this happened!" As geriatricians, we understand that it makes families upset to see their loved ones suffer. However, in many cases they were not, in fact, doing just fine but rather were just getting by. Many seniors have a hard time recovering their strength following a hospitalization. Many will be too weak to go home and will need to go to a nursing home. In others cases, this loss of function is only temporary. Through medical treatment and rehabilitation,

151

some elderly patients are able to return to their previous state of health. For others, the damage suffered is irreversible. Trying to guess which seniors will lose or regain their functional independence is often impossible to predict.

HURRY UP AND WAIT!

Many patients and families think that once they arrive at the emergency room, they will immediately be cared for. Many emergency rooms are quite busy. You might have to wait hours to be seen by a doctor. When you check in at the ER, a nurse will assess how sick your loved one is. It is not first come, first serve. The patients who are deemed to be the sickest are brought back sooner for medical attention. It is important that your loved one tell the nurse all the symptoms she is having. If you don't tell the nurse up front, you may have to wait a lot longer.

Even after you are done in the waiting room, you may spend many more hours being evaluated in the emergency room. During this time, patients are often lying in an unfamiliar environment on an uncomfortable stretcher. For patients with dementia and/or poor vision and hearing, the hospital can be a scary place. The disorientation, lack of sleep, and confusion associated with being in an emergency room are enough to make them delirious. Moreover, lying on a hard gurney can lead to the development or worsening of pressure ulcers.

WHO TAKES CARE OF THE PATIENT?

Most likely your loved one's primary care doctor will not be in the emergency room waiting for him. He will be seen by emergency room physicians who may or may not have access to his medical records.

Even after he is admitted to the hospital, his primary care doctor may still not be there to take care of him. An increasing number of elderly patients are admitted to hospital-based physician groups known as *hospitalists*. The sole job of these groups is to take care of hospital patients. They do not have an office and will not see the patients once he or she leaves the hospital. Hospitalists usually work in shifts, so it is quite common for a person to be cared for by multiple physicians during his hospital stay.

Making sure important medical information is not lost during these multiple handoffs requires developing communication protocols between primary care physicians, nursing homes, emergency departments, and hospitalist physicians. In some hospitals, these protocols work well, and in others they don't.

IT SEEMED LIKE NO ONE WAS IN CHARGE OF THE SHIP!

Many families will complain that a whole bunch of different doctors are seeing the patient, but no one seems to know what is going on. No one seems to want to make decisions and no one can answer all of their questions. While we will never make excuses for those doctors with poor bedside manners, let's discuss some of the other issues at play here. The specialists are asked to provide assistance with regard to a specific medical issue. They will usually defer discussing medical issues that are outside of their specialty. The cardiologist is consulted for his expertise about heart disease. It would be outside his specialty to comment about knee pain or diarrhea.

The problem is that the frail older patient is much different from the younger patient who is usually there because of one medical issue. Many older patients may be suffering from several problems at once. Often these problems are interrelated. Problems with one organ system will have an impact on another system. This is frustrating for patients and families who want to see a doctor, not necessarily a urologist, an orthopedist, or a cardiologist.

So who pulls it all together? In these complicated cases, it will often be the hospitalist or internal medicine doctor who can give you the overall picture of what is going on.

DO BAD THINGS EVER HAPPEN IN THE HOSPITAL?

If a family member needs to be in the hospital, it is because he is very sick and will need to have intravenous fluids, surgery, and so on. Not only are the older patients frailer and sicker, but the treatments performed in a modern hospital are increasingly complicated. When you mix a very sick, frail patient with multiple complicated procedures, there will always be the potential for problems.

Some of the risk is due to problems with the modern hospital system. Patient anxiety, miscommunication among staff, and delays in treatment are important concerns whenever a frail older person is transferred to a hospital. Old medical records are not immediately available and if the patient has never been to that hospital before, there may be no records at all.

The admitting hospitalist physician is usually unaware of the patient's wishes regarding end-of-life issues and aggressiveness of care. Many seniors are not able to communicate effectively due to their weakened state from severe illness or dementia. The family may not be accessible when the hospitalist needs to speak to them. This can all lead to inappropriate testing and therapies. The staff may not know, for example, that a weakened or a demented patient is allergic to a specific drug. When frail elderly patients are admitted to the hospital, they will be exposed to new medications and procedures, all of which can have side effects or complications.

HOSPITALS ARE NOT VACATION RESORTS

The care in a hospital can be very uncomfortable. Patients with pneumonia, for example, will need to have x-rays done and blood drawn frequently. In cases of dementia, seniors may be restrained by the hospital staff so they do not pull out their IVs or fall on the floor. All patients may be woken up by the staff multiple times during the evening to have their pulse, blood pressure, and temperature checked. While the family may be aware of the special individual needs of their loved ones, the hospital has a different focus. The hospital runs on the schedule of the doctor, not the patient. Patients will often be awoken around 5 AM in order for blood work to be drawn, so it can be ready by the time the physicians come to see the patient in the morning.

Many older adults have difficulty adjusting to the disruption of their normal sleep/wake cycle. If the room does not have a window, the patient may not know whether it is day or night.

HOSPITALS CAN HARBOR DANGEROUS BACTERIA!

Hospitals are the places where we send people with serious infections. Many of these patients have been treated with antibiotics before and are at high risk for infections from antibiotic-resistant bacteria. Therefore, putting all these patients in the same building provides an opportunity for bacteria that are resistant to antibiotics to spread from patient to patient (chapter 16).

THE DANGER OF DELIRIUM

We often hear the word *delirium*, but what does it really mean? Delirium refers to an inability to focus or shift attention. It is accompanied by a change in memory and an inability to communicate.

While seniors with dementia (chapter 23) are at an increased risk of delirium, these terms do not mean the same thing.

- Patients with delirium are unable to pay attention and focus when you ask them a question. The patient with dementia is still able to focus his attention when spoken to.
- The behavior, alertness, and memory of patients with delirium can vary from moment to moment. With dementia, the symptoms generally remain the same from day to day.
- Delirium is potentially reversible, whereas most causes of dementia are usually irreversible and the symptoms will get worse over time.

How Serious Is Delirium?

Delirium can cause a variety of problems in the elderly hospitalized patient. Delirious patients often won't eat, won't swallow their medications, and won't exercise. They may pull on their IV lines, catheters, or feeding tubes. In many cases they desperately want to get out of bed, which puts them at a high risk for fall-related injuries. Studies have shown that elderly patients with delirium have longer lengths of stay and a higher risk of death.[1]

How Common Is Delirium?

Delirium is one of the most common complications of hospitalization. About 20 percent of older adult patients will suffer from delirium during hospitalization.[2] The ones at highest risk are those with:

- dehydration
- dementia such as Alzheimer's disease (chapter 23)
- Foley catheters to drain urine from the bladder
- malnutrition
- more than three new drugs added to their treatment plan in the preceding twenty-four hours
- poor vision
- restraints on the arms and legs

Why Is Dementia Such a Strong Factor for Delirium?

Patients with dementia have a 50 percent chance that they will suffer delirium during a hospitalization.[3] This increased risk is not surprising when one thinks of dementia as a state where the brain has a decreased ability to withstand stress. To simplify a very complex and poorly understood disease, we often think of patients with dementia as having a decreased functional brain reserve, just as we think of those with congestive heart failure as having a decreased reserve of the heart or those with emphysema as having a decreased lung reserve. Thus, we would expect that a brain with less ability to withstand stress would be more likely to develop delirium. If your loved one has had an episode of delirium during a recent hospitalization, it would probably be a good idea to talk to your doctor about whether she needs to be carefully evaluated for an underlying dementia.

Medications Can Cause Delirium

In the hospital, the patient will likely receive one or more new drugs. Medications are a major cause of delirium in the elderly.[4] It is essential that a physician or pharmacist review the medications for potentially harmful side effects and problematic combinations. Medications that can cause delirium in the elderly include:

- many older psychiatric medications
- medications with anticholinergic side effects (chapter 8)
- narcotic pain medications (oxycodone, morphine, meperidine, etc.)
- corticosteroids, such as prednisone

In addition to the risk factors listed above, there are many medical illnesses that can make an elderly patient delirious. Some of the more common ones include:

- fecal impaction which occurs when constipation is so severe that the stool gets stuck in the colon. It may appear far-fetched that severe constipation could cause delirium, but it does happen.
- fractures of the hip, pelvis, or spine
- heart attack
- high or low levels of sodium, glucose, or calcium in the blood
- infections (most commonly pneumonia and urinary tract infections)
- low oxygen levels
- low blood pressure
- pulmonary embolus, which is a blood clot that usually forms in the veins of the legs or pelvis then breaks off and gets lodged in the arteries of the lungs

SUMMARY OF THINGS YOU CAN DO TO HELP AN OLDER ADULT WHO NEEDS TO GO TO THE HOSPITAL

- Make sure to bring his glasses and/or hearing aids along.
- Make sure that you have a list of his current medications (including over-the-counter medications).
- If he has a pet, make sure someone can take care of the animal.
- For residents of nursing homes and assisted living facilities, ask the staff if they have a preferred hospital to transfer patients to. Which doctors or hospitalist groups would the staff choose, if they had a choice? Most hospitals have Web sites that describe their facilities. A little prior familiarity with the institution may alleviate some of the fear when a family member is transferred to a hospital.

MANY DISEASES OCCUR IN STRANGE WAYS

Part of the danger seniors face in the hospital is that the doctors may have a hard time diagnosing their illnesses. Trying to pinpoint what is wrong with the ill older adult can be extremely difficult. Because of this difficulty, extra tests are often ordered and serious illnesses take longer to diagnose. The longer it takes to make the correct diagnosis, the sicker the patient will be before he or she receives treatment. Heart attacks and infections (chapter 18) are two common examples of this problem.

HEART ATTACKS

Heart disease is the most common cause of death in the elderly. Many seniors will not complain of the classic squeezing chest pain when they are having a heart attack. In one study, only 37 percent of patients over the age of eighty-five had chest pain during the heart attack. Shortness of breath and fatigue are more commonly seen in older patients with angina pain.[5] Unfortunately, shortness of breath and fatigue are so common that it makes it very difficult to tell who is having a heart attack and who is not. To make matters even more confusing, some patients with heart attacks will exhibit only symptoms, such as abdominal pain, confusion, dizziness, or passing out (*syncope*).

An abnormal electrocardiogram (EKG) is often helpful for diagnosing heart attacks. However, a lot of older adults already have abnormal EKGs. Some of these abnormalities may make it harder for the doctor to tell if patients are having a heart attack. One-third of all heart attacks in older adults are unrecognized.[6] In the frail demented population, this proportion is almost certainly higher, as many cannot articulate their complaints.

OLDER ADULTS ARE AT A HIGHER RISK FOR COMPLICATIONS FROM SURGERY

Older adults are four times more likely to have to undergo surgery than younger adults.[7] When comparing the different age groups, the elderly have the highest rate of death following surgery. We always think from watching movies that the most dangerous time for the patient is when he or she is on the operating table. Actually, this is not the case. Most serious complications occur in the hours and days following surgery.

For the aged, the dangers of surgery involve more than just the tissue damage from the procedure. There are also the effects of the anesthesia, as well as stresses on the aged heart, kidney, and lungs. It is important to weigh the benefits of the surgery against the risk of surgical complications. In addition, infections, bedsores, delirium, and blood clots in the legs are common after many types of surgery. Ask your doctor how often these problems arise among his patients following surgery. You may also want to find out how much experience the doctor has in performing the type of procedure in question.

SHOULD I GET A SECOND OPINION?

This question does not have a simple answer. Every patient and every case is so different that it is almost impossible to make a general recommendation. If it is a complicated or risky procedure, you may want to consider getting a second opinion. Fortunately, Medicare and most HMOs will pay for this.

THINGS YOU CAN DO TO GET READY FOR SURGERY

Note: Always consult with your doctor before starting or stopping any prescription or over-the-counter medication.

- No aspirin, clopidogrel (Plavix), or warfarin (Coumadin), for at least seven days before surgery.

- Stop the Alzheimer's medications donepezil (Aricept), rivastigmine (Excelon), and galantamine (Razadyne) one to two days before surgery.
- Stop smoking.
- Exercise the lungs, either by walking or using an incentive spirometer (see p. 161).
- Stop taking vitamin E and garlic one week before your surgery. Both can potentially impair the ability of the blood to clot.

DON'T BE SURPRISED AFTER SURGERY

We often see patients with dementia whose memory and overall thinking is worse following surgery. This impairment may persist for several months to years following the surgery. Is this due to the drugs used during anesthesia? Is it due to decreased blood flow to the brain during surgery? No one is exactly sure.

MALNUTRITION

Appetite is often decreased when a frail senior becomes acutely ill. It has been shown that when we are ill our bodies produce higher levels of chemicals, such as *tumor necrosis factor alpha, interleukin-1,* and *interleukin-6,* that may cause us to lose our appetites.[8] These chemicals also set off a number of changes in the body that increase the amount of food necessary to meet energy needs.

There are certain things that healthcare professionals do to make one's appetite even worse. Patients with diabetes are usually ordered a diabetic diet and patients with congestive heart failure are ordered a low-salt diet. These bland menus do not help the elderly patient who already has a poor appetite. To make matters worse, many tests, such as colonoscopy, CT scans of the abdomen, as well as most surgical procedures require that the patient be made NPO, or *nils per os,* Latin for *nothing by mouth.* If the patient needs multiple tests and/or procedures or if tests get canceled and rescheduled, the patient can in theory be NPO for several days. Therefore, at a time when the person's energy needs are elevated, she is consuming fewer calories.

The key point to remember is that patients must eat. Food is just as important as medicine. When we explain to patients that they must eat, we often hear, "I'll get to it later, I'm just not hungry now!" Later is not acceptable. The body's energy needs will not wait until later.

PNEUMONIA

Age-related changes to the lungs (chapter 2), underlying lung diseases, and difficulty with deep breathing (due to pain, lying in bed, medications, or surgical incisions) place the older adult patient at a high risk for developing pneumonia in the hospital.

A simple intervention to lower the risk of pneumonia is to get out of bed. Getting patients into a chair or up walking is of paramount importance. Upright posture allows the lungs to expand by about a 15 percent greater volume than when lying in bed. This can also help prevent small areas of the lung from collapsing (*atelectasis*). It is also easier to cough when one is upright.

The nurses may give you a small plastic device (called an *incentive spirometer*) to help you take a deep breath. When you breathe into this device, you may cough a little. That is actually a good sign. It means that you are opening up the small areas of your lungs that have in a sense deflated. If the doctor gives you a spirometer, it is very important to use it.

EXPECT THE UNEXPECTED

Always remember that a variety of problems can occur in the hospital setting. IV sites can get infected. The use of Foley catheters (the tubes that are inserted into the urethra to drain the bladder) can lead to urinary tract infections, as well as discomfort. Side effects to drugs often occur.

SUMMARY OF THINGS YOU CAN DO
TO HELP A FAMILY MEMBER IN THE HOSPITAL

Be a Spokesperson and a Record Keeper

As we stated above, elderly patients often find themselves moving through a complicated healthcare system. Many health care professionals will be unfamiliar with the medical issues of your family member. Patients with dementia and those who are very ill will not be able to tell the doctors their past medical history or talk about what is bothering them. You can help by being the spokesperson, advocate, and record keeper for your family member.

Make a List of All the Drugs

Get a list of all the medications prescribed before and after discharge. You may want to ask the physician if all the medication changes are appropriate or needed.

Grab Those Records

Get a copy of the medical records, including the results of procedures, labs, x-rays, and so on.

Encourage the Patient to Eat

While you are with your loved one, you can do a lot to help by providing encouragement or assistance with eating. Ask the staff if you can bring in any food from the outside that your loved one would enjoy.

Help the Patient Get Out of Bed

Lying in bed can lead to increased weakness that puts the frail elderly person at risk for becoming immobile. You can provide encouragement or assistance with walking and/or sitting in a chair.

Encourage the Patient to Use the Incentive Spirometer

Make sure they take some deep breaths in order to lower their risk of getting pneumonia. We like to tell patients to take a deep breath using this device every time they see a commercial on the television.

Help Keep the Patient Oriented

Keep reminding her where she is and why she is in the hospital. Make sure there is sufficient light in the room during the night. Keep the lights and the window shades open during the day. Put up a large-print calendar.

Keep an Eye Out

Spend as much time as possible in the room to reorient your loved one and to make sure that the IV, Foley catheter, oxygen mask/nasal cannula are not removed or the patient does not try to move in a manner that would lead to a fall.

Take Care of Yourself

We sometimes see family members who will not leave the bedside. Many are fearful that something bad will happen if they are not there. Others may feel guilty. One of the important things we tell families is to make sure they take care of themselves. The patient needs them to be strong. If they are not sleeping well and not eating well, how can they be there for the patient? Some families think that they need to be there all the time. Caring for the elderly family member is a long-term project. While they are in the hospital there is staff that can do a lot of the work, such as bathing, dressing, and so on. When their loved one goes home the hard work will begin. This is why it is so essential that the family caregivers take care of themselves.

Leaving the Hospital

Whenever a frail elderly person is discharged from the hospital, there are a lot of things that need to be coordinated. No matter how hard everyone tries, something often goes wrong. If she is being discharged home there may be a delay getting the medications filled, getting the home health provider to come out to see her, or getting the right home health equipment delivered. Preparing patients to go to a skilled nursing facility is usually even more complicated. The elderly are often so weak at the time of their discharge that they are at a high risk for falls and other problems.

To minimize potential glitches we recommend, if possible, that the transfer to home or to a new skilled nursing facility occur during working hours. On weekends and nights it will be nearly impossible for the nursing home to contact anyone from the hospital (doctors, social workers, therapists) if questions or problems arise.

Part 3
CARING FOR THE FRAIL SENIOR

Chapter 14
FALLS ARE A SERIOUS PROBLEM

"I've fallen and I can't get up!"

BACKGROUND

In the 1990s we saw the commercial of the old lady lying on the floor who pushes a button on her emergency transmitter. The name of the product was Lifecall, and it allowed an elderly person to simply hit a button if he or she fell or were in danger and needed immediate help. This commercial was a little campy in its production and became the source of many jokes. But we should never forget that falls are a very serious problem for the elderly. Below is a list of serious problems that result from falls.

- Bleeding around the brain (*subdural hematoma*)
- Hip fractures
- Lacerations and skin tears
- Psychological trauma
- Fear of further falls
- Social isolation
- Wrist fractures

HOW COMMON ARE FALL-RELATED INJURIES?

Among seniors living at home, only 5 to 10 percent of falls are associated with a fracture, laceration or a need for hospitalization.[1] But the frail elderly are three times more likely to have a fall. Not only are they more likely to fall, they are also three times more likely to have a fall-related injury.

WHAT ARE THE RISK FACTORS FOR FALLS?

As we discuss the risk factors for falls, it is important to remember that most falls do not have one cause but rather are the result of many different factors.

Difficulties with Balance

Maintaining balance while walking is something most of us take for granted. It is actually a complicated process that requires integrating what you see with your eyes, what you feel with your feet, and the balancing mechanism within your inner ear. It also requires that the person have sufficient leg strength. Studies have shown that problems with walking and balance are the biggest risk for falls in the elderly.[2]

With aging, one's eyesight worsens. The inability to see clearly is only part of the problem. There is also a decline in the ability to assess depth perception and to recognize the differences between different surfaces and objects. The elderly patient therefore has more difficulty seeing things, such as the step that leads from one room to the next or the transition from a carpeted to a wooden floor. To make matters worse, when an older adult enters a dark room it may take up to a minute for her eyes to adjust.

Many elderly people have weakness in their lower extremities. This can lead to difficulty with walking and with balance. Over 80 percent of nursing home residents have significant lower extremity weakness and decreased muscle mass in their legs. Most frail older adults, for example, cannot stand up from a chair without using their hands for support.

The Presence of Other Medical Illnesses

Many patients have medical issues that can affect their balance. Falls, for example, are the most common cause of injury among stroke patients. Patients with nerve damage in their feet from long-standing diabetes are at a higher risk as well. Parkinson's disease is another common disorder that can affect balance and increase a patient's risk of falls.

Chronic medical issues, such as pain, arthritis, and seizure, can also contribute to the risk of falls. The sudden onset of an acute illness, such as a heart attack, pneumonia, or a urinary tract infection, may make the person so weak that she is more likely to fall.

Orthostatic Hypotension

Many seniors will have a drop in blood pressure when they stand up after sitting or when they sit up after lying down. The sudden drop in blood pressure can make the person momentarily weak and dizzy. In some patients, the symptoms are worse after a meal as more blood gets pooled in the veins around the stomach and small intestine. This problem, known as *orthostatic hypotension* (OH), can affect over 50 percent of seniors living in long-term care facilities.[3]

The symptoms of OH may be worse in patients who have had strokes or have Parkinson's disease or long-standing diabetes. They may also worsen if the patient becomes dehydrated. Certain blood pressure drugs can also increase the severity of symptoms.

Prolonged bed rest may make the symptoms worse as well. It is therefore essential that the patient recovering in the hospital or the skilled nursing facility increase the amount of time she spends sitting up each day. Just having the patient sit up on the side of the bed for several minutes a couple of times a day can make a difference.

Patients with OH may be treated with medications and dietary changes, such as increasing the amount of salt in the diet and eating smaller meals more frequently. Adjusting their current medications may also help.

Watch Out for Those Medications!

Several studies have shown that older adults who take more drugs are more likely to fall than those who take fewer drugs.[4] There are also specific drugs that may increase the risk of falling: benzodiazepines and many antidepressants are associated with an increased risk of falling. Benzodiazepines (chapter 8) will make one's balance worse. These drugs work in the same manner as alcohol, which we all know can make you tipsy. Many older antidepressants have anticholinergic side effects (chapter 8) that can make orthostatic hypotension worse. They may also increase confusion in patients with dementia. Seniors who take SSRI antidepressants (chapter 22) are also more likely to fall. There is no good explanation for this finding.[5]

Dementia

Dementia puts one at risk for falls. Patients with dementia often get lost or disoriented and can't remember how to get out of a situation or what to look out for. The ability to integrate information regarding shapes, structures, depth perception, and changes in the environment are all impaired in patients with dementia.

Foot Problems

Corns and calluses can make it painful to walk. Other patients may have nerve damage in their feet. Wearing high-heel shoes has also been shown to increase the risk of falls.[6]

The Fear of Falling Can Lead to Further Falls

After a fall, some people are so scared of falling again that they get up from a chair and walk as little as possible. As patients become less mobile, their muscles begin to shrink (*atrophy*) and become weaker, which further increases their

How the Fear of Falling Leads to Further Falls

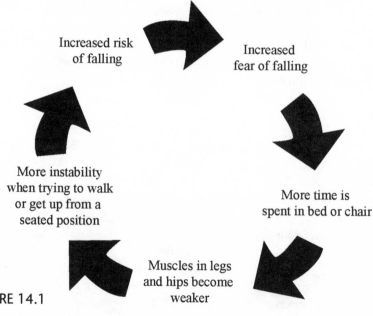

FIGURE 14.1

risk of falling. In addition, restricting one's activities can also increase their feeling of social isolation and depression.

Unsafe Home Environment

This is a major cause of falls among seniors living at home. The older adult must be careful around the bathtub and any stairs or ladders. They must also be cautious outdoors after it rains or snows. Many seniors also have furniture placed in a manner that makes it difficult for them to walk around their home, especially at night. *While there is nothing you can do to guarantee that you'll prevent falls 100 percent of the time, at the end of this chapter we list some steps you can take to reduce the risk of falling in or around the home.*

SERIOUS INJURIES RESULTING FROM FALLS

While most falls do not lead to injuries, plenty do. Osteoporosis and the use of blood-thinning medications are the two biggest risk factors for fall-related injuries. We will discuss osteoporosis at length in chapter 15.

The use of blood-thinning agents is quite common. Aspirin and clopidogrel (Plavix) are commonly given to people who have coronary artery disease or strokes. Atrial fibrillation is an irregular heart rhythm that affects 10 percent of people age eighty and over. The risk of strokes is very high in these patients and many are placed on the blood-thinning agent warfarin (Coumadin) in order to lower the risk. Patients with blood clots in their leg(s) will also need to take blood-thinning medications. In hospitals, heparin and enoxaparin (Lovenox) are commonly used to prevent the development of blood clots in the veins. Even a high dose of vitamin E can thin the blood. With any fall-related injury, the bleeding will be worse if you are taking blood-thinning medications.

What about Head Injuries?

With aging, the veins surrounding the brain become more fragile. As the brain gradually shrinks with aging, these veins are more exposed to shearing forces that can cause them to break. Even a minor head injury can lead to bleeding in the space between the skull and the brain. We call this a *subdural hematoma.* Subdural hematomas can be diagnosed by a CT scan of the head. Sometimes the patient may appear normal after the fall but develops increased confusion over the following weeks to months. If the subdural hematoma gets too big, the patient may get very sick and even die.

HOW CAN YOU TELL IF A FALL IS SERIOUS?

Diagnosing a fall-related injury can be difficult even for the experienced geriatric physician for the following reasons:

- Patients with severe dementia may not remember that they fell.
- After a fall-related injury many older adults may become delirious, making it almost impossible to get an accurate history of what happened.
- The patient may have fallen due to weakness from another illness, such as a urinary tract infection, pneumonia, an electrolyte problem, or even a heart attack.
- Some fractures are small and may not be seen on an x-ray. An MRI or CT would be needed to pick up these more subtle fractures.
- Examining the amount of bruising often does not help. Some patients get very large ugly bruises from such minor events as having their blood drawn or banging their elbow on a chair. In contrast, many serious falls may show minimal to no bruising at all.

SO WHAT SHOULD YOU DO IF YOUR LOVED ONE FALLS AT HOME?

The following are some important points:

- If the person is complaining of leg pain or of general pain when he tries to stand, this may be due to a hip fracture. Do not try to have him walk any further and call 911.
- If the person is not complaining of any pain, you may want to gently try some movements that test how well the hip joint is working. One such movement is flexing the hip by moving the knee gently toward the chest. You can also bend the knee and move the leg outward. If either of these movements causes pain, call the doctor or call 911.
- If the person lands on her head, call 911 and do not let the person get up.
- If the person develops any of the following signs after a fall, it may be a sign of a serious head injury (subdural hematoma) that requires immediate medical attention:

- increased confusion
- loss of consciousness
- nausea
- slurred speech
- vomiting

Sometimes, the symptoms of a subdural hematoma may occur very gradually over the course of several months. Oftentimes there may not even be a documented history of a fall.

TAKE A DEEP BREATH BEFORE YOU ACCUSE ANYONE!

It is very troubling to see your loved one all bruised or with a fracture, especially when no one seems to have an explanation for it. As family or as caregivers, our emotional gut reaction to a fall-related injury is to assume that someone neglected the patient. This type of reaction is reinforced by the stories one hears in the news about hospital and nursing home neglect.

Did the senior fall and forget to tell anyone? Did the staff forget to notify the family? Those large, unexplained bruises or fractures may be due to unavoidable small injuries. Also, just because a senior is not walking anymore does not mean that he cannot fall. He can! For example, it is not uncommon for seniors to fall out of bed, slide out of a wheelchair, or slip off the toilet.

SHOULD THEY BE RESTRAINED?

Some might say, "If a person keeps falling, why don't they tie him down? Why don't they use seat belts in wheelchairs?" On the surface such questions seem to make sense. Restraints are commonly used in the prison system to keep dangerous criminals under control. They are also used in the hospital setting to prevent delirious patients from pulling out their IV or breathing tubes.

Restraints may involve tying the person's arms and/or legs to the bed or chair. Other restraints include special hand mittens, a Posey vest (which wraps around the chest and keeps the body attached to the mattress or chair), a Geri chair (which resembles a baby's high chair), or bedrails.

Medications are also something used to help restrain people, especially demented patients with behavioral disorders. The medications used often include antipsychotics (Haldol, Risperdal, Zyprexa, and Seroquel) and benzodiazepines (Ativan, Xanax, etc.). We discuss these medications in detail in chapters 8 and 24.

While restraints are often used with good intentions, they may lead to a variety of problems. Immobilizing the person will cause the muscles to atrophy and the joints will stiffen. When the restraints are later removed, the patient will be weaker, stiffer, and more likely to fall. The immobility also increases the risk of developing bedsores (chapter 26) and blood clots in the veins of the legs. If the patient's arms are tied down or have mittens on them, then special care is needed to make sure that they receive sufficient amounts of water and food.

Patients with dementia do not have the insight to understand that the restraints are for their own safety. Instead, these restraints often only serve to make the person more agitated. A demented patient may be trying to express something as simple as wanting a sip of water or needing to use the restroom. In other cases something more serious like a heart attack or pneumonia may be involved. If someone is exhibiting new behaviors, we recommend that he be clinically evaluated before considering the use of restraints.

IF RESTRAINTS ARE NOT THE ANSWER, WHAT SHOULD YOU DO?

Falling is a serious problem that needs to be evaluated by a doctor. In some cases, the fall may be the presenting symptom for a variety of acute medical illnesses. After making sure that the patient does not have pneumonia, urinary tract infections, blood electrolyte abnormalities, dehydration, or heart disease, the doctor may recommend one more of the following:

- Physical therapy for muscle strengthening and balance training. Such programs may be helpful for seniors who have recently been ill. The specific exercises employed will likely vary for each program and for each individual. Several studies have shown that tai chi, a Chinese martial art that places emphasis on balance and an awareness of body position, is effective in lowering the risk of falls.[7]
- Stopping potentially dangerous medications—older antidepressants, older antipsychotics, benzodiazepines, and medications with anticholinergic side effects (chapter 8).
- Getting new glasses or having a cataract treated.
- Treating musculoskeletal problems (such as arthritis, foot pain, etc.).

There are other simple preventative measures:

Inside the Home

- Address the issues of poorly arranged furniture, throw rugs, excess clutter, and loose carpeting.
- Improve lighting by keeping the curtains open during the day and install nightlights in the hallways and bathroom.
- Encourage your family member to use the handrails on stairways.
- Add lighting to the top and bottom of staircases.
- Make sure that the person gets up from bed slowly.
- Install alarm systems that are activated when the loved one with dementia tries to get out of bed unassisted.
- Consider a bedside commode if the bathroom is used multiple times during the night.
- Place colored tape at the edge of each step on a noncarpeted staircase.
- Discourage your family member from using ladders and step stools.

In the Bathroom

- Place a nonskid rubber mat in the shower or tub.
- Place a shower chair or bath bench in the shower if your relative is too weak or unsteady to stand while bathing.
- If she must use a bathtub for showering, she may want to try get into the tub by putting her weaker leg in first. To get out of the tub she should do the opposite, stepping out with the stronger leg first.
- Install handrails next to the toilet.

ADVICE FOR CAREGIVERS BEFORE MAKING CHANGES TO THE HOUSE

Talk to your loved one before you begin to make changes around the house. Otherwise, he may feel you are invading his space and trying to take away his independence. Try to include him as much as possible in the process. Check about potential tax credits for home improvements.

Outside

Provide positive reinforcement about using a cane or walker. Many older adults despise these walking aids because it makes them feel "old."

In the winter time, be sure to assist your loved one with outside walking. It is easy to slip on ice. Outdoor sidewalks and stairwells are especially dangerous. Sprinkling salt on any walkways helps prevent ice from forming. Rain can also make for slippery footing.

Make sure the treads on your loved one's shoes are not too worn out. Suggest to her that she consider not wearing high-heeled shoes. They may look nice but they may make her balance worse.

CAN FALLS BE PREVENTED?

While we can adjust some medications, order physical therapy, and make the house safer, we can't prevent all falls. Several studies have shown that if healthcare professionals followed all of the advice listed above they could lower the risk of falls among nursing home and ALF residents by only 20–26 percent.[8] Because the majority of residents still fall despite this aggressive intervention, we believe that it is important to take further steps to prevent fall-related injuries.

WHAT CAN WE DO TO DECREASE FALL-RELATED INJURIES?

Hip Protectors

Hip protectors are large pads worn over the hips that provide cushioning in the event of a fall. They are similar to the pads that football players wear. While some studies have shown that wearing hip protectors may lower the risk of hip fractures, other studies have shown no benefit.[9] In addition, many people find them unattractive and uncomfortable. They may also require some effort to get on and off each day and are often not worn correctly.

Lowering the Level of the Bed

In some cases it may even be advisable to place the mattress on the floor.

Limit the Use of Blood Thinners

Ask your doctor to help you determine whether the benefits of the medication outweigh the risks of injury from falling.

Address Osteoporosis

Medications are available that can lower your risk of wrist, spine, or hip fractures (chapter 15). Talk to your doctor about whether any of these drugs are right for you.

Falls are a common cause of injury in older adults. Falls usually do not have one single cause but rather are the result of a variety of age-related body changes, environmental factors, and medical conditions. While there are things people can do to lower this risk, in many cases seniors will continue to fall in spite of the preventive measures taken by families and healthcare staff. In the next chapter we will discuss the dangers of osteoporosis and what can be done to treat this common disease.

Chapter 15
OSTEOPOROSIS AND BROKEN BONES

"Our body parts, like the parts in an automobile engine, can't work forever."

Aging expert Dr. Leonard Hayflick

Osteoporosis affects millions of elderly people. It is a skeletal disease that causes the bones to become thin and weak. This thinning of the bones occurs gradually over many years. There are no warning signs and you will notice nothing. At a certain point the bones may become so fragile that they can easily break with nothing more than a slight fall.

Osteoporosis is responsible for about 1.5 million broken bones occurring in the United States each year.[1] Half of all women over age fifty will suffer a fracture at some point. In fact, they are more likely to have a bone fracture than a heart attack or cancer.[2]

HOW DO YOU DIAGNOSE OSTEOPOROSIS?

Oftentimes you can tell just by looking at the person that she has osteoporosis. Older men and women who have lost several inches of height since their younger years or who are all hunched over due to spine curvature probably have osteoporosis. Seniors who have had a hip fracture or a vertebral compression fracture almost certainly have osteoporosis as well. In fact, this is how osteoporosis used to be diagnosed before the World Health Organization defined osteoporosis using the DEXA scan.[3]

The DEXA scan measures the bone density of the hip and spine. This scan is relatively easy to perform and not too expensive. Medicare covers the cost of one scan every two years. Getting a scan every two years can help your doctor tell whether your bones are getting weaker. It can also show whether or not the medications you are taking for osteoporosis are working. There are also some bone scan devices that measure the bone density in the wrist and heels. These scans are often cheaper but do not give as accurate information about the density of your hips and spine.[4]

WHAT ARE VERTEBRAL COMPRESSION, OR SPINAL, FRACTURES?

Osteoporosis causes more fractures of the vertebrae than the hips.[5] Many seniors will have one or more small spine fractures and not even know it. Approximately 75 percent of vertebral fractures occur without any symptoms of pain. In other cases there can be severe pain and muscle spasms in the back.

If you are diagnosed with a *spinal*, or *vertebral compression, fracture*, do not become alarmed. It does not mean that you're necessarily going to end up in a

Normal Vertebrae and a Compression Fracture

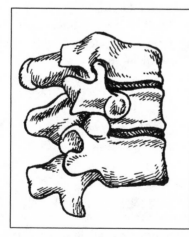 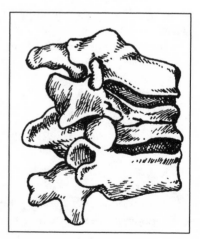

Normal   Compression Fracture

FIGURE 15.1

wheelchair. These fractures are much different than the ones occurring in trauma situations leading to severe damage to the nerves in the spinal cord.

With a vertebral fracture, the square-shaped vertebrae become wedge-shaped (see figure 15.1). This can cause a change in the person's posture. Recurrent (multiple) vertebral fractures can give the person a hunched back and make her shorter. The stooped posture makes it harder for the person to expand her lungs and take deep breaths.[6] You can test this on yourself. Touch your chin to your chest and try to take a deep breath. Not so easy? The stooped posture also makes you more prone to neck pain and shoulder injuries.

If a compression fracture happens suddenly and is very painful, doctors will prescribe pain medications. Several surgical techniques (*vertebroplasty* and *kyphoplasty*) have been developed whereby cement is poured into the collapsed vertebrae and the height is restored.[7] This can be done as an outpatient procedure. Many patients who have this procedure report dramatic improvement in symptoms.

HIP FRACTURES ARE A BIG DEAL

Over 340,000 seniors fracture a hip each year, and 20 percent will die within a year.[8] Despite advances in surgery and rehabilitation, 20 percent will remain completely nonambulatory and about one-third will end up in a nursing home.[9]

Different Types of Hip Fractures

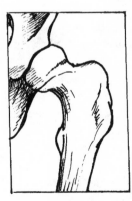 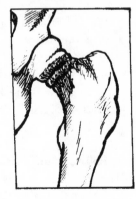 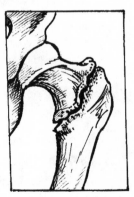

Normal	Femoral Neck	Intertrochanteric
Femur	Fracture	Fracture

FIGURE 15.2

Not all hip fractures are the same. Some are so small that they can't even be seen on an x-ray. Others are quite dramatic. They can occur at one of several locations. Some fractures occur at a spot known as the *femoral neck*, while others occur in an area just below and are known as *intertrochanteric fractures* (see figure 15.2).

Because the fractures can vary in size and location, the treatment options and prognoses may vary. Sometimes the hip can be repaired by using pins to seal the two broken pieces of bone together. In other cases, a hip replacement is needed. This involves replacing the ball portion of the thighbone and the socket that fits into the hip.

Hip fractures are also associated with many complications. Delirium has been shown to occur in 35 to 65 percent of patients following a hip fracture (chapter 13).[10] The emergence of delirium is a complicated and poorly understood process. The hip fracture itself, the medications used during surgery, the increased risk of infection, and the confusion that results as a frail senior moves through the hospital system may all play a role.

Following surgery the person will be put on blood thinners in order to lower the risk of developing blood clots in the legs. Blood clots can cause pain and swelling in the legs. More important, if a clot loosens it can be carried by the blood to the heart and then pushed out into the pulmonary arteries. The clot can block the artery (*pulmonary embolism*) and cause lung tissue to die (*pulmonary infarction*).

DO THE DRUGS USED TO PREVENT AND TREAT OSTEOPOROSIS WORK?

If you have osteoporosis, you should consider getting treatment. Because osteoporosis is a progressive disease, the risk of osteoporosis-related fractures will only increase over time.

The drugs risedronate (Actonel), alendronate (Fosamax), and ibandronate (Boniva) belong to a class of drugs known as the *bisphosphonates*. These medications act to prevent the calcium from leaving the bones. Many studies have shown that these medications can do the following:

- decrease the loss of calcium from the bones
- increase the density of the bones in the hips and spine
- decrease the risk of fractures of the spine and the hips

Unfortunately, taking these medications can be quite complicated.[11] One must have an empty stomach, drink an eight-ounce glass of water with the pill, and sit upright or stand for at least one hour. Fortunately, these medications only need to be given once a week or once a month. The main side effect of these medications is irritation to the stomach and esophagus. In some cases, these symptoms can be quite severe.[12] There is an IV version of Boniva (ibandronate) that is approved by the FDA to be given every three months. Reclast (zoledronic acid) is another bisphosphonate approved by the FDA that is given by IV infusion once a year.[13]

Years ago we used estrogen as a first-line treatment for osteoporosis. Recent data have shown that estrogen may lower the risk of hip and spinal fractures.[14] Doctors are reluctant to use estrogen for osteoporosis as it may also cause a number of side effects, including an increase in the risk of blood clots in the legs, heart attacks, strokes, and breast cancer.[15]

There is, however, another medication called raloxifene (Evista), which was developed by modifying the estrogen molecule in the laboratory. It helps restore bones, and it may even have a protective effect against some breast cancers.[16] However, it may increase the risk of a stroke or of a blood clot forming in the legs.[17]

Another treatment medication that is used is a nasal spray called Miacalcin (calcitonin). Calcitonin is a hormone that is normally produced by certain cells of the thyroid. One of the functions of calcitonin is to decrease the removal of calcium from bones by osteoclast cells.

Teriparatide (Forteo) is a parathyroid hormone that is injected under the skin daily. This drug is not commonly used due to the expense and the need for daily injections. Many doctors do not recommend using this drug for more than two years.[18]

The benefits of these medications vary. Table 15.1 shows that some drugs are FDA approved to prevent osteoporosis in people at risk while others may have a separate indication for use in the treatment of people who already have the disease.

SHOULD I ALSO TAKE CALCIUM AND VITAMIN D?

All patients at risk for osteoporosis should take calcium plus vitamin D. Some calcium supplements have vitamin D included, which helps the calcium absorb better. The National Osteoporosis Foundation recommends that adults over the age of fifty need between 1,200 of calcium and 800–1,000 IU of vitamin D daily.[19]

We are often asked by patients with osteoporosis if taking calcium and vitamin D is enough to prevent fractures. What they are really trying to ask us

TABLE 15.1. FDA-APPROVED DRUG THERAPIES FOR THE PREVENTION AND TREATMENT OF OSTEOPOROSIS[20]

Drug	Dosage	Prevention	Treatment	Use in Men
Actonel (risedronate)	35 mg weekly	Yes	Yes	Yes
Boniva (ibandronate)	150 mg monthly	Yes	Yes	No
Boniva (IV)	every three months	No	Yes	No
Fosamax (alendronate)	70 mg weekly	Yes	Yes	Yes
Reclast (zoledronate)	5 mg IV once yearly	No	Yes	No
Evista (raloxifene)	60 mg daily	Yes	Yes	No
Miacalcin (calcitonin)	200 IU daily	No	Yes	No
Forteo (teriparatide)	injected daily	No	Yes	Yes
Estrogen hormone therapy	dose varies	Yes	No	No

is whether they can take these supplements in place of prescription medications for osteoporosis. The answer is NO! Large studies have shown that the ability of the calcium and vitamin D combination to prevent osteoporosis fractures is at best only around 12 percent.[21] In most randomized controlled studies involving osteoporosis drugs, the patients were all taking calcium and vitamin D in addition to the drug or placebo.

Remember, just because you have started taking a medication for osteoporosis does not mean you are out of the woods. It is recommended that all patients taking osteoporosis medication should have a DEXA scan done every two years. This is to make sure that the medicine is working. If it is not, another drug should be tried.

Chapter 16

WHY IS REHAB SO IMPORTANT?

"Middle age is when your age starts to show around your middle."

Bob Hope (1903–2003)

SEVEN DAYS IN BED MAKES ONE WEAK!

We have been raised to think that when we see a frail older adult who is ill we should let him or her rest and be comfortable. In reality, too much bed rest can actually be a bad thing. Prolonged bed rest may cause the muscles to shrink and weaken. For young adults, a 5–10 percent decrease in muscle strength may not have any dramatic consequences on your daily routine, unless you are a professional athlete. For the frail older adult, that 5–10 percent decrease can determine whether or not he or she will be able to get out of bed, use the toilet, and lead an independent life.

In addition to the loss of muscle mass, the heart and lungs will weaken. Lying flat for days on end can also cause a drop in blood pressure when he or she finally tries to stand up.

REHAB IS AN ACTIVE PROCESS

In many areas of modern medicine the patient assumes a largely passive role. Whether having blood drawn, undergoing surgery, or getting an MRI of the head, the patient's main job is to show up on time and to stay still so the health-care professionals can do their jobs. However, in rehab we don't want you to stay still. We want you moving. Success in rehab is measured by the increase in a patient's ability to perform various physical activities.

In the nursing home, there may be times when we see a resident asking for help and the staff instead encourages him to do it himself. On the surface it may seem as though the staff are being cruel for not providing assistance to someone who is begging for help. However, providing too much help can be even more cruel!

REHABILITATION AFTER AN INJURY CAN BE AN UPHILL BATTLE

Rehabilitation is often difficult for the frail elderly patient. The older patient already has weakened muscles, joints, and ligaments (chapter 2).

Many lack the cardiovascular stamina to do much rehab activity. Others are depressed and lack the motivation. Diseases such as Parkinson's disease and osteoarthritis can make it harder to move around. Patients with advanced dementia are often unable to follow commands or learn new information. Following commands can also be difficult for patients who aren't wearing glasses or hearing aids.

BUT IT HURTS WHEN I EXERCISE!

Many seniors refuse to participate in rehab due to pain. This should not be an excuse to give up. They should talk to their therapist instead of quitting. There are certain types of pain or discomfort that need to be avoided and other types that can be worked through. It's more important to figure out the cause of the pain and what can be done to address it.

- Maybe the person is doing the exercises wrong.
- Maybe medications or other treatments will help with the pain (chapter 27).
- Maybe a cane or walker would help.

Some patients complain, cry, or use profanity during their sessions with the physical therapist. The therapist is not trying to be mean or hurt the patient. If the patient isn't pushed to do more, he or she will never have any chance of recovering muscle strength or flexibility.

WHAT ARE *JOINT CONTRACTURES*?

Some patients with strokes and severe dementia end up with joints that are stuck in a bent position. When a person has one of these locked joints, we say that she has developed a *contracture*. Contractures occur when the muscles shorten over time and actually get stuck in this shortened position.[1]

Contractures can occur in as little as seven days following a stroke and may affect the elbows, shoulders, hands, hips, knees, and feet. Many patients with severe dementia also develop contractures. As doctors we do not know enough about this problem to predict which patients will develop contractures and which ones will not. Stretching the muscles may help to lower the risk of developing contractures. However, simply stretching the muscles a few times a day will not guarantee that contractures will not occur.

Contractures of the feet can cause the foot to get stuck pointing downward. We call this a *foot drop*. An AFO (ankle foot orthotic) boot is often ordered to prevent and correct the foot drop. Patients with contractures of the legs are unable to walk since they cannot extend their legs. When they lie in bed with their hips and knees bent, more of the weight will be distributed to the buttocks, which increases the risk for bedsores. Trying to clean urine and feces from a patient whose hips and knees are locked in a flexed position is very tough. In the situation where the fingers are stuck in a fistlike position, you need to make sure the nails need to be kept short so that they do not dig into the skin of the palm.

Once the senior develops a contracture, it is difficult to reverse. Treatment options have not been studied in the elderly and are often not effective.

WHO DOES THE REHAB?

The *physical therapist* (PT) plays a vital role in a person's rehabilitation program. She evaluates the person's muscle strength, balance, endurance, and flexibility. She then helps design a treatment program to meet the person's needs. The program usually consists of exercises to build strength, stretching exercises to increase flexibility, and balance exercises. In addition to designing and customizing an exercise program, a physical therapist may also use one or more of the following therapies in the treatment of muscle, tendon, and joint injuries:

- electrical stimulation
- heat packs
- ice packs
- massage
- ultrasound[2]

An *occupational therapist* (OT) focuses more on helping a person regain his ability to perform the activities of daily living, such as getting out of bed, using the bathroom, eating, bathing, and getting dressed. The OT will suggest specific strategies and devices to help a person regain some of his lost function.

A *speech therapist* does much more than help people who have lost their ability to verbally communicate due to a stroke or other brain injury. Speech therapists are also actively involved in the evaluation and treatment of patients who have difficulty swallowing (chapter 19).

We like to think of these three healthcare professionals as your rehab coaches. They can provide technical expertise, encouragement, and education. But like an athletic coach, they can't do the work for you. Rehabilitation is an active process. The more effort you put in, the more you will potentially get out of it.

THE NUTS AND BOLTS OF GETTING STARTED IN A REHAB PROGRAM

In order for physical therapists, occupational therapists, or speech therapists to provide care, the physician must first write an order. The rehabilitation therapists can provide therapy only for the part of the body that the physician lists. If the physician prescribes physical therapy for your left hip, the therapist cannot treat your left shoulder as well. That would require a separate order from the doctor.

In order to qualify for Medicare payment of skilled nursing services (at home or at a skilled nursing facility), a minimum of at least one hour of therapy five days a week is required. Though this is far less than the three hours a day required in an acute rehabilitation unit, most frail elderly patients cannot tolerate much more than an hour a day of the combined therapies (physical, occupational, and speech).

Medicare will only pay for rehabilitation services if there appears to be potential for improvement. If someone had a stroke seven years ago and now wants therapy for his weak right arm, it may be hard to justify the rehabilitation services.

By a similar token, Medicare will only pay for rehabilitation services for as long as the patient continues to improve. Once the therapist documents that the patient has reached his *maximum medical improvement*, Medicare will no longer pay for rehab services. If a person becomes passive-aggressive or refuses to participate, there is little chance of improvement and Medicare will stop paying for the services.

WHERE DO I GO FOR REHAB?

Skilled nursing facilities (SNF) are a common setting for rehabilitation. Many seniors are sent to an SNF for rehabilitation following a hip fracture or knee replacement. Others are sent there to recover the strength that they lost while in the hospital. As we stated above, SNFs provide between one and one and a half hours/day of therapy five days a week. They also provide twenty-four-hour nursing care. Skilled nursing facility units are often found in nursing homes and rehabilitation facilities. These units are intended for the frail elderly patient who is medically stable but too debilitated to be treated safely at home.

Options other than inpatient rehab and skilled nursing units are also available to seniors who need physical therapy. Outpatient or home health therapy is typically prescribed for high-functioning patients who have good family support. Outpatient physical therapy usually takes place about three times per week. Transportation to an outpatient rehab facility is not covered by traditional Medicare but may be provided by some Medicare Advantage plans.

DESIGNING THE PROPER REHAB PROGRAM IS NOT SO EASY

Most rehabilitation programs use a combination of muscle-strengthening, balance, flexibility, and endurance exercises. However, no one knows exactly which combination of exercises are most beneficial for complicated frail elderly patients.[3] Every rehab program and every therapist is going to use a different formula of exercises and treatments. Furthermore, it is unclear whether rehabilitation programs that focus on the everyday tasks are more effective than those that focus on resistance training.

Improving the range of motion gives a person more flexibility. This improves one's functioning as much as or more than building muscle strength does. As we will see, for example, in chapter 29, older adults with stiff necks and shoulders will have a harder time driving.

Therapists may also add aerobic exercises to improve endurance. You may have the strength to bend your legs, but without endurance you will not be able to walk up a flight of stairs or down the hallway to the bathroom. For patients who have had falls or strokes, the therapist may focus on improving balance and coordination.

For seniors who cannot walk long distances or climb stairs, physical therapy can still play a role. The therapy can focus on such essential things as moving from a bed to a chair, being able to use a wheelchair, or being able to sit down and get up from the toilet.

There are other benefits to physical therapy besides improving mobility. It has been shown that people receiving physical therapy ask for less pain medication. It also provides an opportunity to address the poor body mechanics that will continue to aggravate the pain. Learning what people can do to minimize the stress on their bodies when they sleep, sit, drive, and exercise is important in the prevention of future injuries. In the short term, getting patients out of bed improves their breathing and may decrease the risk of pneumonia. It may also decrease the risk of falls. (See figure 14.1, p. 168.)

REHABILITATION FOR RESIDENTS WHO HAVE FALLEN OR HAD A HIP FRACTURE

About 350,000 Americans have a hip fracture each year.[4] We cannot overemphasize the importance of physical therapy following a hip fracture or joint replacement surgery of the hip or knee. Without physical therapy the patient is at high risk for not regaining mobility.

Current guidelines recommend starting rehabilitation as soon as possible after a hip fracture, in order to strengthen the muscles supporting the broken hip. Patients whose operation required pinning or screws will be given orders by the orthopedist regarding how much weight can be placed on that leg. Many factors, such as the tightness of the seal that was made during the operation, will determine the orthopedist's orders.

After a fracture your therapist may give you exercises that involve other parts of the body. You may think this is strange, but it makes a lot of sense. If you break your left leg, your right leg and arm need to be stronger in order for you to move yourself around. As we noted in chapter 2, many older people already have weakened muscles. The already weak right leg muscles will get even weaker unless they are strengthened.

When a broken arm or leg is placed in a plaster cast, it needs to be immobilized, which restricts the use of that extremity. That, along with increased bed rest, leads to rapid muscle atrophy (shrinkage). This shrinkage is potentially reversible with physical therapy to help the muscle cells regain their former size. With further disuse, however, the actual muscle cells may be lost.

Only by staying active can the patient maintain muscle strength. When you visit a loved one, remember to only help him with the things that he cannot do. You may think you are being compassionate by wanting to do everything for him, but in reality you are making him weaker and more likely to fall in the future.

THINGS THE FAMILY CAN DO TO HELP!

- Ask the therapist to estimate how much progress to expect for your family member in his recovery.
- Ask the therapist if there are any exercises/activities that you can do with your loved one when you visit.
- Reinforce to your loved one that participating in therapy is extremely important.
- Reinforce to your loved one that good nutrition is essential for regaining muscle strength.
- Take her for a walk when you visit the facility.
- Encourage him to be actively involved in as many of his daily life activities as he can, rather than having everything done for him.

HOW LONG SHOULD REHAB LAST?

Despite the setting, Medicare will only pay as long as the therapist can document that further improvement is expected. For most patients, this usually means several weeks. In the outpatient setting, Medicare has enacted some stringent limits on what it will pay for. While Medicare is getting more stringent, a study published in *JAMA* showed that six months of outpatient rehabilitation led to better outcomes for community-dwelling elderly patients who had a recent hip fracture.[5] While the findings were interesting, we pose the question: Who is going to pay for the extra months of therapy?

The take-home point for this chapter is that in order for a rehab program to be successful, it requires the active participation of the patient. In many cases it also requires the family to get involved as well. The program should involve a variety of different therapies tailored to the patient's overall condition and specific ailment.

Chapter 17
HELPING PATIENTS
MOVE AROUND SAFELY

We want to give you some important pointers regarding how to safely help a frail elderly person with some basic, everyday activities. Before you help move someone always tell the person what you are going to do and encourage the person to help with the movement. Remember to speak in a deep tone with a gentle voice. For patients with dementia, simple one-step commands work best (chapter 24).

SITTING UP ON THE SIDE OF THE BED

If the person needs to get up from the bed, you want to provide help in the safest possible manner. Pulling someone up by grabbing the arms or by grabbing underneath the armpits/shoulders may cause injuries to the shoulders. It is better to have the person turn to one side and then swing the legs over the side of the bed. You can then gently push the person upright.

SLIDING DOWN IN BED

Oftentimes a patient will slide down in bed when the head of the bed is elevated. This may make it more uncomfortable for the patient and may also make it harder to eat. Do not get frustrated if the person continues to slide in the bed after you or the staff have adjusted the patient. This is natural. The important thing is to avoid pulling the patient up in bed by lifting under the arms. It is better to first lower the head of the bed as much as possible. Then have the person bend the knees while you put your hands under the back. Ask the person to push toward the head of the bed while you lift the patient in the same direction. At a facility, the staff will often have a small sheet underneath the patient that can be used to lift a frail elderly person toward the head of the bed. The key word in the above sentence is *lift*. While you shouldn't expect to fully lift a frail older adult off the bed, you don't want to simply drag the person across the mattress, since this could cause damage to the skin (chapter 26).

GOING TO THE BATHROOM IN BED

Some people may be too weak to get out of bed to go to the bathroom. Instead of risking an injury trying to get the patient out of bed, many staff and families want the patient to use a *Foley catheter* (a tube that will drain urine directly from the bladder). Foley catheters come with their own risks (chapter 18) and are often not needed. If you have a bedpan nearby, you can have the person roll to one side. Place the bedpan on the buttocks so when the person rolls onto the back again the bedpan will be underneath the buttocks. When finished, the bedbound patient should try to lift the hips so you can carefully pull the bedpan out.

GETTING OFF THE TOILET SEAT

As we stated in chapter 14, the majority of frail elderly have significant weakness in their legs. Getting up from a low toilet requires a lot of leg strength. If you are assisting someone, never pull the person up by the arms or lift under the armpits. As we noted above, that can injure the shoulders.

Instead, hold the patient by the waist or around the chest. Get close to the patient so that you can keep your back straight and do not have to bend over. Bend your knees and hips. If there are grab bars, have the person hold onto them while you gently lift or push the patient up.

> # WATCH YOUR BACK!!!!!
>
> For caregivers, all this pushing, pulling, and lifting seven days a week can be quite taxing. Caregivers need to be careful how they bend and lift so they don't injure their backs.

WALKERS VERSUS CANES: WHAT'S THE DIFFERENCE?

Walkers and canes act to take some of the weight off of weak and painful legs and hips. They may also help patients having difficulty with balance and coordination. They help stabilize the patient by providing an extra leg (or legs) of support.

Types of Canes

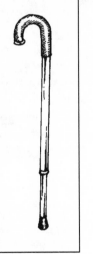
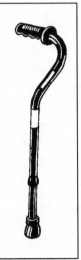
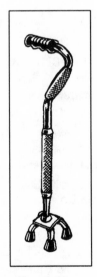

Adjustable Cane   Offset Cane   Quad Cane

FIGURE 17.1

Types of Walkers

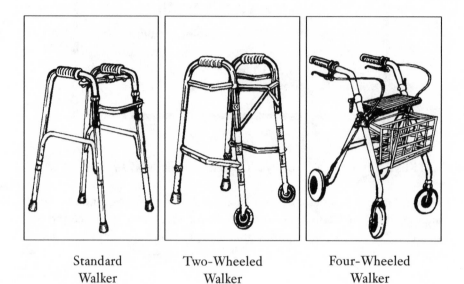

Standard
Walker

Two-Wheeled
Walker

Four-Wheeled
Walker

FIGURE 17.2

Some Points to Remember

No matter what assistive device is used, it needs to be properly fitted. The patient will also need to be educated on how to use the device. While devices may help, don't forget that proper footwear is important. Shoes need to have arch support and good treads on the bottom. Women need to avoid shoes with heels. Glasses and hearing aids need to be worn as well.

Common Assistive Devices
(in order from least to most support)

- single-point cane (figure 17.1)
- quad cane (figure 17.1)
- crutches
- walker (figure 17.2)

Canes

Single-point canes have been used since antiquity to provide support for older adults. Supposedly even Moses used a staff to help him as he walked through the desert for forty years. The canes used by most frail seniors, however, do not resemble Moses' staff. Most canes have rubber tips that help prevent them from slipping. We recommend that you buy an adjustable cane since the height of the cane makes a difference. While using a cane, the elbow should not be straight. It should be bent about fifteen to twenty degrees.[1] Many patients find it easier to use a cane with a pistol-type grip rather than a cane with a curved handle.

Canes can be useful for patients with painful hip or knee arthritis. If the cane is used properly, it can shift 15–20 percent of a person's weight off the bad hip or knee.[2] The cane should be held on the opposite side of the painful or weak leg. If the patient has pain or weakness in the right leg, then the cane should be held by the left hand.

Not all canes are alike. See figure 17.1.

A standard cane is helpful for people with balance problems but will not relieve weight off the hips or knees. The standard cane is useful for people with balance problems. It allows the person with bad vision or nerve damage in the feet to receive sensory input from the floor to the arms.[3] Because of its curved shape, an *offset cane* allows for better weight bearing than a standard cane.

Quad canes provide more support than single-point canes. The disadvantage of a quad cane is that it can be difficult to use on uneven surfaces. We have also found that many patients hate using them because it makes them feel like an "old person."

Walkers

As with canes, not all walkers are alike. Figure 17.2 shows the different types of walkers. A walker can relieve much weight off of an arthritic knee or hip. It can also provide support for people with balance problems. Some walkers have no wheels. Before you take a step you have to lift the walker and move it forward. For patients who have weakness in their arms, this may be quite difficult. Wheeled walkers most often have either two wheels and two points, or four wheels. There are other models now that have three wheels. Some wheeled walkers come with handbrakes, a seat, and/or a basket to place items.

While a walker without wheels may appear to be the most stable, one with two wheels provides a similar amount of stability.[4] A lot of older people absolutely refuse to use one. As with canes, many seniors view the use of a walker as a sign that they are "old."

Aren't All Wheelchairs the Same?

For seniors who can propel the wheelchair themselves, a lightweight model is often preferable to a standard wheelchair. It is important that the wheelchair be adjusted. A poorly fitted wheelchair can be quite uncomfortable for the patient. There are many different types of wheelchairs on the market and numerous accompanying products available. Talk to the physical therapist about which wheelchair would be most suitable for your family member.

Other Assistive Devices

Occupational therapists can suggest a variety of devices to help elderly patients perform the activities of daily living in their home. These include:

- A bedside commode (a portable toilet seat) can be placed by the bed. This is useful when the bathroom is too far away from the bed.
- Grab bars by the toilet help the patient sit down and get up safely from the toilet.
- A shower seat allows the patient to sit in the shower. Many frail elderly are unable to stand while taking a shower.
- Bathtub benches allow people who cannot get into the bathtub to bathe themselves.
- Specialized eating utensils that have large grips are often helpful for patients with severe arthritis in their hands.

To get an idea of the assistive devices available, there is a Web site (www.abledata.com) that is sponsored by the National Institute on Disability and Rehabilitation Research (NIDRR).[5] This site displays numerous products by categories. It also shows pictures of the products and how to contact the manufacturers.

We hope that the information provided in this chapter will allow you or your loved one to remain more independent. The information presented here may also help prevent a serious injury.

Chapter 18
MINIMIZING THE RISK OF INFECTIOUS DISEASES

INFECTIOUS DISEASES ARE A BIG PROBLEM

Infections are very common in the frail elderly. The most common infections that we see involve the urinary tract, the lungs, the skin (either a cellulitis or a pressure ulcer), and the colon. Older adults are also more likely than younger adults to die from an infectious disease. This is due to the older person's

- weakened immune system, which decreases the body's ability to fight off infections
- chronic underlying medical diseases, which make the organs weaker and less able to withstand the stress of the infection on the body
- higher risk of side effects from antibiotics
- poorer ability to tolerate the invasive medical procedures needed to correctly identify and battle the infection
- longer amount of time necessary for the doctor to recognize and correctly diagnose the infectious disease

DIAGNOSING AN INFECTIOUS DISEASE IS OFTEN DIFFICULT

Many signs and symptoms of infection seen in younger patients are less frequent or even absent in older adults. Since childhood we have all been taught that a high temperature is indicative of an infection. Nonetheless, fever may be absent in 20–30 percent of seniors with serious infections.[1] An elevated white blood cell count is often absent as well. Doctors may, therefore, fail to diagnose an infection. Unfortunately, the **real truth** is that patients who lack a fever or a high white blood cell count may have a problem with their immune system and are at a higher risk of dying from their infection.[2]

As we have said often in this book, many illnesses can appear in strange ways in the elderly. For example, we may see a frail older person who comes to our attention because of a fall and it turns out that he had an undiagnosed urinary tract infection or pneumonia that made him weak, thus leading to the fall.

A change in behavior may be the only clue that an elderly person has a serious infection. For example, they may have a decreased appetite, increased aggression, or increased confusion. Recognizing these changes in behavior as signs of an infection can be very difficult even for an experienced doctor. The doctor's job is even harder if the patient has dementia or shows up without anyone who can attest to what the patient's normal behavior is.

Why do these illnesses present themselves in such different ways in elderly people? The **real truth** is that we really don't know why. All we really know is as we discussed in chapter 2, there are many changes in the body as we age.

EVEN TAKING A TEMPERATURE IS NO EASY MATTER

The five main places you stick a thermometer are:

- anus
- armpit
- ear (requires a special electric thermometer)
- forehead strip
- mouth

Which one is the best place? Of the five methods, the rectal temperature is the most accurate. We do not use this method often, as patients and caregivers generally do not like it. When placing a thermometer in the mouth, the patient needs to keep it under his tongue for at least ninety seconds. (Some electronic thermometers work faster.) The patient also needs to keep the mouth closed during this time. Many seniors with dementia cannot follow these simple directions. If the patient will not put the thermometer deep below the tongue or will not keep the mouth closed, then the temperature reading will be lower than the actual temperature.

Getting a body temperature from the armpit is another option. Make sure that the armpit is dry before you take the temperature. Place the thermometer deep in the armpit and have the patient lower the arm so that the elbow is resting on the ribs. The thermometer needs to be left in that position for at least two minutes. (Some electronic thermometers are faster.)

Because some patients may not let you keep the thermometer in the mouth or armpit long enough, many hospitals and nursing homes use an electronic thermometer that is placed in the ear. If the ears are full of earwax, this thermometer is not helpful. Some staff forget to check for earwax. A further option is to place a special strip on the forehead that will read the body temperature of the skin.

You need to be aware that the temperature readings from the mouth, armpit, and ear will be about 0.5–1 degrees lower than the reading you would get using a rectal thermometer, even if the thermometer is used correctly. In some cases the differences can be even greater.

We have all been taught that a normal body temperature is 98.6 degrees Fahrenheit. This was based on a study done in the nineteenth century. Most seniors have a normal temperature that is lower than 98.6°.[3] In addition, a person's body temperature can vary by about one degree during the course of a normal day.

So what is a bad temperature? It depends on whom you ask. Some say 100.0°F, while others think 100.4° or 101.0°F. Still others would say that an increase in a person's baseline temperature of more than 2.0 degrees is not normal. For example, if someone's normal temperature is 97.2°F and the thermometer now reads 99.6°F, he or she may have an infection.[4] Even a low-grade fever can indicate a serious problem. If you have any questions, call your doctor as soon as possible.

DON'T EXPECT THE MICROBIOLOGY LAB
TO HAVE ALL THE ANSWERS!

Samples from blood, wounds, sputum, or urine are collected and sent to the lab to see if there is an infection. Like the forensic specialists on *CSI*, the microbiologists at the lab are highly skilled people who have access to the latest high-tech equipment.

But sometimes the information obtained from the microbiology lab may be difficult to interpret. Our bodies are naturally covered (or "colonized") by bacteria. Using the analogy of a crime scene, you can think of these colonizing bacteria as the innocent bystanders. It is often difficult to tell which bacteria are causing the disease and which ones are colonizing the area but not causing any diseases.

When a sample is sent to the lab, they place it on growth plates in special incubators that allow the bacteria to multiply many times. They can determine which species of bacteria is present. They can then test to see which antibiotics will prevent the bacteria from growing further. They do not test every single antibiotic but instead use one or two from each class of antibiotics.

THE EMERGENCE OF ANTIBIOTIC-RESISTANT BACTERIA

Over the last twenty years, a variety of bacteria strains have emerged that are resistant to many common antibiotics. What this means is that the antibiotics we once used to treat common infections no longer work. How did this happen? The answer is that the bacteria have developed genetic mutations that make them resistant to antibiotics.

How did the bacteria develop these mutations? A typical infection involves many billions of bacteria. In theory, a single bacteria cell can develop a mutation that allows the cell to degrade the antibiotic, pump the antibiotic out of the bacteria, or alter the cell lining (preventing the antibiotic from entering).

If a bacteria cell develops one of these mutations, it will live while the other bacteria cells around it are killed by the antibiotic. Over time the bacteria cells with the resistant mutation will multiply. If the antibiotic is tried again, it will be less effective since there are now numerous bacteria that have the mutation that makes them resistant to the antibiotic. Common examples of these antibiotic-resistant bacteria include *methicillin-resistant Staphylococcus aureus* (MRSA) and *vancomycin-resistant enterococci* (VRE).

Part of the blame for this problem may fall on the doctors who have over-prescribed antibiotics over the past decades. Patients have often been given antibiotics for simple viral infections. Antibiotics can kill only bacteria, not viruses. The misuse of antibiotics over the years has helped select for those bacteria with the genetic mutations that make them resistant to antibiotics.

The end result is that many elderly patients, especially those in a nursing home or hospital, may be colonized with bacteria that are resistant to one or more antibiotics. Like college dorms and prisons, hospitals and nursing homes are confined places that allow bacteria and viruses to easily spread from person to person. When seniors are transferred to different facilities, the most dangerous bacteria can quickly spread to hospitals and nursing homes across a city.

Hospitals try to lower the risk of spreading these bacteria by following the CDC recommendations for *contact isolation*.[5] When a patient is under contact isolation, he is usually in a room either alone or with another person who is also colonized with the same bacteria. People entering the room are advised to wear a disposable gown and gloves.

It is important to remember that not only is the patient colonized with antibiotic-resistant bacteria, but so is much of the room as well. Even if you never touch the patient, staff and visitors can still spread bacteria and viruses. The organisms can move from the patient's body to the bed, other furniture, and even door knobs. It is a good idea to wash your hands before and after visiting the room. If you are not sure whether the patient is under contact isolation, ask the nurse before you enter the room.

SHOULD I USE AN ALCOHOL RUB OR SOAP AND WATER?

They are both effective at removing the bacteria from your hands. Many hospitals and nursing homes are moving more toward using alcohol-based products because they are easier to use. To use an alcohol sanitizer correctly you need to rub it on your hands for twenty to thirty seconds until your hands dry. However, the alcohol does not kill the spores of a bacteria called *Clostridium difficile* (or *C. diff.*) that can cause diarrhea and serious infections of the colon.

SKIN INFECTIONS

The bacteria that infect the skin come from the skin surface. We have all had pimples and boils, which are small infections at the skin surface. A deep infection of the skin is called a *cellulitis*. The skin becomes painful, red, and warm. In some cases swelling can occur, and the patient may even develop a fever.

Some diseases place the older adult at an even higher risk for a skin infection. These include:

- chronic leg edema (swelling with fluid)
- diabetes
- peripheral vascular disease (atherosclerosis of the arteries of the leg)

Untreated, these skin infections will spread. In some cases the infection can be treated with antibiotic pills. In other cases, IV antibiotics will be necessary.

Are these infections contagious? If you come in contact with one of these skin infections, you may not "catch it." However, you need to be careful to take the precautions discussed above so that you don't spread these bad bacteria to other people through contact with your skin or clothing. Remember we said that in a hospital setting, these antibiotic-resistant bacteria can be found not just on the patient's wound but also all over the room.

WHAT IS MRSA?

MRSA stands for *methicillin-resistant Staphylococcus aureus*. This means that the *Staphylococcus aureus* bacteria are resistant to the antibiotic methicillin, which is in the penicillin family.

For many years *Staphylococcus aureus* was treated with antibiotics from the penicillin family. With the emergence of antibiotic-resistant bacteria, the diagnosis and treatment of infections has gotten more complicated. We now often need to send tissue to the lab to see which antibiotics will work to kill the bacteria. If the bacteria is resistant to methicillin, it is likely that it will be resistant to all antibiotics from the penicillin family.

MRSA is not new.[6] In the 1980s and 1990s it was commonly seen among patients who were infected while in the hospital or nursing home. In the last few years, a new variant of MRSA with different genetic mutations has arisen among patients who have never been in a hospital or nursing home. In some areas of the country, up to 50 percent of skin infections involving *Staphylococcus aureus* are now labeled MRSA.

Urinary Tract Infections

A variety of factors place seniors at high risk for urinary tract infections. In women, the loss of estrogen leads to a decrease in vaginal secretions. This decreases the number of normal vaginal bacteria known as *Lactobacilli*. Other bacteria, such as *E. coli*, begin to colonize the vagina. In men, an enlarged prostate results in difficulty emptying the bladder. The remaining urine is more likely to serve as a broth for bacteria to grow.

In young people, the bladder is not a hospitable place for bacteria to live. With aging, urine becomes less acidic and may have less of the proteins known as *bacterial adherence blocking proteins*. The decrease in acidity and the lack of these proteins allows the bacteria to survive and multiply in the bladder.

The use of a Foley catheter increases the risk of a urinary tract infection. A Foley catheter is a small tube inserted into the bladder to help urine drain. It is used in both women and men. Within forty-eight hours, bacteria will start to grow on the tubing. The Foley catheter tubing acts like a highway to shuttle bacteria into the normally sterile bladder. Even if you do your best to keep it clean, in several days, the urine will be loaded with bacteria.

Urinary tract infections are associated with a variety of symptoms. These include one or more of the following:

- back pain
- bloody urine
- change in behavior
- decrease in energy
- painful urination
- fever
- foul-smelling urine
- increased urination
- pelvic pain/discomfort

Unfortunately, diagnosing urinary tract infections can be really tough. Some people may have these symptoms due to disorders other than infections. In other cases, seniors, including all those using Foley catheters, will have lots of bacteria in their urine but may not have an infection. It is often difficult for even doctors to distinguish between patients with lots of bacteria in their bladder from a Foley catheter and those who have a urinary tract infection.

If a male patient has a problem making it to the bathroom, you may want to consider using a condom (external) catheter. This type of catheter is more comfortable and has a lower risk of promoting infections.[7]

PNEUMONIA

Pneumonia is the fifth leading cause of death in the elderly. It is also the most common cause of death in patients with severe dementia.[8]

How Can I Get Pneumonia?

Many family members worry that pneumonia is contagious. There are some rare types of pneumonia that are potentially contagious. These include

Mycoplasma, tuberculosis, and some viruses. Patients with these contagious forms of pneumonia should have a notice on the door warning visitors to wear a mask before entering.

The bacteria that cause most pneumonia do not come from the mold in the air conditioner or from the coughing staff member. In most cases, the real suspects are the bacteria from the person's own mouth.

As healthcare professionals, we often use the term *aspiration* to define the process that occurs when mouth secretions end up going into the lungs. But we have to be careful because the same term can be used to describe when a person vomits and the stomach contents end up in the lungs. In these cases, the stomach contents may cause an intense inflammation of the lung tissues.

If you are confused by the double meaning of the term, you are not alone. Many doctors don't even realize that this term has two different meanings.

Seniors with a greater risk for developing pneumonia include those with:

- Swallowing difficulty due to muscle weakness from a stroke or Parkinson's disease
- Difficulty initiating swallowing due to advanced dementia
- Previous history of pneumonia
- Decreased ability to cough
- History of smoking, which can damage the lining of the respiratory tract that helps to trap and remove bacteria
- Diabetes
- Underlying lung disease, such as emphysema or COPD
- Any medical illness that impairs the immune system
- Poor dental hygiene, which leads to higher amounts of potentially harmful bacteria in the mouth

If these factors come into play or if the amount of bacteria in the aspirated material is sufficiently large, pneumonia may follow. The episode of aspiration that causes pneumonia can be so small and subtle that it is not even noticed.

Many healthy adults aspirate small amounts of mouth secretions as well. In healthy adults, the low number of harmful bacteria, together with forceful coughing and a normal immune system, result in clearance of the infectious material without any harmful consequences.

Diagnosing Pneumonia Is Not Easy!

Many seniors with pneumonia will not have a cough, a fever, or an elevated white blood count. Some may just be extremely tired. We see many patients in nursing homes whose only sign of pneumonia is that they stop eating or become agitated at the staff.

Making matters worse, the chest x-ray that the doctor orders may be difficult to interpret. The x-rays are often of poor quality since the elderly person cannot take a deep breath or may not even be able to stand up. Many seniors may also have underlying heart and lung diseases, which make x-rays even more difficult to interpret.

What Can Be Done to Decrease the Risk of Pneumonia?

Take care of your teeth—since the bacteria that cause pneumonia are found in higher numbers on teeth with poor dentition, the risk of aspiration pneumonia is lower in patients without teeth. One study showed that the risk of pneumonia was lower in elderly patients in institutional settings who get their teeth and tongues brushed three times a day.[9]

Avoid or lower the dose of drugs that will diminish one's alertness, such as benzodiazepines, narcotics, muscle relaxers, antihistamines, and other anticholinergic medications (chapter 8).

Get your Pneumovax shot—elderly patients should receive the vaccine for pneumonia once every five to eight years. Be aware that this vaccine only gives protection against some but not all of the bacteria that can cause pneumonia.

INFLUENZA

While the flu may cause a younger person to miss school or work, it can result in hospitalization and death for the elderly.

The flu strikes nursing homes and ALFs in a wave, where many residents and staff will be infected at the same time. All elderly patients should therefore receive the influenza vaccine (flu shot) every year. The staff at the facilities need to get vaccinated as well.

Some people are against the use of vaccines in children and young adults. Vaccinating the frail elderly is a different issue altogether. We have heard many excuses for not getting vaccinated, such as "I don't get sick," "Vaccines can cause you to get the flu," or "I have never needed to get one before." Not getting a flu shot is a dangerous and foolhardy decision for an elderly person. Many people tell us that they got the flu even though they got their flu shot. It is true that even if you get the influenza vaccine, you can still get sick. However, many other viruses other than influenza can cause similar symptoms.

You may have heard that there is a form of the flu vaccine that is given as a nasal spray rather than as an injection. Such a vaccine uses a live yet noninfectious form of the influenza virus. At the present time this form of the vaccine is not FDA approved for use in seniors.

What about Pills for the Flu?

Thanks to modern medicine, there are medications to take if there is an outbreak of influenza. Tamiflu (oseltamivir) or Zanamivir (relenza) can be taken by a senior to help prevent him from catching the flu. In addition to preventing the illness from spreading, these medications can be used to lessen the symptoms after a senior already has the flu. If these drugs are going to have any benefit, they need to be used within the first two days of flu symptoms.[10]

In the event of an influenza outbreak in a facility, it is recommended that the patients receive one of these two medications even if they were already vaccinated for influenza.[11]

SHINGLES

About one million cases of shingles (herpes zoster) occur each year in the United States.[12] Shingles occurs when the chicken pox virus that was lying asleep in nerve cells for many years reemerges. What makes the chicken pox virus come out of the nerve cells? In many cases, we are not sure. However, we do know that it occurs more often in patients with cancer or in those with weakened immune systems. We therefore see it more commonly in older adults, since cancer is more common and the immune system becomes weaker with aging (chapter 2). Is shingles contagious? It is only contagious to people who have never been exposed to chicken pox virus before. So be careful if you have it. Avoid being near someone who is pregnant or if there are children who have not been vaccinated yet.

Shingles causes painful blisters on the skin that will open and then form crusts. The lesions usually are limited to the area of skin supplied by a single nerve. Sometimes the pain may actually precede the appearance of the skin lesions. It is important to keep the skin lesions clean and avoid scratching them as much as possible. Shingles lesions that get infected with bacteria require antibiotics treatment. Some patients are left with severe pain in the affected area even after the skin has healed. This is known as *postherpetic neuralgia.*

Shingles can be treated with antiviral drugs, such as valacyclovir (Valtrex) or acyclovir (Zovirax). Unfortunately, these medications are effective only if they are taken within the first forty-eight hours of the first symptoms, and many patients do not get to see their doctors within this short period of time.

Is There a Vaccine for Shingles?

In 2006 the FDA approved a vaccine, Zostavax, for the prevention of shingles. In studies involving many thousands of elderly patients, this vaccine has been shown to lower the risk of developing shingles by about 50 percent.[13] It also seems to lower the risk of developing postherpetic neuralgias by 66 percent. It does not offer 100 percent protection. Even after vaccination, you can still get shingles.

The vaccine should not be used in patients whose immune system has been weakened by medications, AIDS, or malignancies involving the bone marrow (leukemias, lymphomas). In October 2007 the Centers for Disease Control and Prevention (CDC) recommended that all persons sixty years or older should have this vaccine regardless of whether they have already had zoster herpes.[14] At the time of this writing, the cost of this vaccine is not covered by Medicare.

DIARRHEA

Severe diarrhea can cause a lot of problems. It can cause the body to become dehydrated and to lose too much potassium. Medications, intolerance to certain foods, fecal impaction, and a wide variety of intestinal diseases are some of the common causes of diarrhea.

Infections of the Colon Can Also Cause Diarrhea

Many bacteria can cause diarrhea. In most cases, it resolves in a day or two. If it does not resolve quickly, the doctor can have a sample of the stool tested to see if white blood cells are present. If they are present this tells us that there is an inflammatory process going on in the body such as an infection. Many families will ask why we are not giving the patient an antidiarrheal agent, such as Lomotil (diphenoxylate hydrochloride/atropine sulfate), for diarrhea symptoms. The reason is that rushing to give an antidiarrheal agent without testing for *Clostridium difficile* or other causes of infection can be dangerous as it can make the infection worse.

Clostridium difficile

Clostridium difficile (*C. difficile*, or *C. diff.*) is a bacteria responsible for about three hundred thousand cases of diarrhea yearly in the United States.[15] In severe cases, the patient can die.

Many millions of people already have this bacteria living in their colons. When the bacteria is residing in the colon but not causing an infection, we say that the patient is *colonized*. About 30 percent of hospitalized patients and between 4 and 20 percent of nursing home residents are colonized with *C. difficile*. Less than 3 percent of healthy adults are colonized.

The bacteria is spread from a person's anus to his or her hands after a bowel movement. Now think of all the things you touch during the day. By not washing the hands carefully, a patient can spread *C. difficile* to whatever she touches. The bacteria can be found on bed rails, bedpans, windowsills, floors, toilets, telephones, and on the hands of hospital workers. Visitors and health-care workers can then touch any of these things and then accidentally put their fingers in their mouths. Studies have shown that *C. difficile* can be cultured from the hands, clothing, and even the stethoscopes of healthcare workers.[16]

The seniors at the highest risk of getting an actual infection from this bacteria are those who are ill, those who have recently received antibiotics, those with a feeding tube (chapter 20), and those who use antacids or proton pump inhibitor stomach pills (Nexium, Prilosec, AciPhex, Protonix).[17]

What Are Some of the Signs and Symptoms of *C. difficile* Infections?

Seniors may exhibit one or more signs/symptoms:

- abdominal pain or cramping
- diarrhea
- elevated white blood cell count
- fever
- increased confusion
- weakness, nausea, anorexia, dehydration
- white blood cells on a smear of the stool

We usually test for *C. difficile* infection by sending a sample of the patient's stool to the lab to look for the presence of the *C. difficile* toxin (a substance produced by the bacteria when it is actively infecting the colon). Testing for this toxin can be a bit tricky and for that reason we usually like to send more than one stool sample.

Treating *C. difficile*

If left untreated, this infection of the colon can be life-threatening. In recent years, mutated versions of this bacteria have emerged that can produce up to eighteen times more toxin.[18] Fortunately, good antibiotics are available. The antibiotics commonly used are metronidazole (Flagyl) or vancomycin pills. The IV version of vancomycin is not effective as it will not get to the bacteria living in the colon. With proper treatment, fever usually resolves within one day and diarrhea within six days of starting treatment.

Even with appropriate antibiotics, symptoms may recur in 20 percent of patients. This happens because the antibiotics kill only the bacteria and not the spores. Some of the spores may not grow for one to two weeks after the antibiotics have stopped. This is no reason to get alarmed. Another course of antibiotic pills usually does the trick. These relapses can occur up to three weeks following treatment.

Steps Staff Can Take to Prevent the Spread of *C. difficile* Infections

- Hand washing between treating all patients
- Use of disposable gloves and gowns if the person is known to have *C. difficile* infection
- Environmental cleaning and disinfection including the use of an agent that will kill the spores. Remember, the whole room is going to contain the spores.
- Use of antibiotics only when appropriate. The antibiotics can also kill the normal bacteria in your colon, which then allows the *C. difficile* bacteria to grow more easily.

STEPS CAREGIVERS CAN TAKE TO PREVENT INFECTIOUS DISEASES!

1. Do not visit the nursing home or hospital if you have the flu or any other respiratory illness.
2. Wash your hands before and after visiting a patient's room.
3. When visiting relatives with pneumonia, encourage them to sit up and get out of bed (unless there is a medical reason to the contrary). Encourage them to use their incentive spirometer.
4. Follow all recommendations regarding respiratory and contact isolation.
5. Encourage your loved one to get the flu and pneumonia vaccines.

As we discussed, the elderly are not only at a higher risk for developing infections but they are also more likely to die from infection. The continual emergence of antibiotic-resistant bacteria will continue to represent a major concern for patients and healthcare professionals alike in the years to come.

Chapter 19

HOW *NOT* TO LOSE WEIGHT!

We are fortunate to live in a nation where food is plentiful. The downside, not surprisingly, is that obesity has become a major health epidemic in America. What is, however, more surprising, is that malnutrition is such a common problem in our frail elderly population.

Before we go any further, we need to define the term *malnutrition*. Malnutrition, or undernutrition, refers to the medical problems that result from the insufficient intake of food. How common is this problem? About one out of six seniors is technically malnourished and many more have difficulty eating.[1]

WHY IS MALNUTRITION SO DANGEROUS?

The most obvious danger is the loss of weight. It is not just the loss of weight, but rather the loss of muscle mass that will make the person weaker. In many cases the person can become so weak that she will have a harder time getting out of bed, walking, and taking care of her basic needs.

It may seem somewhat obvious that malnutrition can:

- weaken the immune system
- lower the bone marrow's production of red blood cells
- increase the risk of developing pressure ulcers (bedsores)
- increase the risk that wounds will not heal properly
- increased the risk of death

The **real truth** is that we do not know whether these consequences are a result of malnutrition. In some cases they may be, while in others the development of the problems listed above may be due to the fact that the person is very sick. People who are very sick often do not have much of an appetite.

TIME TO THROW OUT THE MISCONCEPTIONS

Malnutrition and *starvation* are terms that many people associate with abuse or neglect. It conjures up images of suffering children in Africa or prisoners of war. Politicians and lawyers may highlight malnutrition and dehydration as evidence that nursing home residents are suffering from abuse and neglect. Some people, including many healthcare professionals, will say that malnutrition occurs because the caregiver, nursing home, or hospital staff simply did not take the time to feed the patient.

Anyone who has tried to feed an elderly person with no appetite can tell you that it is one of the most frustrating experiences imaginable. We see many families that become resentful or angry at the patient for not eating. Caregivers will often complain that the patient "just won't eat," or that he or she "can eat, but is just being stubborn."

Such oversimplifications do not reflect the **real truth**. We are not saying that cases of neglect do not occur. What we are saying is that in a number of these cases, malnutrition is far more complicated than some bad cooking or someone forgetting to feed the patient. Malnutrition in this special population is a complicated problem involving a variety of poorly understood age-related organ changes, medical illnesses, and psychiatric disorders. Psychological and social issues often play a role as well.

WHAT ARE THE AGE-RELATED ORGAN CHANGES THAT PLACE THE ELDERLY AT SUCH A HIGH RISK?

In chapter 2 we discussed the changes of the mouth and gums that occur with aging. Faulty dentures and poor dentition can often make it both difficult and painful for elderly people to eat certain types of foods. Decreased saliva production is another mouth problem that can affect many older adults. Some drugs (chapter 8) are notorious for causing the side effect of dry mouth. Decreased saliva can make it difficult to adequately chew and swallow many types of food.

Normally the stomach relaxes and expands when we begin to eat. This relaxation process allows more food to be held in the stomach. As you get older, this reflex mechanism of the stomach gradually becomes impaired. Gastrointestinal problems (constipation, heartburn, acid reflux, etc.) are extremely common and can have a profound impact on a person's appetite. Think about how you felt the last time you had diarrhea or really bad indigestion.

There also may be a loss in the ability to smell and taste. One large study found that more than 62 percent of seniors over the age of eighty had a decreased ability to smell.[2] Furthermore, with normal aging there appears to be a decrease in the sensation of hunger.

WHAT COMMON MEDICAL ILLNESSES ARE ASSOCIATED WITH WEIGHT LOSS AND MALNUTRITION?

- AIDS
- cancer
- chronic infections
- congestive heart failure
- COPD (chronic obstructive pulmonary disease)/emphysema
- poorly controlled diabetes
- poorly controlled thyroid disease
- renal failure

HOW DO THESE MEDICAL ILLNESSES AFFECT THE APPETITE?

The type of malnutrition seen in the frail elderly patient is more complicated than that of a person who is on a voluntary hunger strike. This is an important point that even many healthcare professionals often forget! The body of the person on the hunger strike will adapt to the lack of food by slowing down its metabolism in order to conserve energy. By contrast, the older adult who has an acute life-threatening or chronic illness(es) is in a state where inflammation is occurring in one or more parts of the body. Recognizing patients with *cachexia*—described as failure to thrive—can be difficult. Many frail elderly patients without an obvious disease are also in this state of cachexia. As a result, metabolism is actually greatly increased. The breakdown of protein and muscle increases dramatically.

While we know very little about the molecular details, we do know that chemicals produced during inflammation, called *cytokines*, are involved.[3] The names of the cytokines that appear to play roles are *tumor necrosis factor-alpha* (TNF-α), *interleukin-1* (IL-1), *interleukin-6* (IL-6), among others. These cytokines work to set off dozens of changes in the body. For example, the body begins to have difficulty metabolizing glucose, protein, and fats. The body starts to break down the muscle tissue to extract protein to use as fuel. The appetite diminishes and the person feels tired. It is strange but true that at a time when your body's need for food is increasing, these cytokines are shutting down your appetite.

What confuses even a lot of doctors is that many patients with cachexia do not appear to be underweight. In some cases these patients are even overweight. So even though they have extra fat, their body is still responding to the cytokines as discussed above.

Patients with cachexia are also at high risk for poor wound healing after surgery and at high risk for pressure ulcers. While aggressive nutrition may be attempted, high-calorie diets alone for reasons we don't understand are in many cases ineffective at shutting off and reversing these cytokines.

Oftentimes, hospital patients are not eating as they await procedures or recover from illnesses. This makes them even more nutritionally depleted by the time they arrive back at home or at the nursing home. As we stated in chapter 9, many frail older adults are leaving the hospital much earlier than in years past. They therefore may be in the state of cachexia when they leave. Other illnesses, such as severe arthritis and strokes, may make it difficult for the patient to perform routine activities associated with eating, such as grocery shopping, cooking, and so on.

CAN MEDICATIONS DECREASE APPETITE?

In some cases, the medications used to treat a number of common medical conditions may affect a person's appetite. Many books and medical journals provide lists of potential appetite-reducing drugs that are so long it seems as though every medicine known to man is on it. To be fair, we prefer to say that these drugs "may be associated with malnutrition" rather than "cause malnutrition." This is because in many cases there is no evidence that these medications actually cause elderly people to lose their appetites or to lose weight. Our experience has been that the most common medications to be concerned about are:

- antidepressants such as citalopram (Celexa), duloxetine (Cymbalta), escitalopram (Lexapro), fluoxetine (Prozac), paroxetine (Paxil), sertraline (Zoloft), venlafaxine (Effexor)
- digoxin (Lanoxin)
- narcotics such as codeine, hydrocodone, morphine, oxycodone[4]

Some drugs can affect the senses of smell and taste. Others may decrease saliva production. Still others can cause side effects that decrease the patient's desire or ability to eat. In chapter 8, we discuss how anticholinergic medications can decrease saliva production. Verapamil and narcotics can cause constipation. Potassium pills and NSAIDs (such as ibuprofen and naproxen) may cause heartburn or abdominal pain.

If you or your family member is on one of these medications, do not get upset. Please do not yell at your doctor! They are all very good medications that may be needed to treat important medical illnesses.

DOES DEMENTIA INCREASE THE RISK OF MALNUTRITION?

The majority of patients with dementia eventually lose their appetite and the ability to feed themselves. It is so common that weight loss and lack of appetite are considered to be important clinical features that help define the time period when a patient has progressed to the advanced stages of Alzheimer's disease.

We have heard many people say that the weight loss is not due to the dementia but is due to the fact that the caregivers or the staff do not take the time to feed the patient. The **real truth** is complicated. Some patients will absolutely refuse to eat unless they are hungry, and in many cases they never seem to be hungry. Because this illness damages the brain, you can't logically explain to patients that their health is at risk if they are not eating. The patients with severe dementia have already lost the brain cells that allow them to think logically.

Patients may also fail to recognize edible objects as food. Others may have difficulty handling eating utensils. Some clench their teeth or spit their food out, making mealtime a very stressful experience for the caregiver. We have even seen patients who will pocket chewed food between their cheek and gums for hours. Advanced dementia is associated with a variety of behaviors that make it difficult for the seniors to effectively chew their food and initiate an effective swallow.

It may take a while to figure out how to get the person to chew his food and swallow. In some instances, even the experts may be at a loss. Remember, these patients are suffering from a neurological disorder that will continue to get worse over time, so what worked in the past may not work in the future.

WHAT ABOUT DEPRESSION?

The loss of appetite is a very common symptom of depression. Screening patients for depression is important whenever an older adult loses his appetite. In many cases, treating the depression can improve the appetite. In other cases, some antidepressant medications may make the appetite worse.

SOCIAL ISSUES CONTRIBUTING TO MALNUTRITION?

A variety of psychological and social issues, such as social isolation, poverty, lack of transportation, and elder abuse may also be contributing factors to this problem. Issues of abuse and self-neglect run across all ethnic and socioeconomic groups. Howard Hughes, for example, was the richest person in the United States when he died in 1976. At the time of his death he was six-foot four inches tall and weighed only ninety pounds.

HAVE YOU THOUGHT ABOUT YOUR SWALLOWING LATELY?

We hope your answer is no! We swallow so often during the day that we take it for granted. If you are eating a hamburger, you don't just take a bite and swallow. The piece of hamburger in your mouth must be chewed until it is all mushed up into a lump that we call a *bolus*. Once the bolus is formed, it must be pushed to the back of your throat before you can start to swallow. This is a voluntary process that is under the control of the individual. Once you start to swallow, the bolus must be moved from the back of your throat into your esophagus. At this point the muscles of the pharnyx and esophagus take over and the process becomes involuntary. The whole swallowing process involves many different muscles, which must all work together without any thought.

As we discussed, patients with advanced dementia often have trouble swallowing. Many patients with strokes and Parkinson's disease also have difficulty swallowing. Other problems that lead to difficulty swallowing include the presence of a tracheotomy tube or cancers of the throat, mouth, or esophagus. People with difficulty swallowing may complain of:

- coughing or choking when they try to eat or drink
- drooling
- the feeling that food is getting stuck in their throat
- losing weight

People with swallowing problems are at an increased risk for pneumonia. This was the reason that Pope John Paul II had recurrent lung infections toward the end of his life. In chapter 18 we discussed in great detail how aspiration leads to lung infections.

How Are Swallowing Problems Evaluated?

If you or a family member is experiencing these problems, talk to a doctor. You may be referred to an otolaryngologist (ears, nose, and throat specialist) who can evaluate the muscles of your throat and your vocal cords to make sure they are working correctly. The doctor may also refer you to a gastroenterologist who may want to insert a tube with a small camera to look at your esophagus and stomach. This procedure allows the gastroenterologist to look for blockages that can cause you to feel as though food is getting stuck in your throat when you swallow.

Another option is a modified barium swallow test (also known as *videofluoroscopy*), which can evaluate whether food or water is going into your lungs when you swallow (aspiration). This test is performed by a speech pathologist in the radiology department. The patient swallows small amounts of liquid, applesauce, pudding, and cookies that have been mixed with a white liquid called barium. The barium can be seen on a moving picture x-ray that allows the speech therapist to easily visualize the patient's ability to swallow and whether aspiration is present. Depending on the results of this test, a speech pathologist may be able to develop an individualized plan of care tailored to the needs of the patient. This plan may involve exercises to strengthen weak swallowing muscles. He may also recommend changing the thickness and texture of the patient's food.

TRYING TO TELL IF THE PATIENT IS MALNOURISHED IS VERY DIFFICULT!

If the patient appears to be skin and bones, then making the diagnosis is not so hard. As physicians we would like to make a diagnosis before it gets to that point. One thing we can do is get the patient on the scale. Documenting a patient's weight over time allows us to see whether he or she is gradually losing weight, perhaps slowly enough to otherwise go unnoticed.

There are no ideal body weights in the elderly. Charts listing ideal body weights or ideal *body mass indexes* (weight in kilograms/height in meters^2) have not been established for the elderly. Part of the problem is that it is difficult to get accurate heights of seniors because many:

- have *kyphosis* (hunched back) from osteoporosis (chapter 15)
- are bedridden
- have contractures in their hips or knees that prevent them from fully extending these joints (chapter 16)
- have lost some of the arch in their feet

There is no lab test that will tell you whether a senior is malnourished. Many doctors will test blood levels of the proteins *albumin* and *prealbumin* in order to help assess the nutritional status of the patient. Dieticians and many doctors think these two proteins are markers of protein stores in the body. Albumin is a protein made by the liver that circulates in the blood. Prealbumin is not a precursor of albumin. The **real truth** is that it is really a protein that binds to thyroid hormone in the bloodstream. This protein, like many proteins, will be found in lower levels when a senior gets sick and is in the cachexia state.[5] Remember, however, that no lab value alone can make the diagnosis of malnutrition.

HOW MUCH PROTEIN DOES A PERSON NEED TO EAT PER DAY?

Estimates as to the amount of protein per day that a person needs may vary. The first thing you need to do is to figure out your weight in kilograms (kg). Take your weight in pounds and divide by 2.2 kg/lb. A target of 0.8 to 1 gram of protein per kilogram per day is a safe bet. For patients with malnutrition and evidence of muscle wasting, at least 1.3 to 1.5 grams per kilogram of body weight per day may be needed.[6]

HOW MANY CALORIES A DAY DOES A PERSON NEED?

There is a special formula that dieticians use to calculate how many calories the person needs per day. It takes into account the person's gender, age, height, and weight.

If you do not like complicated formulas, we have something easier to use that has been validated in a recent research study. Take the patient's weight in pounds and divide by 2.2. This gives you the person's weight in kilograms. You can then take this number and multiply it by 30.

For example, if a person weighs 132 pounds:

132 lbs ÷ 2.2 kg/lbs = 60 kg
60 kg × 30 calories/kg =1,800 calories per day

Adjustments to this formula may need to be made if the patient is extremely obese, extremely underweight, or has eaten very little for an extended period of time (weeks to months). In both cases, you will need the assistance of a dietician or a physician to help you figure this out. In addition, people with chronic medical illnesses should talk to their doctor about the foods and/or diet plans they should be avoiding.

ARE THEY SPENDING ENOUGH TIME HELPING THE PERSON EAT?

We have seen many cases where families have accused nursing homes, ALFs, or even other family members of neglecting their loved one. You can't simply assume that the reason for weight loss is neglect. In fact, two studies have been done where researchers gave nursing home residents all the extra help they could need with their meals. Even with this intense intervention, 60 percent showed no significant improvement in the amount of food that they ate.[7] Instead of making accusations, it may be a good idea to ask the caregivers or nursing home staff what problems they encounter when they try to feed the person. Have they consulted with a dietician for advice in the evaluation and management of this problem?

WHY DO SO MANY FRAIL ELDERLY PATIENTS BECOME DEHYDRATED?

Water is the most important part of any diet plan. Patients may live for several months with no food because they can use their muscle and fat cells as energy sources. Without water, most people will get seriously ill in a few days. When we think of someone who is dehydrated, we often have a vision of someone stranded in the desert or being tortured in a prison. The word *dehydration*, like *starvation*, can elicit a strong emotional response. When we hear about elderly patients becoming dehydrated, the natural inclination may be to assume that the patient is being abused or neglected.

However, there are many factors that may place frail seniors at risk for dehydration:

- Age-related changes in the brain that decrease the thirst drive. The frail elderly do not get as thirsty as younger people on a hot summer day or when they exercise.

- With the loss of lean muscle mass (see chapter 2), there is less water stored in the body of the elderly patient.
- Kidney function is often impaired (see chapter 2), which means the kidney is less effective at holding on to water and electrolytes.
- There is a higher risk of infections and acute illnesses that will increase their need for additional fluids.
- There is a higher chance that they will be on a water pill (diuretic) for either congestive heart failure or hypertension.

How Much Fluid Do Seniors Need?

A useful way to estimate this amount is to take the patient's weight in pounds and divide it by 2.2. This will give you the weight in kilograms. You can then multiply this by 30 to give you the number of milliliters of water needed per day. Dividing this number by 1,000 will give you the volume in liters. For example:

For a 165-lb man ÷ 2.2 pounds per kg = 75 kg
75 kg × 30 ml water = 2,250 ml
2,250 ml ÷ 1,000 ml per liter = 2.250 liters per day

This is the total amount of fluid normally needed per day. If the resident is having fevers, diarrhea, vomiting, or liquids oozing from a wound, then the amount of fluids needed may increase substantially.

What about Eight Glasses of Water per Day?

Many seniors are convinced that they need to drink eight glasses of water a day. We are not sure where this idea came from, but in most cases eight glasses are not needed. Our 165-pound man needs 2.25 liters of fluid per day. The key here is the word *fluid*. Notice that we did not say 2.25 liters of water. Much of the food we eat is largely water. Drinking an additional eight glasses a day will make you go the bathroom a whole lot. If you have a bad heart or kidney issues talk to your doctor about how much fluid you need per day.

How Could This Person Have Been Allowed to Become Dehydrated?

In many cases, dehydration is considered a *sentinel event*—both dangerous and preventable—that must be reported to state regulatory agencies.

However, dehydration can be very difficult to assess in frail elderly patients. In many cases, even the doctors cannot tell if such a patient is dehydrated.[8] Patients with dementia will not be able to tell the doctor if they have diarrhea, increased urination, fever, or a decrease in their water intake. Some seniors who are dehydrated appear to be OK, while others who are not dehydrated look as though they were.

WHAT CAN WE DO ABOUT MALNUTRITION?

The first thing your doctor needs to do is to address any dental or gastrointestinal problems. Broken teeth or poorly fitted dentures may need to be addressed by a dentist. A variety of over-the-counter medications are available to treat heartburn and esophageal reflux symptoms. Your doctor may address constipation by advising you to increase fluid intake, limit or avoid constipating medications (such as narcotics or verapamil), and use one or more medications to treat constipation. If the person is depressed, an antidepressant that does not suppress appetite may be helpful.

TWO IMPORTANT POINTS TO ALWAYS REMEMBER ABOUT THE MANAGEMENT OF MALNUTRITION

- There is usually no simple solution.
- Patients and families need to be aware that appetite and weight loss will not always improve.

INTERVENTIONS IN THE MANAGEMENT OF MALNUTRITION

Interventions to treat this poorly understood and complicated problem can be broken down into five categories:

- diet modification
- drugs to stimulate the appetite
- feeding tubes (this will be discussed at length in chapter 20)
- nutritional supplements
- speech therapy evaluation

Altering the Diet

Many healthcare professionals do not realize that the first step in addressing a poor appetite involves asking the patient one simple question: *What do you like to eat?* We usually ask our patients to make a list. Don't worry if it includes "naughty foods" like bacon-double cheeseburgers, milk shakes, and double-fudge chocolate brownies.

It has been our experience that caregivers find this hard to accept. We live in an age where the media inundate us with information that we all must eat a well-balanced diet that is high in fiber and low in cholesterol. We are not arguing with that. A healthy diet is very important for middle-aged and healthy elderly patients. Unfortunately, rules need to be bent for frail patients who are not getting enough calories.

Doctors often order special diets for patients with specific diseases. For example, low-salt diets are often ordered for seniors with advanced congestive heart failure, and low-fat, low-calorie diets are ordered for people with diabetes. As we discussed earlier, there is a loss of taste with aging. But for some reason, many elderly develop a craving for sweets and carbohydrates. So cutting back on sweet food (as we do for many patients with diabetes or congestive heart failure) can have a big impact on appetite. If a person is not eating, such restrictive diets lose their intended purpose. While you don't want to discard all health and nutrition goals, it can be helpful to be more flexible with diet.

Other Diet Modifications

Dieticians will often suggest behavior modifications such as eating with others rather than alone. Some seniors eat more when they take meals in a dining room rather than alone in their room. A dietician may also recommend "finger foods" for patients with dementia who have lost the ability to use the fork and knife.

WHAT CAN THE SPEECH THERAPIST DO?

As previously mentioned, speech therapists are trained to do a lot more than just work with children who have speech problems. They are essential in the evaluation of patients with a swallowing disorder. They will assess the patient to see:

- the strength of the facial muscles and chewing muscles
- the strength of swallowing muscles
- whether the patient coughs while drinking or eating

A speech therapist can develop an exercise program to help strengthen the swallowing muscles. Just like a physical therapist is the rehab expert for an athlete with a knee injury, you can think of the speech therapist as the rehab expert for those people who have weakness in the muscles involved with swallowing. They may also provide a variety of tips for making feeding both easier and safer.

NO THIN LIQUIDS

Common sense would say that it is easier to drink water than it is to eat a hamburger. For the person with difficulty swallowing, the hamburger is actually a lot safer. When you chew the hamburger, it forms a big lump (*bolus*) that you move to the back of your throat. When you swallow, the food stays clumped together as it goes down the esophagus. Water, on the other hand, cannot be chewed into a lump, so it splashes around as the patient tries to move it to the back of the throat. When the person swallows, part of it may go into the esophagus and part may go into the lungs. Now that you understand this, don't be surprised when the patient is put on a no-thin-liquids diet.

A no-thin-liquid diet means that the person should not drink any water, juice, soda, tea, or coffee, unless it has been thickened with a product such as *Thick-it* or *Thick and Easy*. We have seen many patients who are supposed to be on these diets continue to get water, coffee, or juice from their families, who don't realize the importance of this safety measure for their loved ones. We can't begin to tell you how many times we have seen the families either forget or feel guilty and give the patient water or juice when no staff is around.

WHAT ELSE CAN BE DONE TO DECREASE THE RISK OF CHOKING ON FOOD?

Standard interventions include one or more of the following:

- Eating soft foods that are easy to chew
- *Compensatory feeding strategies* (e.g., reducing the bite size, keeping the chin tucked and the head turned while eating, and swallowing repeatedly)
- Sitting up when eating. You can test this strategy sometime if you try eating a hamburger while sitting up and then while lying down on your

back. You will notice that it is harder to swallow when lying down. For the older person at risk for aspiration, this is an important intervention that we often overlook. It is usually best for frail seniors to be out of bed and sitting up in a chair while eating.

NUTRITIONAL SUPPLEMENTS USUALLY DON'T WORK!

Nutritional supplement drinks, such as Boost, Ensure, or Sustacal, are often ordered in addition to the meals. The idea is that these drinks will provide the extra calories needed to gain muscle mass. Unfortunately, research shows that it's not so simple. A landmark research study (which was also a randomized, placebo-controlled study) revealed that without an exercise program, these supplements do not improve muscle strength or physical frailty.[9] What this may mean is that the state of cachexia, which we discussed earlier, cannot be cured with just a nutritional supplement.

In other studies it seemed that the calories consumed from supplements were often at the expense of regular food intake. It is believed that the residents felt full after drinking the supplements and ate less of their meals.[10] In fact, there is research suggesting that the frailest seniors are the ones most likely to use nutritional supplements *instead of* rather than *in addition* to their meals. In other words, the patients who need the calories the most are the least likely to benefit.[11] If supplements are going to be used, make sure they are taken between meals rather than with the meal.

ISN'T THERE SOMETHING THAT YOU CAN GIVE TO IMPROVE HER APPETITE?

There are three medications that are commonly used. These medications are cyproheptadine (Periactin), megestrol acetate (Megace), and dronabinol (Marinol). Many dieticians will strongly recommend the use of one of these drugs. Unfortunately, none of these medications appears to be a magic bullet that will completely address the problem. And there are very few studies looking at the use of these three medications in the frail elderly.

All three drugs are associated with side effects. Cyproheptadine is an old antihistamine that is associated with the anticholinergic side effects of dry mouth, blurry vision, urine retention (especially in men), constipation, tachycardia, and confusion (chapter 8).[12] Because of these potentially dangerous side effects, we don't recommend this medication.

Megace (megestrol acetate) is a drug that was engineered by modifying the female hormone progesterone. This modified hormone is the most popular appetite stimulant used in the elderly. Megace has been shown in many studies to increase appetite and weight in patients with AIDS and cancer.[13]

Studies looking at the use of this drug in the nursing home population have not been able to clearly show an improvement in appetite, weight, muscle mass, or survival.[14] One study of this medication in frail elderly patients has even suggested that it may actually cause muscle wasting.[15] Is it safe? Megace may place nursing home residents at an increased risk of developing blood clots in their legs.[16] This drug may also make diabetes worse and can affect the adrenal gland as well.[17]

Marinol (dronabinol) is a pill form of THC, the active ingredient in marijuana. Anyone who has watched a Cheech and Chong movie knows that one of the effects of marijuana is an increase in appetite (aka, the munchies). This medication is approved by the FDA as an appetite stimulant in patients with HIV. At the time of this publication, the FDA has not approved this medication for increased appetite in the frail elderly. Our experience has shown that frail elderly patients need to be started at 2.5 mg once daily in order to minimize the potential for the side effects of dizziness and sedation.[18]

ARE THERE ANY OTHER POTENTIAL APPETITE STIMULANTS?

Another medication commonly used is the antidepressant mirtazapine. Mirtazapine is not so popular among younger patients because many find that it makes them sleepy. Others dislike it because they gain weight. While the associated weight gain might make this medication unappealing to a young woman with depression, it may be a godsend for the older patient with no appetite and difficulty sleeping.[19] Because it can cause some sedation, we recommend starting at a low dose, and of course consult a physician before using it. The general recommended starting dose is 15 mg a day. We generally like to start our patients at 7.5 mg at night. While some seniors may eat more when taking mirtazapine, it is not FDA approved as an appetite stimulant.

Studies involving small numbers of healthy older adults have shown that the use of growth hormone and testosterone may lead to an increase in muscle mass, energy level, and weight gain. The use of these medications for the frailer elderly who are not eating is poorly studied and potentially dangerous (chapter 5).

WHY CAN'T WE JUST USE A FEEDING TUBE?

Feeding tubes are often recommended by doctors for patients who cannot or will not eat enough calories or drink enough water. While it may seem like a simple solution, it really isn't. The next chapter will discuss the indications, complications, and ethical issues associated with feeding tubes.

THINGS YOU CAN DO TO HELP AT HOME

- If you are helping to feed a loved one, be patient!
- Wait for the person to swallow the food before giving her the next spoonful.
- Make sure she is wearing her glasses and hearing aid during mealtimes.
- Keep noise to a minimum.
- Reduce potential distractions.
- Make sure that the food looks good.
- Remember that the human touch is important when feeding. Don't let the person eat alone.
- Always try to give choices with meals and snacks.
- Consider small, frequent meals or adding frequent snacks.
- Focus on serving foods that are high in calories.
- Don't restrict the diet to only healthy foods.
- Focus on food that is easy to chew.

THINGS YOU CAN DO TO HELP AT THE NURSING HOME

- Ask the staff if it is OK to bring food from home for the resident.
- Don't leave dentures on food trays and do not wrap them in napkins. They can get lost.
- Make sure the resident is sitting up in a chair while eating and not lying in a bed.

Chapter 20

THE TRUTH ABOUT FEEDING TUBES

In chapter 19 we discussed how many seniors with dementia continue to have a poor appetite despite diet modifications, nutritional supplements, and appetite stimulants. Even with a team effort, healthcare professionals often have no simple solution in these cases.

How do families make sure that their loved one receives her food, water, and medications? How do nursing homes avoid getting in trouble for allowing the resident to lose weight or become dehydrated? Modern technology has given us another option for addressing this issue—the feeding tube.

These tubes act as a bypass track to move food into the stomach. Stomach tubes were invented in the early 1980s for children and young people with throat and esophagus problems who were no longer able to swallow. These patients wanted to eat but could not. In other words, they were for people who wanted to live and knew that without proper nutrition they would wither and die. In the twenty-first century, this technology has been adapted for use among malnourished elderly patients. At least 30 percent of all stomach tubes now placed are in people with end-stage dementia.[1]

Although these tubes deliver food and water, it is considered a medical treatment, not a basic part of normal care. In 1986 the American Medical Association issued a policy statement that classified artificial nutrition and hydration as a "life-prolonging medical treatment."[2] This is where the controversy around feeding tubes has arisen.

WHAT ARE THE DIFFERENT TYPES OF FEEDING TUBES USED?

A thin *nasogastric tube* (from the nose to the stomach) is often used to provide nutrition for up to several weeks. Use of these nasogastric tubes (also known as Dobhoff tubes) is not a long-term solution for seniors who do not eat. Many patients find them uncomfortable. Passing the tube through a nostril down into the stomach can be a frightening experience and can cause gagging. Nasogastric tubes can make swallowing uncomfortable and can even lead to increased nausea. They are so uncomfortable that patients with delirium and dementia often pull them out. If left in too long these tubes can also cause sinus infections and even pressure ulcers in the nose.

If nutritional support is needed for a longer period of time, then percutaneous endoscopic gastronomy (*PEG*), or a *stomach tube*, may be needed. A bag of fluid is attached to a tube that runs through the abdominal wall and through the stomach wall. A *percutaneous endoscopic jejunostomy* (*PEJ*) differs from a PEG in that the tube extends from the stomach into the small intestine. PEGs and PEJs, however, are not suggested for seniors with rapidly progressive or incurable diseases, such as end-stage cancers.

Placing a PEG or PEJ requires making a hole through the abdominal wall and then through the wall of the stomach. Because of their wide tubing, PEGs allow the patient to be fed over a few minutes. In many cases the liquid can just be poured into a bag and it will drain by gravity into the stomach. PEJs, on the other hand, are much thinner tubes that can only handle about 100 ml of fluid per hour. A mechanized pump that regulates the rate of flow is often required.

This is an important point because many seniors dread getting a feeding tube. We have heard from many older adults that the idea of being tied up to a feeding tube makes them feel like a freak. Many patients are only receiving feedings during part of the day. For the remaining hours the short amount of tubing that extends outward from the abdominal wall can be clamped. We reassure our patients that when they wear a shirt over their stomach, it will be very hard for people to even notice they have a feeding tube.

DO FEEDING TUBES MAKE A DIFFERENCE?

Feeding tubes have been shown to be effective medical therapy for younger patients with acute strokes, other neurological diseases, and cancers of the mouth, esophagus, and stomach. Based on a review of the medical literature, the use of these tubes in seniors with advanced dementia:

- will not prolong their life. The majority will still die within one year of beginning tube feeding.
- will not decrease their chances of getting pneumonia.
- will not improve nutritional markers such as protein levels or body weight.
- will not prevent or help heal bedsores (chapter 27).[3]

As healthcare providers we do see individual cases of residents with severe dementia who are able to live for years after a feeding tube is placed and may in fact gain weight. However, in the majority of cases, the findings listed above appear to be true.

WHY HAVE FEEDING TUBES BECOME SO POPULAR IN THE FRAIL ELDERLY?

Many caregivers turn to doctors for guidance about whether or not a feeding tube should be used on their loved one. The majority of doctors, however, do not know that studies have shown a lack of benefit from feeding tubes in the demented elderly.[4]

It is not just doctors who are at fault here. There is much pressure on nursing homes to prevent malnutrition. The amount of feeding that a person with dementia receives can be quite erratic. Time availability of family or nursing home staff may vary. The resident may refuse to eat even if there are no time constraints. For a nursing home that is under regulatory pressure to make sure patients don't lose weight, the feeding tube offers a solution whereby they can, in theory, show they have provided a consistent amount of nutrition.

Not only are the nursing homes under regulatory pressure, but they are under financial pressure to use feeding tubes as well. Patients requiring tube feeding get reimbursed at a higher daily rate than those who do not. Not only do they bring in more money, but these residents require less staff support than someone who needs to be fed by mouth.[5]

WHAT ARE THE POTENTIAL COMPLICATIONS WITH FEEDING TUBES?

Many residents may get diarrhea from either the tube feeding or from the liquid solution used to deliver medications through the tube. Infections can occur at the site where the tube inserts into the stomach.

Pneumonia is the most common cause of death among patients with dementia who have feeding tubes. Sometimes the term *aspiration pneumonia* is used when these patients get ill. A family, upon hearing the term *aspiration* may think that the mishandling of the tube feeding somehow contributed to the pneumonia. The confusion in terms is discussed at length in chapter 18.

COMMON PITFALLS WE ENCOUNTER WITH TUBE FEEDING

Failure to get an adequate amount of water is a concern with tube feeding. In addition to the tube feeding formula, patients also need to get water put in the tube. The amount of water needed varies for each person. What we have seen is that many patients receive none or just a few ounces a day. The lack of adequate amounts of water can lead to a state of dehydration where the patient becomes dizzy or weak. Blood pressure may drop and the concentration of sodium in the blood may rise.

When a feeding tube is inserted, standard nursing protocols state that the head of the bed should be elevated by at least 30 degrees while the food is running into the tube. The idea here is that elevating the head of the bed will help prevent the tube feeding from going up from the stomach into the throat, where it can potentially end up in the lungs (aspiration is discussed in chapter 18). The problem is that when you elevate the head of the bed you are increasing the amount of pressure around your tailbone and buttocks. This can increase the risks of developing a pressure ulcer (chapter 26).

USING THE TUBE TO GIVE MEDICATIONS

All medication pills need to be crushed before being placed in the tube. The more the pills are crushed, the better. Try to get the pills into a powder consistency. Then take the powder and dissolve it in about an ounce of warm water. It is a good idea not to mix medications. It is also recommended to flush the tube with an ounce of water before and after each medication. If the patient needs several medications, it can be quite time consuming to flush after each medication. The amount of fluid used in all these flushes can be substantial if the patient receives many medications. Talk to your doctor about what will work best for you and your loved one. Some medications come in a liquid form, which may be easier to push through the tube. These medications also may be more expensive than the pill form.

WARNING! Before you start crushing all the pills, check with the pharmacist or your doctor to make sure that it is safe to crush the pills. Some are made in a manner that releases the medication slowly. By crushing one of these *extended release, controlled release,* or *sustained release* tablets, the person with the feeding tube may be rapidly exposed to a large amount of medication. We have seen situations where people with feeding tubes were given crushed-up, high-dose blood pressure pills only to have the blood pressure drop dangerously low soon afterward.

You should also check with the pharmacist to see which medications should be given on an empty stomach and which should be given with food. If the medication needs to be given on an empty stomach, then stop the feeding for at least thirty minutes prior to giving the medication.

WHAT IF THE TUBE GETS CLOGGED?

Fluid should easily flow through the tubing. If you have to force it in, then there is a problem. Most likely the tubing is clogged. Because of the smaller diameter, the PEJs are more likely to get kinked or clogged up with tube feeding or medication fragments.

We used to recommend flushing the tubing with 5–10 cc of soda water to unclog it. However, it's been found that this can potentially damage the tube.[6] Instead, push 5–10 cc of warm water in the tubing and then clamp the tube (the clamps are attached to the tube). After five minutes, you can try to flush with water until the clog in the tubing clears. If this doesn't work, call the doctor!

LET'S THINK ABOUT SOME OF THE ETHICAL ISSUES!

There was a ninety-five-year-old woman with dementia. After nutritional supplements and medications failed to increase her weight, her caregiver asked that we place a feeding tube in her. Two years later, her caregiver died. Without a healthcare surrogate, she ended up living for an additional six years in which time her dementia progressed to the point that she was completely bedridden and contracted in a fetal position. She was admitted to the hospital several times. Was it ethically justified to "maintain her nutritional status"?

Many people question the ethics here, because the lack of appetite is part of the natural course of this slowly progressive illness. Before tube feedings were available, the lack of appetite and weight loss was simply accepted as part of end-stage dementia. In the twenty-first century, weight loss and dehydration have become interpreted as signs of poor care. We need to ask ourselves: Do we really want to prolong the end stages of Alzheimer's disease?

How much of a workup should we do on a ninety-five-year-old person with dementia who refuses to eat? How many medical procedures do we want to subject the patient to? Are you helping the patient or prolonging her suffering?

Unfortunately, we have no clinically significant treatments for the underlying Alzheimer's disease (chapter 24). Nursing interventions to improve the appetite and promote weight gain can be extremely time consuming and often ineffective despite the best of intentions. Without a better understanding of the mechanisms by which some seniors appear to just wither away, the debate over whether to use a feeding tube in the frail elderly will continue.

Chapter 21

TAKING CARE OF
OLDER ADULTS
WHO ARE INCONTINENT

Urinating is a very complicated process that most of us take for granted. Urine is formed as the blood is filtered through the kidneys. Urine then flows down the ureters into the bladder, where it is stored until it is time to urinate (figure 21.1).

There are nerve fibers in the body that tell the bladder wall muscles to contract and others that tell it to relax. There are other nerves that give the signal to let the urine pass out from the bladder into the urethra. There are also nerves that support the muscles at the bottom part of the pelvis to keep the bladder in place.

While much of this runs on autopilot, we all know that we can force ourselves not to urinate. Anyone who has had to wait in line to use a bathroom after drinking a pitcher of beer can tell you that the brain has control over the urinating process... well, maybe some control!

Many older adults have difficulty holding their urine, a problem called *urinary incontinence* (UI). There is not really a good definition for this disorder, but if a person believes that she has a problem holding her urine, then she has UI.

UI MEANS MORE THAN JUST SOILED CLOTHES!

The poor hygiene associated with urine-soiled clothes can lead to skin irritations and an increased risk of getting bedsores in seniors who are bed bound

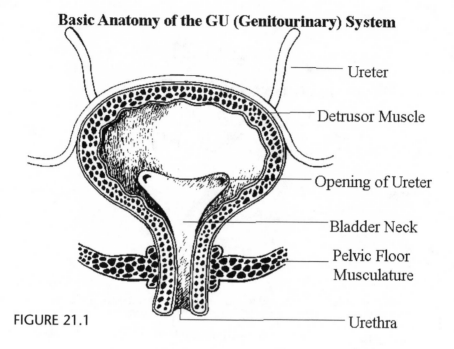

Basic Anatomy of the GU (Genitourinary) System

— Ureter

— Detrusor Muscle

— Opening of Ureter

— Bladder Neck

— Pelvic Floor Musculature

FIGURE 21.1 — Urethra

(chapter 26). In the past, doctors thought that the soiled clothes could increase the risk of getting urinary tract infections, but we no longer believe this to be the case.

The psychological and social impact of this problem can be devastating. Many seniors are so embarrassed by this problem that they don't even want to discuss it with family members or their doctor. Fewer than half of all women who think that their incontinence is a problem will seek help from their doctor.[1] So instead of trying to seek help for this problem, they isolate themselves. They may avoid any social interactions out of fear that they will smell of urine. Forget going to a party or going to see a movie. They become so fearful about having an accident that they just remain at home. In addition, the thought of relying on other people for assistance with toileting, cleaning, and changing garments can decrease a person's self-esteem. For people who have been independent their whole lives, this can be a major source of humiliation.

WHAT ARE THE MAJOR RISK FACTORS?

Whenever we evaluate a person with UI, we always want to address both those factors that may be temporary and those that are chronic in nature. Below is a list of the temporary factors that can give you UI or make it worse. It is important to realize that many seniors have more than one risk factor:

- decreased estrogen levels, resulting in
    - atrophic vaginitis (the shrinkage and drying of the vaginal tissue)
    - shrinkage of the pelvic floor muscles that support the bladder
    - delirium (discussed in chapter 13)
- excess urine production (either from the use of diuretics, caffeine, or excess drinking)
- restricted mobility (for people who are either restrained or who are too frail to get to the bathroom easily)
- severe constipation
- urinary tract infection

HOW DO WE EVALUATE URINARY INCONTINENCE?

Because multiple factors often contribute to the patient's problem, a full assessment is needed!!! The first step in evaluating urinary incontinence is to get an understanding of the frequency, timing, and amount of urine involved in the UI episodes. The doctor will also want to know if there was anything that brought on these symptoms or made them worse.

After getting a detailed history of symptoms, the doctor will then want to check a sample of urine to see whether infection, diabetes, or kidney disease is contributing to the problem. The staff may also use a Foley catheter or an ultrasound machine to see how much urine is still in the bladder after the patient has tried to urinate.

Before we get into the diagnosis and treatment of the specific types of UI, it is important that the following steps be taken:

- avoid alcohol
- avoid coffee, black tea, chocolate, and caffeinated sodas
- avoid fluids late in the day
- avoid green tea, which contains xanthine, a compound very similar to caffeine

- avoid, if possible, the use of diuretics (water pills)
- treat any urinary tract infections
- treat elevated blood sugar levels
- use pads, diapers

We cannot overemphasize the significance of these steps. Any drugs or surgeries will not work unless you take the above steps! That being said, let's move on.

WHO WANTS TO WEAR A DIAPER?

The answer is no one! There is a strong social stigma around the use of adult diapers; we tend to associate wearing a diaper with being an invalid or a baby. On one of the opening monologues to an episode of *Seinfeld*, Jerry talks about how a person's first birthday and last birthday are the same. In both cases, the person doesn't know any of the people there, needs help blowing out the candles, and is wearing a diaper.

Although people hate wearing them, adult diapers and pads allow a person to move around without constantly worrying about soiling their clothing. Some helpful tips:

- Absorbent pads need to be changed several times a day.
- Clean the skin during diaper changes with premoistened wipes. Some have ingredients that may help with odor.[2] Baby powder or cornstarch can minimize skin irritation.
- Even though the patient is wearing the pad, you still want to encourage him or her to use the bathroom every two hours while awake.
- Putting underwear over the pads may help to address the self-esteem issues associated with wearing an adult diaper.

FUNCTIONAL INCONTINENCE

Many frail seniors have UI that is not due to any problem with the bladder. These patients have what we call a *functional incontinence*. The person has a disease or problem that prevents him from using the bathroom. Examples of things that can cause this functional incontinence include:

- the bathroom is too far away
- being restrained to a chair or bed
- dementia or delirium
- physical impairment (arthritis, strokes, etc.)
- severe depression

The treatment for people with a functional incontinence involves addressing the steps listed on pages 235 and 236. Using a bedside commode (which can be purchased at any equipment supply store) may help those patients who can't get to the bathroom in time. In addition, many facilities use a regimen known as *prompted voiding*. Every two hours during the day the patient is assisted to the bathroom. By getting the patient out of bed throughout the day, this regimen may also help maintain their physical function. What about during the nighttime? We are not sure whether continuing the prompted voiding schedule at night is helpful. Getting them up every two hours at night may keep them dryer, but it may ruin their ability to get some decent sleep.

URGE INCONTINENCE

People with urge incontinence complain that they must urinate often. And when they feel that urge, OH BOY! It becomes a mad dash to the toilet. This can happen during the day as well as the night. It is most often due to overactive muscles in the bladder wall. This is seen in both men and women with very sensitive bladders. It may also occur in some people who've had strokes or have Parkinson's disease. These illnesses may lead to damage in areas of the brain that normally tell the bladder that it is not time to urinate.

Treatments for Urge Incontinence

Bladder Retraining

The patient is instructed to urinate only according to a timetable. Initially, the patient will urinate every hour regardless of whether she feels the need to urinate. Every few days the interval between toileting is increased by fifteen- to thirty-minute intervals. The goal is to gradually get to two and a half to three hours between toileting.

Kegel Exercise

Kegel exercises are an important treatment for women with either urge or stress incontinence. This treatment is not normally done in the nursing home or in the primary care physician's office because it requires the expertise of specially trained staff.

In a nutshell, Kegel exercises involve having the woman draw in her perivaginal muscles and anal sphincter without contracting her abdominal, buttocks, or thigh muscles. These exercises need to be done thirty to eighty times per day for at least six weeks. In some cases, vaginally inserted cones may serve to help make these exercises more effective. As you can imagine, this could be upsetting to discuss with many elderly women.

Medications

The medications used to treat urge incontinence (overactive bladder) act to relax the muscles in the bladder wall. The muscle-relaxing medications approved by the FDA are:

- darifenacin (Enablex)
- oxybutynin (Ditropan), oxybutynin XL (Ditropan XL)
- solifenacin (Vesicare)
- tolterodine (Detrol), tolterodine LA (Detrol LA)
- trospium (Sanctura)

All of these medications are about equally effective for treating an overactive bladder.[3] They all have anticholinergic side effects, which are listed below and discussed in greater detail in chapter 8.

- blurry vision
- confusion, hallucinations, delirium
- constipation
- dry mouth
- inability of men with enlarged prostates to empty the bladder
- tachycardia
- urinary retention

The anticholinergic effects of these five drugs may not be the same. Talk to your doctor about which one is best for you. Your doctor will use these medications only when the benefit of the drug outweighs the potential risk. In order to maximize the benefit, you want to make sure that the drugs have the best chance of working. Therefore, they should not be used until all of the steps listed on pages 235 and 236 have been followed.

One Final Note on Urge Incontinence

We have taken care of many patients who frequently have the urge to urinate at night. Jumping out of bed at night to make a mad dash to the toilet is a recipe for falls and other injuries. There are four steps you can take to minimize the risk:

1. Install a nightlight so the path from the bed to the toilet is not poorly lit.
2. Rearrange any furniture obstructing the path to the bathroom.
3. If the distance from the bed to the bathroom is too far, consider getting a bedside commode. This is a portable toilet that can be placed next to the bed.
4. Avoid the use of sleeping pills.

STRESS INCONTINENCE

Stress incontinence involves the leakage of small amounts of urine with any activity that increases abdominal pressure, such as laughing, sneezing, or coughing. The increased abdominal pressure squeezes on the outside of the bladder and causes urine to leak out. The ability of the bladder to hold urine inside will decrease in older women whose vaginal tissue and pelvic muscles have thinned out due to lack of estrogen. Some elderly women have pelvic muscles and ligaments that are so weak that the uterus, rectum, or bladder actually prolapses (protrudes) into the vagina whenever they laugh, sneeze, or cough.

The treatments for stress incontinence involve one or more of the following:

- Surgery, especially for women whose bladder prolapses into the vagina.
- The use of a *pessary*, which is a custom-fitted plug that is inserted into the vagina and helps to keep the bladder from dropping down into the vagina. These devices need to be removed and cleaned regularly.
- Duloxetine (Cymbalta) is an antidepressant that has been shown to

decrease the number of episodes of stress incontinence. However, duloxetine is currently not FDA approved for this indication.

- Kegel or biofeedback exercises. Biofeedback uses electronic or mechanical instruments to give information to the patient about her pelvic, abdominal, or bladder activity. It is often used in conjunction with other behavioral techniques, such as Kegel exercises.[4]

WHAT ABOUT ESTROGEN?

Estrogen has been shown to have a variety of effects on the urethra and genital tissues. It thickens urethral and vaginal walls. It also improves underlying connective tissue and the blood supply.[5]

Estrogen can be used in a variety of ways. There are pills, vaginal creams, and even vaginal rings. With the estrogen creams, a small amount of the cream can be applied to the vagina several times a week.

While the creams may help, estrogen pills for some unknown reason can actually make the symptoms worse.[6] Estrogen pills have fallen out of favor in recent years out of concern that they may increase the risk of heart attacks, breast cancer, and uterine cancer.[7]

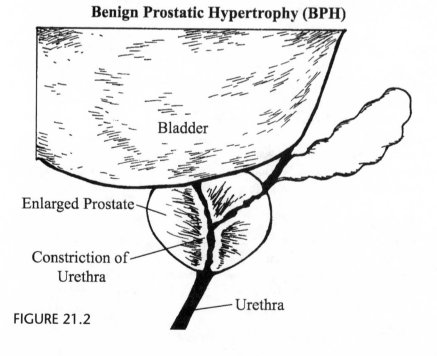

Benign Prostatic Hypertrophy (BPH)

FIGURE 21.2

OVERFLOW INCONTINENCE

With overflow incontinence, the bladder is unable to empty and the patient will frequently urinate in small amounts day and night. Overflow incontinence may occur when there is an obstruction of the urine leaving the bladder. This obstruction can be due to *benign prostatic hyperplasia* (BPH) (figure 21.2), or due to a narrowing of the urethra (the tube that urine flows through when it leaves the bladder). Overflow incontinence can also happen when the bladder muscles are not contracting due to diabetes or a spinal cord injury. Sometimes there is no apparent reason why the bladder will not contract.

The main treatment options for men with BPH are either a surgical correction of the obstruction, medications, or the use of a Foley catheter. A variety of surgical procedures exists for men with enlarged prostates. Talk to your doctor about which one is best for you. Medications are also available. The two main categories of drugs used to treat BPH are listed below:

Alpha-Blockers	**5-Alpha-Reductase Inhibitors**
terazosin (Hytrin)	finasteride (Proscar)
doxazosin (Cardura)	dutasteride (Avodart)
tamsulosin (Flomax)	
alfuzosin (Uroxatral)	

Recent studies have shown that the combination therapy of alpha-blockers (terazosin, doxazosin, tamsulosin, and alfuzosin) and a 5-alpha-reductase inhibitor is better than treatment with just one drug.[8]

DOES SAW PALMETTO HELP?

There have been many studies looking at the effectiveness of the herbal product saw palmetto in lessening the urinary symptoms in men with enlarged prostates. While the herb has been shown to be very safe, it has not been shown to be any more effective than taking a placebo.[9]

ISN'T IT EASIER JUST TO USE A FOLEY CATHETER?

A Foley catheter is a small tube that is inserted through the urethra into the bladder.[10] Once it is inserted, a small balloon is inflated at the tip to keep the tube in the bladder.

Normally, the bladder does not have a lot of bacteria growing inside. When you insert a tube that extends from the outside into the bladder, bacteria now have easy access to the bladder. Because of this easy access, the risk of urinary tract infections rises dramatically.

Cleaning the bag with a bleach or vinegar solution will not get rid of all the bacteria. Antibiotics may kill most of the bacteria, but new bacteria will colonize the tubing and they will become harder to kill. Frequently changing the catheter will not lower your risk of a urinary infection.

Therefore, the decision to use a Foley catheter should not be taken lightly. It should not be used simply to make it more convenient for the staff or families. In nursing homes, the government monitors the percentage of residents with urinary catheters as an indicator of the quality of care at each facility. The thought here is that good nursing homes will use Foley catheters less often. It should also be noted that some patients will pull on their Foley catheters, which can damage the urethra, since the Foley has a hard inflatable tip to prevent it from slipping out once it is in place.

WHAT IS A CONDOM CATHETER?

Some men will use another type of urinary catheter that does not go inside the penis. The condom catheter fits over the penis just like a regular condom. There is a small hole at the end that attaches to tubing that drains the urine. These condom catheters are often more comfortable than those that are placed directly inside the bladder. There is also a lower risk of getting a urinary tract infection.[11] Because the tubing does not go into the bladder, it will not drain the bladder in men who are unable to empty their bladders due to an enlarged prostate or a neurological injury. The condom catheters often fall off and can cause some irritation to the skin at the head of the penis. Despite these drawbacks, condom catheters should be used instead of Foley catheters whenever possible.

Urinary incontinence is a topic that many patients and healthcare professionals do not enjoy talking about. Treatments are available, so it's important not to keep quiet if you or a loved one is suffering from this problem.

Chapter 22

DEPRESSION CAN BE
A REAL BUMMER

"If you live to be 100, you've got it made. Very few people die past that age."

George Burns (1896–1996)

Ten percent of all seniors seen by primary care doctors are suffering from clinical depression.[1] Not only is it common, but it is often difficult to diagnose. Television shows often give a distorted view of this disorder. Hollywood usually portrays the depressed person as someone who is sad, crying all the time, and does not want to talk to anyone. The depressed TV character just wants to be left alone.

Among seniors, depression does not often follow this script. Older adults often show up at their primary care physician's office with medical complaints rather than saying that they feel sad. They may mention physical symptoms, such as joint pain, back pain, muscle pain, weakness, or abdominal pain. In many cases, they may be quite talkative and even quite animated.

They may also complain of anxiety symptoms, such as difficulty sleeping, agitation, difficulty concentrating, irritability, and fatigue. The important thing is to recognize that all of these symptoms may really be manifestations of depression.

I CAN'T REMEMBER ANYTHING!

When a person comes to see us complaining that his memory is no good, Alzheimer's disease is not the first thing to come to our minds. More likely, the person is depressed. As geriatricians we see this problem so often that we always first need to rule out depression whenever we are evaluating a person complaining of memory loss. Severe depression can look so similar to dementia that some people call it *pseudodementia*. Telling the difference between the two can be hard even for an experienced physician.

DIAGNOSING DEPRESSION

The standard criteria for the diagnosis of major depression involves having five or more of the following for a greater-than-two-week period:

- fatigue
- feeling sad
- feelings of worthlessness
- guilt
- lack of energy
- loss of interest in activities that were previously enjoyable
- sleep disturbance—insomnia or sleeping too much

Diagnosing depression in patients with dementia is really tough. People in the late stages of dementia are not able to answer questions that involve deep insight into personal issues, such as guilt and worthlessness. Instead, seniors with dementia may exhibit a variety of other signs. Indications to be on the lookout for include:

- behavioral disturbances
- agitation, hand wringing
- slow movements and speech
- multiple medical complaints
- daytime and nighttime variation in mood
- anxiety
- worrying
- tearfulness
- lack of reactivity to pleasant events

- easily annoyed
- appetite loss, weight loss
- lack of energy
- thoughts of extreme pessimism and suicide

DEPRESSION NEEDS TO BE TREATED!

Aside from ruining one's quality of life, depression can have a major impact on one's health. Studies have shown that depressed patients are less likely to comply with treatment of their medical illnesses.[2] Do you really think that those who are severely depressed are going to care that their blood pressure was 141/94 or that their LDL cholesterol was 167? Of course not! We have taken care of many patients who are so depressed in the hospital that they will not eat or participate in their rehabilitation. On the other hand, we have seen other depressed seniors who may want to go to the doctor or emergency room more frequently.

Identifying older adults with depression and intervening is crucial to decrease the risk of suicide among elderly white men. Another inaccurate portrayal from movies and TV is that suicide is something that primarily affects rock stars and other young people with drug or criminal issues. When looking at the actual statistics, this is not the case. Elderly white men are at the highest risk, and no other population group is even a close second. The risk of suicide continues to rise for white men even past the age of seventy-five.

ARE ALL NURSING HOME RESIDENTS DEPRESSED?

There is a perception out there that nursing homes are such miserable places that everyone living there must be depressed. That certainly is not the case. It is true that people living in nursing homes are more likely to be depressed than those who are healthier and living at home. However, let's look at the numbers. Studies have actually measured the percentage of nursing home residents who are depressed. The number falls somewhere between 6 and 20 percent.[3] Depression affects between 1 and 2 percent of the general adult population. The percentage rises to about 10 percent among seniors who seek medical attention from a primary care physician.[4] Since nearly everyone in a nursing home is suffering from a number of chronic medical problems, the question is whether the higher rate of depression in the nursing home is due to the person's medical problems or to being stuck in a long-term care facility. The other major point to remember is that the majority of residents are not depressed.

BEFORE WE DISCUSS TREATMENT . . .

Depression needs to be thought of as a treatable chronic illness, like high blood pressure or diabetes. As with diabetes, patients will need long-term treatment. Getting older adults to accept treatment can be difficult. In years past, depression was often viewed as a sign of mental weakness, and this view persists.

Many older adults are hesitant to utilize mental health services due to the stigma associated with mental illness. They may think that psychiatric treatment is only for "crazy people." Others will try to convince everyone that there is nothing wrong with them and explain it away by saying:

- "You would be depressed too if you were in my situation!"
- "What do I have to look forward to?"

SOME THINGS YOU JUST CAN'T TREAT!

Dr. Golden had a patient who explained to him that "growing old just isn't fun." What she was referring to was the loneliness that many older adults face. Some books talk about "healthy aging" and highlight older adults who are healthy and active. While we smile when we see active seniors enjoying their later years, the **real truth** is that for millions, the "golden years" are a time of loneliness. According to the US Census Bureau, 59.2 percent of women and 21.6 percent of men over the age of seventy-five are widowed.[5] Many older adults are geographically isolated from their children. Others may not have had any or have actually outlived them.

What about your friends? Starting in your seventies, your friends will die faster than you can make new ones. Some other friends will move out of town to be with family or to go to a nursing home.

It is important to keep these issues in mind. Many geriatric and gerontologic experts advise seniors that they need to make some new friends and find new interests and activities. Such simple advice may be condescending, but it beats drugs. All communities have outreach programs for seniors. Many religious groups sponsor activities for their older members as well. In spite of this community support, finding new interests is tough for those people who have poor hearing and vision, bad arthritis, urinary incontinence, no car, and a limited budget.

ALCOHOL AND BENZODIAZEPINES ARE NOT THE ANSWER!

The benzodiazepines listed in table 8.1 (see p. 105) should not be used for more than a week or two in patients with anxiety or insomnia symptoms, since these pills can make the underlying depression worse.

Remember that these drugs work by a mechanism that is similar to alcohol (chapter 8). You wouldn't dream of drinking a six-pack as a way to treat your depression. But when you take a benzodiazepine, you are pretty much doing the same thing. By taking this drug you are in a sense masking, not treating, the underlying depression.

We have all seen our friends do some really stupid things while drunk. When they sober up, they often try to blame the bad behavior on the alcohol. While we can't blame it entirely on the alcohol, we do know that it acts in a way that makes you lose your normal inhibitions. For the older adult with depression, taking benzodiazepines increases their risk of falling, becoming confused, getting into an accident, or just acting inappropriately. For elderly white men, the loss of inhibition can increase the risk of suicide. Moreover, don't forget that these pills are all very addictive.

WHAT ABOUT PROZAC?

Fluoxetine (Prozac) is a very popular medication used to treat depression. As geriatricians, we don't recommend this medication for seniors since it can inhibit the breakdown of a variety of other commonly used drugs, such as:

- benzodiazepines
- beta-blocker heart medications (atenolol, carvedilol, labetalol, meto-prolol, propranolol, timolol, etc.)
- calcium channel blocker hypertension medication (amlodipine, dilti-azem, nifedipine, verapamil)
- haloperidol (Haldol)
- NSAIDs (ibuprofen, naproxen, celocoxib, etc.)
- phenytoin (Dilantin)
- tricyclic antidepressants (amitriptyline, desipramine, doxepin, and imipramine)
- warfarin (Coumadin)[6]

WHAT ARE THE OTHER POPULAR DRUGS TO TREAT DEPRESSION?

Paroxetine (Paxil) may interfere with the breakdown of some drugs, such as tricyclic antidepressants, Haldol, or beta-blockers.

Escitalopram (Lexapro), citalopram (Celexa), and sertraline (Zoloft) appear to be well studied and well tolerated in the frail elderly population. These can be given once a day and appear to have minimal risk of interactions with other drugs, as compared to fluoxetine or paroxetine.

All of the drugs listed so far belong to the same class known as *serotonin selective reuptake inhibitors* (SSRIs). They work to increase the level of the neurotransmitter serotonin in the brain. These medications have become popular because they are much safer than the medications that were used to treat depression in the 1970s and 1980s. The side effects of SSRIs can include insomnia, upset stomach, diarrhea, and headache.[7] In rarer cases these medications may cause a low-sodium level in the blood.[8] Probably the most frustrating for patients is that the SSRIs make it more difficult for both men and women to have orgasms.

To minimize the risk of side effects in the elderly we start the SSRIs at very low doses. We then increase the dose slowly every two to three weeks. As always, discuss any drug regimen with your doctor before initiating or changing a drug regimen.

THESE PILLS DON'T SEEM TO WORK!

Patients and families often become frustrated that these medications don't seem to be working. However, you must remember that frail elderly patients are often started on very small doses. So if they are not working, take a deep breath before flushing the pills down the toilet. To give them a fair chance to work, the person may need to be taking a higher dose (prescribed by a doctor) for four to six weeks before deciding the medication is not helping the depression.

OLDER IS NOT ALWAYS BETTER!

The SSRI medications are generally quite mild compared to the older antidepressants, such as amitriptyline (Elavil) and doxepin, which have many bad anticholinergic side effects (chapter 8). In addition, these older drugs are bad for your heart.[9]

Sometimes we use these older medications in low doses for patients with pain due to irritation of nerves (chapter 27). The doses used for pain control are six- to eightfold lower than the doses used for depression.

Another medication commonly used is the antidepressant mirtazapine (Remeron). We mentioned this medication in chapter 19, as it is often prescribed to patients with a poor appetite. As we stated earlier, this medication is not so popular among younger patients because many find that it makes them sleepy and gain weight. However, some older depressed persons may actually benefit from these drug side effects. It also has no sexual side effects.[10]

Because it can cause some sedation, we recommend starting at a low dose and giving it at night. The general starting dose is 15 mg a day. We generally like to start our elderly patients at 7.5 mg a day.

Several studies have shown that bupropion (Wellbutrin) works as well as the SSRIs. Bupropion has also been shown to have fewer sexual side effects than the SSRIs and may be helpful in patients who are trying to quit smoking. This drug is not too popular for the frail elderly because it can ruin their appetites. People with a history of seizures should avoid taking this drug.[11]

Duloxetine (Cymbalta) works on both the neurotransmitters serotonin and norepinephrine. It is well studied in the elderly. It has been shown to be helpful in the treatment of pain due to damaged nerves.

Venlafaxine (Effexor) also works on both serotonin and norepinephrine. Although it is well studied in the elderly, we have found two additional problems with this medication: (1) it can raise the blood pressure and (2) patients can get flulike symptoms if they suddenly stop taking it.[12] Like the SSRIs, both duloxetine and venlafaxine have sexual side effects.

HOW LONG DO I NEED TO TAKE THESE MEDICATIONS?

While some may try to stop medications after feeling better for six months to a year, it has been our experience that the majority of patients will need to be on these medications indefinitely.

I AM ON MEDICATION AND IT IS NOT WORKING— WHAT DO I DO NEXT?

We encounter this problem often. Several options exist for the physician:

- Increase the dose of the medication
- Add a second medication

- Switch to another medication
- Add psychotherapy

WHERE CAN I FIND A GOOD PSYCHIATRIST?

Finding physicians with expertise in geriatric psychiatry issues may be difficult in many areas around the country. Finding someone well trained at geriatric counseling or psychotherapy may be even harder to find. You can try the membership list for the American Association for Geriatric Psychiatry. You can access this list at http://www.gmhfonline.org/gmhf/find.asp.

WHAT ABOUT ELECTROSHOCK THERAPY?

Most people are terrified at the thought that they or a family member would need electric convulsive therapy (ECT), which is commonly referred to as electric shock therapy. We all remember the horrible scenes of Jack Nicholson in *One Flew over the Cuckoo's Nest* getting ECT. In reality, patients do not suffer as he did in that movie. During the treatment, the person is given surgical anesthesia medications to sedate and paralyze their muscles. The patient will not feel or remember a thing.

Despite its terrible image, ECT is the most effective treatment for major depression. More people will get better from this treatment than from any drug on the market. ECT is used for those who have not benefited from or are unable to take antidepressant medications. It may also be indicated for people who are so ill (suicidal, in a catatonic stupor, refusing food and fluids, etc.) that the most rapid treatment is needed.

ECT may be associated with several problems. Many patients become confused right after the treatment. In elderly patients the period of post-treatment confusion can persist for several hours or even days. There is often a temporary inability to recall information learned after the treatments have begun. Some patients may also forget things that happened before the course of treatments. In some cases the memories come back, and in other cases they don't.

THINGS YOU CAN DO TO HELP!

- Reinforce the importance of treatment for depression.
- Ask if your loved one has any thoughts about committing suicide.
- Ask the doctor if the antidepressant medication needs to be increased.

Depression is a serious illness that can have a major impact on a person's health and quality of life. If you feel that you or your loved one is depressed, talk to your doctor. Do not try to treat this on your own without professional help.

Chapter 23

CAN DEMENTIA BE PREVENTED OR TREATED?

"By the time you're eighty, you've already learned every-thing. You only have to remember it."

George Burns (1896–1996)

By age eighty-five, 35 percent of people will have a diagnosis of dementia (also known as *senile dementia*).[1] In chapter 1, we discussed how the eighty-five and over age group is now the fastest growing segment of the population and that more Americans will suffer from dementia in the years to come. Many of these seniors who are diagnosed with dementia will unfortunately need nursing home care.

In order to begin our discussion about dementia, we need to clarify a few issues.

IS DEMENTIA THE SAME THING AS ALZHEIMER'S DISEASE?

In the real world, these terms are often used interchangeably by healthcare professionals. Alzheimer's disease is the most common type of dementia, but other types do exist.

WHAT DOES IT MEAN TO BE DEMENTED?

When we think about a person with dementia or Alzheimer's disease, we often think about someone who has no memory. The lack of memory is the most obvious sign, but to make the diagnosis of dementia requires memory loss plus one or more of the following:

- Impairment in language skills (difficulty finding words, wrong tones in speech).
- Inability to perform skilled movements, such as writing or tying shoelaces.
- Difficulty with activities that involve planning, organizing, sequencing, and abstracting ideas. These activities would include balancing the checkbook, preparing a meal, using the telephone, and driving.
- Visual-spatial impairment. This means that they have difficulty understanding what they see with regard to size and shapes. It is most apparent when they are asked to draw a design or to identify particular shapes.

Our purpose here is to discuss the major categories of dementia, as well as the latest research in the treatment and prevention of Alzheimer's disease. In the next chapter we will discuss the behavioral disorders associated with dementia.

No matter what type of dementia your loved one may have, it is important to understand that the family still has an important role to play. In the nursing home, for example, the residents of families who visit often and communicate with staff are less likely to have untreated or undiagnosed medical issues. No one knows your loved one better than you. In many cases you may be able to recognize when your family member is having a problem way before any healthcare professionals do. On the other hand, the changes that occur with early dementia can be so subtle that many family members and friends may not even notice that a problem exists.

CLUES THAT A LOVED ONE MAY HAVE DEMENTIA

- asking the same question over and over
- having a lot of difficulty paying the bills (and not because of a lack of money)
- no longer clean and well groomed
- house is dirty
- can no longer remember phone numbers or important dates

- refrigerator that is either empty or full of rotten food
- getting lost in places that used to be familiar
- not taking medications correctly
- receiving one or more driving tickets or has recently having been in an automobile accident
- having difficulty picking the right words to say

BUT SHE REMEMBERS EVERYTHING FROM YEARS AGO!

We hear this comment frequently from family members who do not understand that their loved one has dementia. The ability to retain new information is lost early in dementia. While your grandmother might not remember what you told her five minutes ago, she will remember explicit details about her childhood, college years, and so on.

HOW CAN YOU TELL IF YOU HAVE DEMENTIA?

This is a question we're often asked by patients in our clinics. Others will make statements such as "My memory is shot" or "I am forgetting everything!" Seniors often worry that they are becoming more forgetful. Many are fearful of getting Alzheimer's disease. The majority of the time the person is not demented but is in fact suffering from depression.

It is almost impossible for you to self-diagnose yourself with dementia. Most of the time, patients who truly suffer from dementia are unable to tell that they have a problem. They usually describe their memory as "pretty good" or "just fine."

HOW CAN YOUR DOCTOR TELL IF YOU HAVE DEMENTIA?

Getting a History

Evaluating a patient with dementia involves getting a detailed history from family or friends. A family member or friend who knows the patient well should be present at the time of the evaluation. You cannot get an accurate history from the patient alone. Patients with dementia are unable to remember details or recognize subtle changes in their behavior and thinking.

The doctor will need to ask family and friends questions such as "When did your loved one begin having trouble performing her duties at work? Is she having trouble doing the math to pay the bills correctly? Is she able to drive or go to a store without getting lost?"

Screening Tests May Include One or More of the Following

Many healthcare providers will use one or more short tests to see if the patient is likely to have dementia. These include questions such as "What year is this?" "What city are we in?" "Can you draw the face of a clock at ten minutes after eleven?" The inability to answer some of these questions may raise a red flag that the patient has a memory problem. Sometimes, patients get offended that we are asking them such "easy" questions. They are the lucky ones!

Your doctor may also order one or more of the following tests to see if there is a medical reason other than Alzheimer's disease that could explain the memory loss:

- Homocysteine level—high homocysteine levels may increase the risk of a stroke and for developing dementia.
- TSH—this measures how well your thyroid is working
- Vitamin B12 levels—patients with low vitamin B12 levels may suffer from memory problems.
- VDRL—this is to check if you have neurosyphilis (which is now very rare in the United States).
- CT or MRI of the brain—your doctor may also order a CT or MRI of the brain. These scans can tell whether there are tumors, strokes, normal pressure hydrocephalus, or bleeds in the brain that could explain the memory loss.

WHAT IS ALZHEIMER'S DISEASE?

It is very important to remember that Alzheimer's disease is diagnosed based on the physician's evaluation of the patient. The only way to be absolutely certain someone has Alzheimer's is to do a tissue biopsy of the brain. In other words, we would have to remove a piece of brain tissue. Certainly, not a simple operation. Rather than subjecting patients to this invasive procedure, doctors make an educated guess by carefully examining the patient and ruling out other causes of memory loss.

When we look under the microscope at the brains of people who have died with Alzheimer's disease, we see that several distinct parts of the brain have lost a lot of nerve cells. We also see specific findings known as *neurofibrillary tangles* and *beta-amyloid plaques*. These findings were first noticed by Louis Alzheimer in 1906. After a hundred years of research, we are just beginning to understand how these tangles and plaques form and kill nerve cells.

The clinical course generally progresses slowly. Half of all patients will die within three to six years of the onset of dementia symptoms.[2] Since these people are in their seventies, eighties, or nineties, the cause of death is often due to diseases other than dementia. Although we say the disease is progressive, the rate at which people decline can vary greatly. Some may progress more rapidly while others may live for another ten to fifteen years.

What Are the Stages of Alzheimer's Disease?

We generally think of Alzheimer's disease as having three stages (mild, moderate, or severe). While we list the signs of each, you should realize that these are not well-defined categories. There are no distinct cut-offs between these categories. People with Alzheimer's disease may exhibit symptoms from more than one category at a time.

The signs of *mild* disease include:

- Changes in personality
- Confusion about the location of familiar places and objects
- Difficulty remembering things from a few moments ago
- Difficulty using the right words in sentences
- Loss of spontaneity and sense of initiative
- Poor judgment
- Repeatedly asking the same question over and over
- Trouble handling money

With moderate disease, more parts of the brain are affected. Behavioral problems start to emerge. The signs of *moderate* disease include:

- Difficulty with reading, writing, and numbers
- Difficulty organizing thoughts and thinking logically
- Hallucinations, delusions
- Inability to learn new things
- Increased memory loss
- Loss of impulse control (using profanity or undressing at inappropriate times)

- Perceptual-motor problems (such as trouble getting out of a chair, setting the table, or recognizing the depth or differences between objects)
- Problems recognizing friends and family members
- Repetitive statements or movements
- Restlessness, agitation, anxiety, tearfulness, wandering

The signs of *severe* disease can include one or more additional signs:

- Difficulty swallowing
- Inability to get out of bed without assistance
- Inability to talk
- Inability to walk
- Increased sleeping or a lack of sleep
- Lack of bladder or bowel control

It is therefore not surprising to see patients at the severe stage suffer from complications such as recurrent infections, weight loss, falls, fractures, pressure ulcers, and contractures (see chapter 16).[3]

Is Alzheimer's Disease Inherited?

It can be. There is ongoing research relating to the genetic and environmental factors responsible for causing this disease. While genetics may play a role, no one gene is responsible for this disease. Most research seems to show that many genes may be involved.

It appears that a small percentage of cases are actually inherited. In these cases, the disease usually develops at a younger age (late fifties and sixties).[4] People who develop the disease at an older age (late seventies, eighties, and nineties) probably did not inherit any Alzheimer's genes from their parents. "But both my mother and my grandmother developed dementia in their eighties," someone might say. This still doesn't mean that you have inherited a risk factor for Alzheimer's disease. Remember, just by making it to age eighty-five, you have a 35 percent chance of getting dementia.

Is There a Genetic Test for Alzheimer's?

There is a popular genetic test that looks at the gene that encodes one of the proteins involved in the metabolism of cholesterol. This protein is known as *apo E.* Just as people can have different eye colors, people can have one of three different types of apo E (apo E2, apo E3, apo E4). Apo E3 is the most common type seen in the population. Studies have shown the apo E4 protein is found in a higher percentage of patients with Alzheimer's than among the general population.[5]

So Who Should Get This Test?

Probably nobody. We do not recommend this test because about 40 percent of people who have apo E4 will never get Alzheimer's disease.[6] In addition, many people with Alzheimer's disease have the apo E2 or the apo E3 protein. This test does not help us diagnose Alzheimer's disease, nor will it tell us if you are going to have dementia. There is as of yet no specific test for Alzheimer's disease, though research in this area continues in earnest.

Is Alzheimer's a Fatal Disease?

Alzheimer's disease is a disease of the nerves of the brain that continues to worsen over time. People do not die of brain failure, per se. They will usually die from complications of the disease. These complications include pneumonia, urinary tract infections, falls, and so on. Others will die from other unrelated illnesses, such as cancer or congestive heart failure.

WHAT ARE THE OTHER TYPES OF DEMENTIA BESIDES ALZHEIMER'S DISEASE?

While Alzheimer's disease is the most common form of dementia, other types do exist.

Lewy Body Disease

Lewy body disease is sometimes referred to as *Parkinson's dementia*. An examination of the brains of these patients under the microscope reveals abnormal structures called Lewy bodies. They are also seen in a certain segment of the brain in patients with Parkinson's disease. We usually make this diagnosis without having to open someone's skull to take a biopsy. A doctor will make this diagnosis by noticing a gradual loss of memory and two or more of the following:

- fluctuating memory, attention, alertness that seems to be better at times and worse at others

- features of Parkinsonism (rigid arms, stooped posture, hand tremors, slowed speech, lack of facial expression)
- recurrent visual hallucinations

Other features that may support the diagnosis include falling, passing out (syncope), and severe illness following even a small dose of certain antipsychotics. In addition to visual hallucinations, many people with Lewy body disease will have some of the behavioral problems that we will discuss in more detail in the next chapter. Despite these differences, the **real truth** is that in many cases it is very hard for a doctor to tell the difference between a patient with Lewy body disease and Alzheimer's disease, and some patients could have both.

The hallucinations and other behaviors need to be treated with the correct antipsychotic medication. Treatment with the wrong antipsychotic may make the Parkinson's symptoms worse and may place the person at a risk for a severe illness involving high fevers and even death. To minimize these risks, quetiapine (Seroquel) is the antipsychotic often used to treat these patients.[7]

Vascular Dementia

Vascular dementia is sometimes referred to as *multi-infarct dementia*. This type of dementia is caused by one or more strokes. Strokes are blood clots that block one of the arteries supplying blood to the brain. The specific artery that gets clogged will determine which part of the brain tissue dies. Blood clots or hardening of the arteries can arise due to the presence of atherosclerosis of major vessels, diseases of the heart valves, or irregular heart rhythms (atrial fibrillation, atrial flutter, etc.). A stroke may also result in a weak arm or leg, which increases one's risk of falling.

Tobacco users and patients with diabetes or hypertension are at a very high risk for this type of dementia. As it turns out, the majority of patients with dementia seem to have features of both a vascular dementia as well as Alzheimer's disease.[8] We use the term *mixed dementia* to refer to these cases.

Some Less-Common Causes of Dementia

Normal pressure hydrocephalus can cause dementia, an awkward pattern of walking (as though one's feet are stuck to the floor), and urinary incontinence. Most patients do not exhibit all three conditions.

Fifty percent of these cases are associated with a variety of head injuries. The head injury may be so slight that the patient and family may not even remember it. A CT or MRI of the head will show very large fluid-filled areas of the brain, known as *ventricles*. The treatment for normal pressure hydrocephalus is to insert a tube into the brain that will drain the spinal fluid into the abdomen. In some cases this surgical intervention will completely or partially improve the symptoms. In other cases it may not work. This procedure is also associated with an increased risk of infection and bleeding in or around the brain.[9]

Subdural hematoma is a bleed that develops between the brain and the skull (chapter 14). A subdural hematoma can occur after a serious head injury. People who take blood-thinning medications may be at higher risk. If it is severe, the skull will need to be opened and the blood drained out.

Vitamin B12 deficiency is commonly seen in older adults and is associated with many neurological and psychiatric problems. Measuring vitamin B12 levels in the blood is not the definitive test for B12 deficiency. This is only a screening test. There are some cases of people who have low levels in the blood but are not vitamin B12 deficient. There are also some people with normal blood levels who are actually vitamin B12 deficient. If your doctor has a strong suspicion for vitamin B12 deficiency, he might want to check the methylmalonic acid and homocysteine levels in the blood. These levels are elevated with vitamin B12 deficiency.

Injections of vitamin B12 usually correct neuropsychiatric abnormalities. We usually give the injection once a week for four weeks and then once a month thereafter. If the person takes a 1,000-microgram vitamin B12 pill daily, that may work. However, simply taking an over-the-counter B-complex pill will not be good enough, as it does not contain enough B12.

Hypothyroidism is due to a thyroid gland that is not making enough thyroid hormone. Patients may appear slow in their thought, speech, and actions. They may also seem confused. This disorder is easy to diagnose with a simple blood test that measures the thyroid-stimulating hormone (TSH). If the TSH level is high, the thyroid levels will be low, and the person will be given thyroid hormone pills to take daily.

WHAT DOES MILD COGNITIVE IMPAIRMENT MEAN AND HOW IS IT DIFFERENT FROM DEMENTIA?

Some seniors are diagnosed as having *mild cognitive impairment*. What this means is that their memory is comparatively worse than other people their age with a similar educational background.[10] The memory impairment is not as bad as those who have dementia. In addition, there is no:

- difficulty finding the right words to say
- difficulty balancing the checkbook, preparing a meal, using the telephone, and driving
- difficulty integrating visual input with regard to size and shapes

Some researchers now think of mild cognitive impairment as a transition between normal aging and dementia. Some even use the term *predementia* to describe mild cognitive impairment.[11] The majority of patients with mild cognitive impairment will eventually develop Alzheimer's disease.

MEDICATIONS TO TREAT ALZHEIMER'S DISEASE AND OTHER DEMENTIAS

Providing early treatment for Alzheimer's has been based on the observation that once a mental function is lost, it becomes almost impossible to regain. Therefore, you want to preserve what you have for as long as possible. The **real truth** is that at the present time there really are no treatments that can stop the gradual progression of this neurological disease.

Acetylcholine Phosphodiesterase Inhibitors (Aricept, Exelon, and Razadyne)

In the last ten years a variety of medications have become available for the treatment of patients with Alzheimer's disease. The most commonly used class of drugs are known as *acetylcholine phosphodiesterase inhibitors.* Simply put, with Alzheimer's, there is a loss of nerve cells in specific parts of the brain. Some of these nerve cells transmit signals to other nerve cells using a substance known as *acetylcholine.* As these neurons die, there is less acetylcholine to transmit signals. The acetylcholine phosphodiesterase inhibitors act to slow down the rate that the remaining acetylcholine gets broken down by the body. Donepezil (Aricept), rivastigmine (Exelon), and galantamine (Razadyne) all fall into this class of medication. All three are approved by the FDA for the treatment of Alzheimer's disease that is mild to moderate in severity. These medications all work about the same.

How Effective Are These Drugs?

Many research studies have been done to try to answer this question. Looking at all of these studies, we see that patients who take these medications perform slightly better on psychological testing than those who took a placebo.[12] In figure 23.1 you see that the patient with dementia who receives no medication continues to worsen at the same rate, while the patient who was given the medication, in theory, has a slower rate of decline.

In theory, by delaying the progressive nature of Alzheimer's disease, this medication can help patients maintain their remaining function and stave off nursing home placement. Unfortunately, these changes are so small that they are often clinically insignificant. These drugs do not prevent the destruction of the brain cells that occurs with Alzheimer's disease. As a result, the use of these drugs has come under increased scrutiny by some doctors and researchers who question whether the benefit is worth the cost.[13] Depending on your Medicare Part D drug plan, these drugs can be expensive.

It has been difficult for us to explain to families that even if the medication is working, they will likely not see any improvement. Only a small percentage of patients will improve when they take these medications. This differs greatly from the effect of medications used to treat high blood pressure, high cholesterol, or diabetes. If the person taking the pill for hypertension sees no decrease in the blood pressure readings, the doctor will likely add a second drug. With Alzheimer's disease, we can only hope that the rate of decline slows down.

Potential Benefit of Alzheimer's Disease Medications

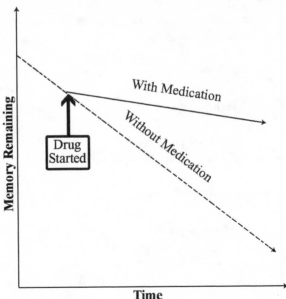

FIGURE 23.1

Things to Remember Regarding These Medications!

- can cause nausea, abdominal pain, vomiting, and diarrhea, as well as anorexia
- may also increase gastric acid secretion, which is particularly of concern for people with an increased risk of stomach ulcers
- Make sure that the person is not on an anticholinergic medication (see table 8.2, p. 108). Anticholinergic medications counter the effects of acetylcholinesterase inhibitors and should be avoided in patients with Alzheimer's disease.

Memantine (Namenda)

In the last few years, a new medication called memantine has become available. Memantine works through a different mechanism than acetylcholinesterase inhibitors. *Glutamine* is the main stimulatory neurotransmitter in the brain. Overstimulation of glutamine on receptors known as NMDAs may lead to brain cell damage. Memantine acts to block the glutamine from binding to NMDA receptors. Like the other drugs discussed above, the ability of this drug to slow the rate of progression of dementia is slight at best.[14] This drug is currently approved by the FDA for the treatment of only moderate to severe dementia. Fortunately, this drug has been shown thus far to be very safe.

After slowly increasing the dose over four to five weeks, the patient will take this medication twice a day. A large study has shown that patients with moderate to severe Alzheimer's disease who were already taking the maximum Aricept dose did better when memantine was added.[15]

Do These Medications Work for Mild Cognitive Impairment?

The most current research suggests that these drugs do not delay the onset of Alzheimer's disease in patients with mild cognitive impairment.[16]

What about Ginkgo Biloba?

Ginkgo biloba has been used in China as an herbal medicine for more than five thousand years, but has been studied scientifically for only two decades. Studies have been done to see if this herb has any effect on memory. Some studies show a benefit while more carefully designed ones show none.[17] Ginkgo is generally very safe to use.

In theory, ginkgo may have some effect on the ability of the platelets in your blood to effectively form clots. Most research, however, has shown that this effect is not clinically important.[18] Despite the lack of evidence for an increased risk of bleeding, ginkgo should still be used with caution in patients who are already on blood thinners, such as warfarin (Coumadin), heparin, enoxaparin (Lovenox), aspirin, and clopidogrel (Plavix).

What about Over-the-Counter "Memory Pills"?

There are many advertisements on the Internet and radio for products that claim to improve memory. Nonetheless, there are no products that have ever been shown to improve memory. Many of these products contain stimulants, such as caffeine, which can increase blood pressure and heart rate. For patients with dementia, they can also increase anxiety and agitation. Products containing ginseng or vitamin E may increase the risk of bleeding if the patient is already on blood-thinning medications.

What about Omega-3 Fatty Acids (Fish Oils)?

There have been large studies showing that a low intake of fish and low blood levels of omega-3 fatty acids are more commonly seen in patients who develop dementia.[19] At the present time, however, there is no good evidence showing that taking omega-3 fatty acids lowers the risk of developing or slows the progression of Alzheimer's disease.

What about Vitamin E?

Vitamin E (μ-tocopherol) acts as an antioxidant, and early research had shown that a high dietary intake of vitamin E is associated with a decreased risk for developing Alzheimer's disease. While research from the mid-1990s showed that vitamin E was effective in slowing down the damage from Alzheimer's disease, more recent studies suggest that vitamin E does not reduce the risk of developing dementia.[20]

What about Folate?

At the present time the use of folate has not been shown to restore memory, prevent further memory loss, or help prevent strokes.[21]

> Do not forget that all vitamin and herbal products are regulated as food supplements, not as medications (chapter 4). The quality and quantity of active ingredients in an herbal product can vary quite considerably among different brands and even among different batches from the same manufacturer.

PREVENTING VASCULAR DEMENTIA

Patients with a history of strokes or heart disease need aggressive medical care. This may involve taking:

- blood pressure–lowering medications
- blood-thinning agents
- cholesterol-lowering agents

PREVENTING OR DELAYING ALZHEIMER'S DISEASE

What about Estrogen?

In the 1990s many people were excited about the use of estrogen replacement therapy as a means of preventing Alzheimer's disease in women. At that time, estrogen replacement therapy was a wonder treatment that could also lower a woman's risk of heart disease and treat osteoporosis. You were considered to be a bad doctor if you did not put your postmenopausal patients on hormone replacement therapy. Ten years later, it appears that none of these benefits turned out to be true.

The belief that hormone therapy is beneficial in preventing dementia was based on studies that looked at populations of women who used estrogen replacement therapy. It seemed that the women who took estrogen had a reduced risk of Alzheimer's disease. When studies were done with people who were randomized to receive either estrogen therapy or a placebo, the results did not show a clear benefit. Estrogen replacement therapy does NOT appear to prevent or delay the progression of Alzheimer's disease.[22]

What about Blood Pressure Medications?

There appears to be a strong relationship between poor blood flow in the small blood vessels of the brain and the development of Alzheimer's disease. Doctors are now quite aggressive about treating older adults with a type of blood pressure drug known as an *angiotensin-converting enzyme inhibitor* (ACE-I) (lisinopril, enalapril, captopril, etc.). Although some encouraging preliminary research exists, it is not clear at this time whether this class of drugs can slow down the damage to the brain that occurs with Alzheimer's disease.

What about Cholesterol Medications?

The need to lower cholesterol is important. Reducing cholesterol may lower the risk of a stroke by reducing the amount of blockage in the arteries that supply blood to the brain. At the present time there is strong evidence to suggest that taking statins (cholesterol drugs Zocor, Lipitor, Crestor, etc.) reduces the risk of developing Alzheimer's disease.[23] However, further studies will be needed before doctors can tell patients with certainty that these drugs can prevent Alzheimer's disease.[24]

How Important Is It to Stay Active?

Studies have shown that physical activity is associated with a slower rate of decline in memory. There are other studies that suggest it may help protect against developing dementia. Studies using rats have shown that exercise may decrease the amount of amyloid deposits. Amyloid deposits appear to be involved with the damage that occurs to the brain with Alzheimer's. Whether this applies to humans remains unknown.

What about Keeping the Person "Intellectually Active"?

We are often asked by families if it is a good idea to keep the person's brain stimulated. People who participate in intellectually stimulating activities and are more socially engaged with family, friends, and the community have a slower rate of decline and a lower risk of becoming demented.[25]

Studies have also shown that older adults with mild dementia who participated in mental skills training were able to function better than those who did not. A wide variety of memory-enhancing brain exercise products are commercially available.[26] The problem is that no one is sure of exactly which mental exercises will work best to prevent Alzheimer's disease or delay it from getting worse.[27] While much exciting research exists, many experts believe that it is premature to recommend specific products.

Activities such as crossword puzzles or reading books may be fine. But we suggest avoiding overstimulating activities, such as a poker marathon in a Las Vegas casino. We actually had a family who tried this with their demented grandma. Between the time changes, the lack of sleep, and all the commotion in the casino, grandma became very agitated and confused. The family ended up having to take her to a local emergency room for help controlling her behavior. Overstimulation can cause the patient with dementia to become disoriented and may lead to many behavioral problems that we will discuss in the next chapter.

What about an Alzheimer's Vaccine?

The development of a vaccine that can prevent Alzheimer's disease from occurring is something that scientists at many universities and corporations are actively researching. No vaccine currently exists. The **real truth** is that you should not hold your breath waiting for this vaccine to be developed. Under the best-case scenario it will be decades before such a product is available.

WHAT CAN WE EXPECT?

We hear this question quite commonly from families who are caring for people with dementia. The course of this disease is often so slow that many health-care professionals tend to forget it is a progressive neurological disease. Over the course of time, one or more of the following things will happen:

- contractures of the knees and hips
- decrease in appetite
- difficulty sleeping
- inability to eat without assistance
- inability to get out of bed without assistance
- increased likelihood of falling
- loss of the ability to hold urine
- loss of the ability to speak
- pneumonia

Pneumonia is an extremely common natural event in patients with advanced dementia. Fifty percent of death certificates of persons dying with dementia report pneumonia as the final cause of death.[28] In the United States most of these terminal patients are treated with aggressive medical care.

However, it is difficult to predict which illnesses the person with dementia will eventually get. Sometimes a person may seem quite stable until an acute illness occurs. A frail elderly person with a urinary tract infection or pneumonia may recover from the illness but may not seem quite the same afterward. The dementia may seem worse, as if the person took a major step backward. Will the person's mental capacity ever recover? In some cases, the person's mental capacity may return, in other cases it may not. We cannot fully explain or even predict why this happens.

SO WHAT CAN YOU DO?

There is no cure for Alzheimer's disease and most other dementias. Most of the current treatments do not really work. There is still a lot that the family can do to help. In order to maximize the brain function that has not been destroyed, the following disorders need to be addressed:

- Addiction to alcohol, benzodiazepines, and narcotics
- Chronic pain
- Depression
- Poor hearing and vision
- Sleep disorders
- Use of anticholinergic medications (chapter 8)

Chapter 24

TREATING THE
BEHAVIORAL PROBLEMS
ASSOCIATED WITH DEMENTIA

Many families need to prepare themselves for what to expect as their loved one loses her memory. As the severity of the dementia increases, at least half of all patients will develop one or more behavioral problems.[1] Behavioral problems are a major reason why families are no longer able to take care of their loved one at home. It is not surprising that in the nursing home setting, approximately two-thirds of the residents are demented, and 90 percent will have one or more behavioral issues.[2]

SO WHAT ARE THESE DEMENTIA-RELATED BEHAVIORS?

- Accusing people of stealing from them or hurting them
- Agitation—shouting and using profanity, hitting, scratching, spitting, or biting
- Being very demanding and uncooperative
- Depression
- Extreme anxiety
- Hoarding various items, such as food, medication, and so on
- Saying the same thing over and over
- Staying up all night long
- Using sexually inappropriate language and actions
- Wandering off and getting lost
- Hallucinations—hearing or seeing things that do not exist

TRYING TO FIGURE OUT WHAT'S GOING ON CAN BE HARD

If you or I were to become angry, we would hope it would be for a good reason. Perhaps someone stole something from you or maybe someone insulted a family member. The person with dementia may become agitated for no apparent reason. In some cases, the agitation may be due to:

- Disorientation after moving to a new home or apartment
- Hunger or thirst
- A need to go to the bathroom
- A need to remove clothes that are soiled with urine or feces
- A new acute illness (pneumonia, heart attack, etc.)
- Overstimulation by noise or light
- A side effect of a new medication
- Untreated pain

Sometimes families note that the agitation becomes worse in the late afternoon or early evening. The term *sun-downing* is sometimes used to describe this problem. Although geriatricians see this problem all the time, little is known about what causes sun-downing or how to treat it.

SO IF WE DON'T KNOW WHAT'S GOING ON, THEN WHAT ARE WE SUPPOSED TO DO?

Trying to care at home for a person with dementia who has behavioral problems is extremely difficult and taxing. In order to deal with these behavioral problems, at least one of three things must change: the caregiver, the environment, or the patient. Of the three, the patient is the least likely to change. Why do we say that? Well, the person with dementia has a damaged brain and that is something that is not going to change. The impairment in brain function does not allow the person to perceive his or her environment correctly. The disease also impairs the ability to respond correctly to the actions of other people.

Environmental factors in the home or facility that can make behavioral problems worse include:

- Change(s) in the daily routine
- Confinement to a space with no safe place to wander
- Glaring or dim lighting

- Noise
- Sensory overload (hearing and visual stimulation)
- Sleep deprivation

WHAT CAN THE CAREGIVER DO?

There may be things that the caregiver can do to modify how they act when dealing with a person who has dementia. Such interventions/strategies include:

- Follow a routine—try to maintain a regular schedule with regard to nighttime sleep, naps, meals, bathing, and exercise. These activities should all occur around the same time each day.
- Try to distract—if the person with dementia becomes upset over something that is unrealistic, try to avoid further conflict by changing the topic. Don't waste time arguing with a demented person. It will accomplish nothing.
- Be flexible and patient—do not get into an argument over eating and sleeping times. Although you want to establish a routine, these things can always be done a little later.
- Speak slowly, in a low-pitched voice.
- Speak in a calm, reassuring voice.
- Break up complicated tasks into small, successive steps.
- Encourage light exercise daily.
- Make sure the drapes are open during the day. Ideally, the person should get some sunlight daily.
- Provide time orientation using an easy-to-read clock.
- Treat any pain.
- Music therapy—calming music or music that is familiar to the person with dementia works best.
- Make sure that the person has a regular toileting schedule. This will help keep the patient drier and less anxious.

As the dementia continues to destroy more brain cells, the person with dementia will understand less and less of what is going on around him and will also have a harder time articulating his concerns. The US Department of Health and Human Services published a brochure titled *Alzheimer's Disease: Unraveling the Mystery*, which makes this point very well:

To a person who cannot remember the past or anticipate the future, the world around them can seem strange and frightening. Sticking close to a trusted familiar caregiver may be the only thing that makes sense or provides security. Taking off clothes may seem reasonable to a person with AD who feels hot and doesn't understand or remember that undressing in public is not acceptable.[3]

Trying to reason with a person who suffers from dementia can be a futile experience. These people unfortunately have already lost the function of the parts of the brain that deal with reasoning. If you are going to try to reason with him, keep it simple. Try to use simple words and short sentences. Distraction techniques work better. For example, we had a patient who always looked out her window and saw motorcycles parked outside. She was continuously fixated about riding the bikes. She would often be found wandering, trying to get out of the facility so she could go ride the bikes. Reasoning did not work. Blocking the window in her room did the trick.

Sometimes a simple change on the part of the caregiver works, but in other cases the behaviors do not go away. These behaviors are often the result of multiple complicated factors. As a caregiver, do not blame yourself if these behavior problems do not go away.

WHAT CAN THE DOCTOR DO?

We have taken care of numerous patients whose families are at their wit's end trying to manage disruptive behavior. In order to help the doctor figure out the possible cause of a certain behavior, it is important to make a careful note of the following:

- When during the day does this behavior occur?
- How long does it last?
- What seems to bring about this behavior?
- Where does this behavior occur?

The doctor should check the medications that the person is taking. Some medications can make the behavorial problems worse. These medications include benzodiazepines, muscle relaxers, antihistamines, and medications used to treat Parkinson's disease.

The doctor may also order blood work, looking for signs of an infection or of a blood electrolyte abnormality. In some cases, the doctor may even order an x-ray or a CT scan.

HIRING AN AIDE

Some families choose to hire a private companion to help watch the person at home for several hours a day. This gives the family time to go to work, run errands, or take a break. In certain cases this extra expense may well be worth the money.

Hiring an aide may also be a good idea for the nursing home resident who has a lot of behavior problems. For example, if the resident becomes delusional and aggressive in the late afternoon and early evening, then an aide may help to provide extra supervision during those hours. The aide can make sure the patient doesn't wander off, which reduces the risk of falling. Sometimes, just having someone nearby can provide a sense of reassurance to an anxious resident.

ISN'T THERE A PILL FOR THESE BEHAVIORAL PROBLEMS?

It is important to consider medications when nothing else works. Drugs may be needed if the aggression raises concerns for the safety of the patient or the staff.

In many cases, there is no magic pill to fix these behaviors. Our understanding of brain function is still quite limited. None of the drugs actually "fix" the brain damage that is responsible for the abnormal behavior. While many books discuss ways to fix these problems, the reality is that simple solutions often don't exist!

SOME WON'T EAT!

Feeding a severely demented patient can be extremely difficult. Some patients will absolutely refuse to eat unless they are hungry. In chapter 18 we discussed many factors that contribute to this problem. Medications to stimulate appetite usually do not work.

What about trying to convince the person to eat more? Good luck with that! Trying to explain the importance of eating using logic to a person with dementia will fall on deaf ears. Patients with dementia will at some point lose the brain cells that allow them to understand and participate in logical discussions.

SOME ARE LOOKING FOR THEIR FAMILY!

Alzheimer's destroys the short-term memory long before long-term memories are lost. A person with dementia will forget what you told him two minutes before but will remember many of the details of a remote past. Therefore, we are not surprised when we hear families describe how the patient with Alzheimer's disease keeps looking for his long-deceased parents. Others will be looking for a deceased spouse. In these situations, it is better to remain calm and try to redirect the patient to do something else.

SOME WILL WANDER!

Some people with dementia are prone to wandering. Some may be looking for their childhood home or another place they lived in the past. If they are not watched, they can walk out of their apartment, home, or long-term care facility and potentially injure themselves. We have even seen cases of people with dementia who have wandered off and ended up in jail, the emergency room, or even dead. If you have a family member who could wander off while at home, it may be a good idea to tell the neighbors. This way they can alert you or the police if they see your loved one wandering. Some people recommend that the person wear an ID bracelet.

If the person needs to be moved to the nursing home, you need to tell the staff about this potential problem. Nursing homes may have one or more interventions to address this issue. The more common measures include placing such residents on floors with locked doors and with elevators that require special codes to enter and exit. As long as the hallway doors are locked, the residents can walk up and down the halls as much as they like. The use of electric ankle bands or wristbands that signal the doors to lock are also used in some facilities. Other interventions involve the use of motion detectors in the hallways or alarms that will go off when the person tries to get out of the bed or chair.

SOME ARE ANGRY!

For those people with dementia who need medication to treat their agitation, several different types of drugs may be used to treat aggressive behavior. At the present time, there is no FDA-approved treatment specifically for agitation associated with dementia. Benzodiazepines are the most common medication used for agitation. Examples of benzodiazepines are:

- alprazolam (Xanax)
- clonazepam (Klonopin)

- diazepam (Valium)
- lorazepam (Ativan)
- temazepam (Restoril)

This class of medication is discussed at length in chapters 8 and 25. Some seniors may actually get even more agitated when they are given a benzodiazepine. You can think of these medications as acting like alcohol. When some people get drunk they get tired and sleepy. Others get nasty, belligerent, or wild.

Because of the dangers associated with the use of benzodiazepines, there has been a great effort in the psychiatric community to find other drugs that would act as mood stabilizers. Many psychiatrists are using antiseizure drugs (such as valproic acid) as an alternative. Divalproex is a version of valproic acid that stays in your system much longer. Whether seizure medications are good mood stabilizers is unclear at the time of this writing. Some studies show a positive effect and others show none.[4] In our experience, it has helped some patients while it had no effect on others. If the doctor prescribes one of these medications, make sure that the drug levels in the blood are checked at least every six months to make sure the dose is not too high.

In some cases, an antipsychotic medication may work. The most commonly used antipsychotics are risperidone (Risperdal), olanzapine (Zyprexa), and quetiapine (Seroquel). Some patients may still be receiving older medications, such as haloperidol (Haldol). These medications were developed for treating schizophrenia. For some patients they seem to reduce the amount of aggressive and agitated behavior, while for others it does not seem to help.

Several years ago there was some evidence that the medications used to treat Alzheimer's disease, such as donepezil (Aricept), may help. Recent studies, however, have failed to show any benefit of these medications in the treatment of those people with dementia who are agitated.[5]

AND SOME COMPLETELY ACT OUT!

Another type of problem occurs when patients display psychotic behavior. We refer to seniors as being psychotic when they display one or more of the following symptoms:

- delusions
- hallucinations
- paranoia

While some people may hallucinate (see or hear things that do not exist), others may have delusions. Delusions are false beliefs that may guide a person to act in an unusual manner. The delusion that we most commonly encounter is the belief that people are "stealing my things." Other delusions may involve beliefs that someone is trying to harm them or that they are living somewhere else. This can be quite distressing to the person with dementia, who honestly believes what she is saying.

Fifty percent of people with Alzheimer's disease will exhibit psychotic symptoms during the course of their illness.[6] Psychosis is also commonly seen in people with Lewy body dementia and Parkinson's disease. In many cases the drugs used to treat Parkinson's disease can have the unwanted side effect of causing psychosis.

How do you know when someone with dementia is telling you something that is true? The **real truth** is that this is a tough question to answer. On the one hand, you do not want to ignore real complaints. The frail elderly are an easy target for crooks and con artists. Con artists know that many elderly are lonely and have memory problems in addition to hearing and vision problems. At the same time you don't want to falsely accuse anyone.

It is natural to become upset and angry when you hear your loved one making an accusation of wrongdoing. The idea of someone taking advantage of your loved one is enough to make most families enraged. While we can't speak for the specifics of your own personal experiences, in many cases there has been no theft. In the hospital or nursing home, it is still a good idea to discuss your concerns with a nursing supervisor. The supervisor may be able to help identify which employees were working on the shift in question. By the same token, if you are the one being accused, try not to get insulted or take it personally.

USING ANTIPSYCHOTIC DRUGS TO TREAT PSYCHOTIC BEHAVIOR

The newer antipsychotics are less likely to cause the abnormal facial movements and muscle rigidity seen with older agents, such as haloperidol (Haldol).[7] The most commonly used antipsychotics are olanzapine (Zyprexa), risperidone (Risperdal), and quetiapine (Seroquel).

These antipsychotic drugs are approved by the FDA for the treatment of schizophrenia. However, the FDA has not given any of these medications an official indication for the treatment of behavioral problems in people with dementia. In fact, the FDA has never approved any drug for the treatment of any behavioral problems in patients with dementia.

Do these medications work in people with dementia? In some cases they do an excellent job, and in other cases they have no effect. The largest study showed no difference between olanzapine, risperidone, quetiapine, and a placebo.[8]

If a person has already tried one or two medications without any improvement or has experienced significant side effects, it is still not unreasonable to switch to a different drug. This is because each of the drugs binds with different strengths to about ten different receptors in the body and nervous system.

DO ANTIPSYCHOTICS HAVE SIDE EFFECTS?

Some common side effects that you may encounter with these drugs:

- Zyprexa (olanzapine) is associated with weight gain, increased cholesterol levels, increased blood sugar levels, and worsening diabetes.[9]
- Risperdal (risperidone) may cause sedation or the blood pressure to drop when the user stands up.[10]
- Seroquel (quetiapine) can cause sedation. If the person has Parkinson's disease or Lewy body dementia, this is the safest antipsychotic to use.[11]

THE NEW ANTIPSYCHOTICS CAN INCREASE YOUR RISK OF DYING!

This was the conclusion of the FDA after reviewing seventeen studies involving the use of the newer antipsychotic medication in the treatment of behavioral problems in patients with dementia. The FDA was concerned that demented patients who took an antipsychotic medication seemed to have a higher risk of death when compared to those who didn't. No one really understands what is responsible for this observation. The FDA now requires that all prescriptions for antipsychotics must have a prominent warning label on the package insert.[12]

SO WHY WOULD DOCTORS RECOMMEND THESE "DANGEROUS MEDICATIONS?"

Many experts in the field think that this label is unfair because the results of seventeen different studies were combined. These studies were all different with regard to the drugs and dosages used. The bad results could have been explained by the increased death and strokes reported in just one or two of the studies.

As a matter of principle, we do not use these medications unless they are absolutely necessary. If the benefits of treating the abnormal behavior outweigh the potential risk of a medication's side effect, then we recommend proceeding with medication therapy. In many cases we have found these medications to be lifesavers for patients whose behavior threatened their well-being and that of their family or nursing home staff.

Why can't we just use the older antipsychotics? That would be nice, especially as the older ones are so much cheaper. There are two problems:

- The older drugs actually have more side effects. Older antipsychotic medications, such as Thorazine, can cause anticholinergic side effects. Haloperidol can cause involuntary movements that may mimic Parkinson's disease or appear as nonstop mouth twitching.[13]
- The supposed increased risk of dying is the same for the old drugs as well as the new ones.[14]

SOME WILL SAY SHOCKING THINGS!

Peope with dementia may say shocking things. Sometimes they can be quite rude. Always remember these people no longer have the brain cells that allow them to understand that what they say is wrong. It is not helpful to scold them or argue with them, as that will not accomplish anything. In some cases, the person can pick up on the tone of your voice and may actually become more agitated.

HOW DO WE DEAL WITH SUN-DOWNING?

As noted earlier, this term refers to the worsening of behavioral symptoms at night with improvement in behavior during the daytime. We are not sure why this occurs for so many nursing home residents and homebound people with dementia. Nor does there exist a clear strategy to deal with this problem. In some cases a low dose of an antipsychotic drug may help. Other types of medications, such as melatonin, antidepressants, and benzodiazepines, have been studied without great success. A variety of other interventions can also be tried. These include optimizing daylight exposure during the day and the use of a nightlight during the evening.

AND SOME JUST WON'T GO TO SLEEP!

Many people with dementia will wander at night and then sleep during the day. This scenario is often unbearable for caregivers. The normal sleep cycle is controlled by what we refer to as our *circadian rhythm*. The circadian rhythm can be thought of as our internal twenty-four-hour time clock that controls the cycle of sleep and waking. The circadian rhythm is regulated by several areas of the brain. One of these areas is damaged with the onset of Alzheimer's disease.

So what can be done to fix this problem? This is another tough question for which we do not have a good answer. Chapter 25 discusses at length what can be done to address sleeping problems.

Several medications are used in people with dementia despite the lack of FDA approval. Trazodone (Desyrel) is recommended by many experts for patients with dementia who need sleep medication. Trazodone is an antidepressant, but the dose used for sleep (25 mg) is far smaller than the dose used for depression (150–200 mg). Mirtazapine is an antidepressant that is commonly used in patients with dementia. The medication seems to work best for those patients with insomnia and poor appetite. Quetiapine is an antipsychotic drug that causes sleepiness. As mentioned repeatedly, no drug should ever be taken that is not prescribed by the person's physician.

GRANDMA WON'T GET OUT OF BED!

Some families will tell us that their loved one just wants to sleep all day. In this case, several things need to be checked:

- Is the patient taking drugs that cause sleepiness, fatigue, or confusion?
- Is the patient depressed? (See chapter 22.)
- Is there a thyroid problem?
- Is there an electrolyte imbalance? (Sodium and glucose levels may be abnormal.)

BEING A CAREGIVER FOR A PERSON WITH DEMENTIA IS NOT EASY

Many family members are not prepared either mentally or financially for their new responsibilities. Some even become resentful of the financial and social sacrifices they must make in order to take care of their loved ones. Many caregivers may be too ill themselves to take care of a spouse with dementia. Children may feel overwhelmed trying to care for a demented parent while trying to focus on their own jobs and families. Studies have even shown that spouses of people with dementia are more likely to suffer from depression and anxiety disorders than those who do not have this burden.[15]

TIPS FOR THE CAREGIVER

- Take advantage of community resources for adult daycare, support groups, meals on wheels, or respite care.
- Make sure you take care of yourself. If you get sick, who is going to take care of your loved one?
- Talk to your doctor if you think you are having symptoms of depression (feeling hopeless and guilty, having difficulty sleeping, difficulty concentrating, or having a poor appetite).
- Ask other family members to help.

THINGS YOU CAN DO TO MAKE THE HOUSE SAFER FOR THE PATIENT WITH DEMENTIA

- Install automatic shutoffs on appliances, such as irons and stoves.
- Install nightlights.
- Install smoke detectors.
- Make sure the house is well lit.
- Minimize cluttering of furniture.
- Remove any firearms from the house.

For many families, dealing with their loved one who is acting out can be physically overbearing and psychologically draining. Do not feel guilty if you feel that you can no longer manage to care for your loved one with dementia.

Taking care of a patient with dementia who exhibits behavioral problems is one of the most difficult problems that we face as geriatricians. In some cases, we can quickly get these behaviors under control, which improves the quality of life for both the patient and the caregiver. In other cases, it may take us several tries before we make any progress. Often times we must settle for coping with symptoms that are less unbearable rather than totally fixed.

Chapter 25

DIFFICULTY SLEEPING

Growing old, as noted earlier, is associated with a variety of age-related changes and chronic illnesses. One of these changes—poor sleep—can have a major impact upon the quality of life of seniors. It can lead to increased fatigue, confusion, and depression.

GROWING OLD AFFECTS THE QUALITY OF SLEEP

Normally, sleep is divided into two stages: *REM (rapid eye movement) sleep* and *non-REM sleep*. REM sleep is associated with dreaming. Non-REM sleep is broken into four stages. Stages 1 and 2 of non-REM sleep are associated with light sleep, while stages 3 and 4 represent the deep-sleep stages that are associated with feeling rested when a person wakes up in the morning. With aging there is a gradual decrease in the amount of time spent per night in REM sleep as well as in the deep stages of non-REM sleep.

WHY DO SO MANY OLDER ADULTS SUFFER FROM INSOMNIA?

The term *insomnia* is used to describe patients who have a difficulty falling asleep, staying asleep, or going back to sleep. More than 35 percent of older adults have difficulty falling asleep.[1] More than 25 percent have difficulty maintaining their sleep. In the majority of cases, their trouble sleeping is due to other diseases and conditions (see table 25.1).[2] In fact, many older adults may be suffering from more than one factor listed in this table.

TABLE 25.1. FACTORS THAT LEAD TO INSOMNIA IN THE ELDERLY

- Caffeine, nicotine, diet pills
- Excessive napping during the daytime/excessive time spent in bed
- Lack of bright-light exposure during the day
- Medical disorders
  - Arthritis/chronic pain
  - Benign prostatic hypertrophy (BPH)—an enlarged prostate will cause some men to wake up multiple times during the night to urinate
  - Chronic obstructive pulmonary disease (COPD)/emphysema
  - Congestive heart failure—may cause shortness of breath or cough when the patient tries to lie down
  - Dementia (see chapter 24)
  - Heartburn and gastroesophageal reflux disease (GERD)
  - Parkinson's disease
- Medications
  - Albuterol
  - Decongestants (e.g., pseudoephedrine)
  - SSRI antidepressants (e.g., fluoxetine, sertraline, citalopram)
  - Theophylline
- Noisy environment
- Psychiatric disorders (depression, generalized anxiety, substance abuse)
- Sleep disorders (sleep apnea, restless leg syndrome)[3]

SLEEP DISORDERS

What Is Sleep Apnea?

A person with sleep apnea has many periods of breath-holding spells (apnea) that occur throughout the night. During an episode of apnea, the patient is not breathing due to either a closure of the upper airway (obstructive sleep apnea) or a lack of stimuli from the brain to order one's body to breathe (central sleep apnea.)

Central sleep apnea is usually related to medical conditions such as strokes. Obstructive sleep apnea is often related to obesity and is caused by obstruction of the throat by enlarged tonsils and/or the tongue. In many cases, the tongue relaxes during sleep and falls in the back of the throat, which prevents air from being allowed into the lungs. The oxygen level drops. The brain actually senses the falling oxygen level and sends a stimulus for the patient to have a brief arousal to restore normal breathing.

A person with sleep apnea may have many breath-holding spells that will completely fragment and disrupt a night's sleep. The person may think that she is sleeping all night long, but in reality the sleep is constantly disrupted. As a result, the person may complain of falling asleep throughout the day, always feeling tired or having an inability to concentrate, memory problems, and even depression.

Does Your Loved One Have Sleep Apnea?

If you notice any of the following, you need to tell the doctor:

- excessive daytime sleepiness/fatigue
- loud, frequent snoring
- stops breathing or gasps for breath during sleep
- wakes up from sleep feeling tired and unrefreshed
- wakes up with a morning headache

If you have one of these symptoms, it does not mean that you definitely have sleep apnea, but you need to talk to your doctor. If your doctor thinks you may have sleep apnea, an overnight sleep study may be ordered to determine the type and degree of the apnea. The doctor may also send you to see a physician who specializes in sleep disorders.

Central sleep apneas are usually treated with medications and with attempts to resolve the underlying cause. Obstructive sleep apnea is usually associated with obesity, and the following recommendations are usually made for this condition:

- CPAP mask—A CPAP (continuous positive airway pressure) mask is a special, tight-fitting mask that fits over the mouth and nose. It is worn during sleep and blows air into the lungs in order to help keep the air passages open. It is often poorly tolerated by seniors, especially those with dementia.
- Limiting medications that are sedating—benzodiazepines (see chapter 8) are not only sedatives but are also muscle relaxers. They can relax the

muscles of the air passages, which can make them in a sense more floppy and harder to open for air to easily flow through.
- Surgery—most frail seniors are not candidates for surgery as they are at high risk for complications due to their frailty.
- Weight loss—this, however, might be difficult to achieve or not desired in the frail older adult (chapter 19).

What Is Restless Leg Syndrome?

We give patients a diagnosis of restless leg syndrome when they complain of one or more of the following:

- Creepy-crawly sensations in the limbs, primarily in the legs (but occasionally in the arms and trunk)
- Involuntarily jerking of the legs
- An overwhelming urge to move the legs
- Symptoms that are more severe during periods of rest and at night
- Symptoms that are relieved by movement of the leg

Ten percent of people over the age of sixty-five have this problem.[4] Restless leg syndrome is usually associated with involuntary jerking of the legs, known as *periodic limb movements in sleep* (PLMS). PLMS symptoms make it difficult both to fall asleep and to stay asleep. Persons with PLMS have numerous brief arousals throughout the night provoked by involuntary limb movements. This problem can lead to feelings of daytime tiredness or fatigue.

Many things can cause restless leg syndrome and PLMS. Some of the more common medical conditions that can cause this disorder include iron deficiency, anemia, diabetes, folate deficiency, and end-stage kidney disease. It can be made worse by certain drugs, such as antinausea agents, calcium channel blockers (used for high blood pressure), some over-the-counter antihistamines, phenytoin (Dilantin), major tranquilizers, antidepressants, as well as tobacco, alcohol, and caffeine.

The drugs of choice for treating restless leg syndrome are actually drugs that are used to treat Parkinson's disease (ropinirole and pramipexole). While other drugs are sometimes used, ropinirole and pramipexole are the only two drugs approved by the FDA at the present time for the treatment of restless leg syndrome.[5]

DRUGS ARE NOT THE ONLY ANSWER

Many patients ask their doctor for a pill that will help them sleep. Before even considering using drugs, it's a good idea to begin addressing the problem by avoiding the things that can sabotage a good night's sleep. A good night of sleep starts with good sleep "hygiene." The following are some tips for good sleep hygiene:

- Avoid alcohol.
- Avoid caffeine products, especially in the late afternoon and evening time.
- Avoid watching TV in bed or sleeping with the TV on because it is actually a stimulating medium that keeps people awake.
- Consider a white-noise machine to help decrease the amount of sleep interruptions.
- Drink a glass of milk.
- Establish a regular nighttime routine. In other words, try to go to bed and wake up at a regular time.
- Get regular exercise in the late afternoon.
- Limit fluid intake at night.
- Limit napping to about one hour a day.
- Stay out of the bed if you are not sleeping.
- Stop smoking.
- Take a warm bath/shower at least an hour before bed.
- Try not to get anxious about not sleeping.

These factors play a role at any age, but in the elderly they are particularly important since the elderly are additionally affected by the age-related factors discussed at the beginning of the chapter. We cannot overemphasize the significance of addressing these issues before starting any medication. All studies showing the effectiveness of a sleeping pill have been carried out in people who were already following the above recommendations.

Is It Okay to Take a Nap?

It is important for seniors to maintain a normal sleep-wake cycle. This means that the nighttime is for sleeping and the daytime is for being awake. Some seniors find that if they nap, they are more alert and have more energy for the rest of the day.[6] Seniors who nap during the day do not lose out on sleeping at night. However, napping should be limited to an hour or two per day.

What about a Glass of Milk?

This is not an old wives' tale. Milk contains an amino acid called *tryptophan* that can make people sleepy. Other foods that contain tryptophan include turkey and fish.

Avoid Caffeine

Caffeine is a stimulant and may interfere with sleep. Caffeine will also make you urinate more. Avoid all caffeine products at night. This includes coffee (decaf as well as regular), tea, and chocolate.

Don't Hide in the Dark

It has been shown that many frail seniors only get about five minutes of sunlight a day. Drapes and curtains should be kept open during the day. If a person is unable to go outside for twenty to thirty minutes per day, then there are light boxes that can be bought that will mimic sunlight. The use of these light boxes has been shown to be helpful in patients who seem to fall asleep too early at night and awaken too early in the morning.[7]

Is It Safe to Take a Sleeping Pill?

Many patients and families request that we prescribe something for sleep. As the old saying goes, be careful what you wish for. There are problems with all sleep medications. Some are in fact quite dangerous in the frail elderly (chapter 8).

Some prescription sleeping medicines are addicting. This applies to the benzodiazepines. Examples of benzodiazepines are:

- alprazolam (Xanax)
- chlordiazepoxide (Librium)
- clonazepam (Klonopin)
- diazepam (Valium)
- lorazepam (Ativan)
- temazepam (Restoril)

As we stated in chapter 8, the long-acting benzodiazepines (clonazepam, diazepam, and chlordiazepoxide) should never be used in the frail elderly population. Alprazolam, lorazepam, and temazepam have been shown to be effective as short-term aids for older adults who are having difficulty falling asleep. By short term we mean a period of less than two weeks. Research has shown that these medications do NOT have any benefit in the treatment of chronic insomnia.[8]

Because of the changes to the body that occur with aging, benzodiazepines will stay in the system much longer than in a younger person.[9] If an older patient takes a pill at night, she will still be affected by the medication the following morning. The lingering effects may impair the memory and increase confusion. The ability to drive safely may also be compromised after awakening the following morning.

Benzodiazepines can help you fall asleep, but the quality of sleep may be impaired. Using a benzodiazepine decreases the amount of time that the user is in deep (restful) stages of sleep. Since seniors already spend less time in the deep phases of non-REM sleep, their use of a benzodiazepine can be a big problem. Moreover, after two to three weeks, patients may become tolerant to the effects of the drug.[10] They will then need higher doses of the drug to get the same benefit. Some patients even develop a "rebound insomnia" when the medication wears off.

Remember that these drugs are addicting and increase the risk of falls. If you have undiagnosed sleep apnea, these drugs can make your symptoms worse.

Avoid Chloral Hydrate?

Chloral hydrate is an old drug that has been around since the nineteenth century. It is very cheap and comes in a liquid form. Many people have overdosed and some have died on this drug, especially if they were drinking alcohol or taking other sleeping pills.

Stay Away from Over-the-Counter Sleeping Pills?

Many nighttime cold, flu, or allergy medications containing diphenhydramine or chlorpheniramine can be purchased without a prescription. These over-the-counter medications may cause troublesome side effects in older adults.

Taking these medications may cause dry mouth, blurry vision, difficulty urinating (more common in older men), constipation, and an increased heart rate. Older adults with Alzheimer's disease may experience increased confusion and worsening of memory. Also, persons with restless leg syndrome could have worsening of the leg movements with the use of these drugs.

Table 25.2 is a list of the common over-the-counter drugs containing diphenhydramine or chlorpheniramine that you may find in your local drug store. Particularly for seniors, do not take any of these medications without first asking your doctor. Be aware that this list does not include all over-the-counter medications containing these ingredients—your pharmacy may stock other brands of cold/flu/allergy medications that contain diphenhydramine or chlorpheniramine. The pharmacist can assist you in identifying medications not included on this list.

TABLE 25.2. OVER-THE-COUNTER DRUGS CONTAINING DIPHENHYDRAMINE OR CHLORPHENIRAMINE

- Alka-Seltzer Plus (Cold/Nose & Throat)
- Alka-Seltzer PM
- Allergy Relief, Allergy Sinus Relief
- Bayer PM Extra Strength
- Bayer Select
- Bayer Select Maximum Strength Night Time Pain Relief
- Bayer Select (Allergy Sinus/Flu Relief)
- BC Allergy Sinus Cold/Multi Symptom Cold Powder
- Benadryl
- Contac Day & Night Allergy/Sinus, Contact Day & Night
- Dristan
- Excedrin PM
- Formula 44 Cough Mixture, Vicks Formula 44M Cough, Cold & Flu
- Goody's PM
- Sudafed Sinus Nighttime Plus Pain Relief
- Sudafed Cold & Allergy, Sudafed Plus, Sudafed Sinus & Allergy
- Theraflu Cold Medicine, Nighttime Strength
- Theraflu Flu, Cold & Cough
- Tylenol Allergy Sinus, Tylenol Cold Night Time, Tylenol Flu
- Vicks 44 Cold & Flu

What about a Shot of Whiskey?

Many people will have one or more drinks to help them go to bed. The problem is that alcohol, like benzodiazepines, will lower the amount of time that you spend in the deep, restful stages of sleep.[11]

ARE THERE ANY DRUGS THAT ARE SAFER?

Zolpidem (Ambien)

Because of the concerns regarding the use of benzodiazepines, many doctors like to prescribe zolpidem (Ambien) instead. This medication will start to work in about thirty minutes and does not last as long in the body as a benzodiazepine. Unlike benzodiazepines, it has no effect as an antianxiety drug and does not act as a muscle relaxer, either. It does not appear to disrupt the pattern of REM and non-REM sleep.

Like the benzodiazepines, this drug is not FDA approved for the long-term treatment of insomnia. The long-term use of this medication may lead to some withdrawal effects. The most common side effects include drowsiness, dizziness, and nausea.[12] Although the drug comes in a 5 mg and a 10 mg dose, the 5 mg pill is probably safer.

There is a newer version of the drug called Ambien CR. The CR stands for controlled release. In other words, the breakdown of the pill is slower, which in theory will allow it to work longer in your body. In low doses the CR form has been shown to be safe in seniors.[13]

Zalepon (Sonata)

Another drug that can be used is zalepon (Sonata).[14] This medication begins to work very quickly. It is metabolized by the body much quicker than the benzodiazepines or even zolpidem. Because this drug starts to work quickly, it is designed to help the person having difficulty falling asleep. Zolpidem and alprazolam, on the other hand, should be taken thirty to sixty minutes before one even goes to bed. Zalepon is metabolized quickly, so there should be much less confusion and tiredness the following morning. This medication is not addictive and has no apparent withdrawal effects. However, zalepon is not often prescribed since it is very expensive compared to other drugs.

Eszopiclone (Lunesta)

Eszopiclone has been shown to improve sleep in elderly patients.[15] This medication is not addictive and does not have any major side effects. Eszopiclone was the first drug approved by the FDA for chronic insomnia.

Melatonin

Many people have read that melatonin is a natural supplement that can be taken to improve sleep. Melatonin is a hormone made by certain cells in an area of the brain called the pineal gland. These cells release the melatonin at night, with the levels peaking between 2 and 4 AM.

We are not exactly sure of its precise role, but we do know that it seems to help regulate the body's natural daily clock. This internal clock gets signals from sunlight and darkness to help regulate the daily need to be awake and to sleep.[16] There is a dramatic decrease in the amount of the melatonin produced by the brain with aging. It is unclear that this age-related decrease in melatonin levels is associated with sleep problems.

So do melatonin supplements help with sleep? We are not sure.[17] There have been studies both in the healthy elderly and in Alzheimer's patients, showing that the use of melatonin at night can improve the quality of an elderly person's sleep. Unfortunately, the studies all used different preparations and dosages of melatonin. To make matters even more complicated, other studies have shown no benefit at all. Therefore, the possible benefit, safety, and potential drug interactions of melatonin use in the elderly is unknown at the present time.

Ramelteon (Rozerem)

This prescription medication works by binding to the same receptors in the brain as melatonin. By binding to these receptors, this medication works on the part of the brain that regulates the body's natural sleep-wake cycle. Ramelteon has been shown to slightly decrease the amount of time it takes for seniors to fall asleep.[18] This medication is nonaddicting and has no antianxiety properties. Ramelteon is not even listed as a controlled substance by the US Drug Enforcement Agency. It is also approved by the FDA for the long-term treatment of insomnia. Benzodiazepines, Sonata, and Ambien are classified as controlled substances by the Drug Enforcement Agency (DEA).[19] The prescribing of controlled substances is strictly regulated and monitored by the DEA.

Valerian

Valerian is an herbal supplement that has been shown to help people fall asleep. The doses used in these studies ranged from 400 to 900 mg. Before you rush out and buy this product, bear in mind that this supplement has not been studied in frail elderly patients. Therefore, we can make no comment here on how safe or effective it is for seniors.

Chapter 26
WHY DO PEOPLE GET BEDSORES?

First, let's clear up some of the confusion around the terms *bedsores, pressure ulcers*, and *decubiti*. All of these terms mean pretty much the same thing. Still, as we shall see, *pressure ulcers* are often caused by many factors, only one of which is pressure. *Bedsores* are wounds that can often occur in patients who sit in a chair for too long.

Regardless of what you want to call them, these wounds are very commonly seen among elderly people during the course of a nursing home or hospital stay. Seniors at especially high risk are those who are bed or chair bound, in a poor mental state, malnourished, severely ill, immobile, or unable to hold their urine.

Many people will point to the development of a bedsore as a sign of poor care or even neglect. The occurrence of pressure ulcers in a nursing home or hospital is considered a *sentinel event* by Medicare.[1] A sentinel event is defined as an "unexpected event that caused a patient serious harm or death." Among hospitalized patients, pressure ulcers are viewed by Medicare in the same light as doing surgery on the wrong site or leaving a sponge inside the patient after surgery.[2] The people who give accreditation to nursing homes also look at the percentage of people who have pressure ulcers as one way to compare the quality of care between different facilities.

Unfortunately, nursing homes that admit a lot of patients with bedsores for wound care will therefore have a higher number than those who do not. The government only sees how many you have, not if they initially occurred in the facility.

Therefore, we are not surprised that many families and even some health-care professionals become quite alarmed when they see a patient whose bedsores were "allowed to happen." We believe that people should not be so quick to judge.

In some cases the ulcers may be an unwelcome result of modern medicine's success in prolonging life among older adults who are very sick. Despite our best efforts, these vulnerable seniors have an increased risk of developing pressure ulcers. While we will discuss some of the major risk factors, remember that doctors cannot predict with absolute certainty which patients will develop pressure ulcers.

WHAT ARE THE FACTORS INVOLVED IN THE DEVELOPMENT OF BEDSORES?

Age-Related Skin Changes

One of the biggest and often overlooked risk factors for pressure ulcers derives from changes that occur with aging to the largest organ in the body: the skin. The outer layer of the skin is known as the *epidermis*, and the inner layer is known as the *dermis*. A variety of changes occur to both layers with normal aging (chapter 2). The skin thins and loses some of its blood supply. The cells of the skin also lose some of their ability to regenerate.[3]

Environmental Factors

When we use the term *environmental factors*, we are not discussing global warming or the depletion of the ozone. Instead, we are referring to four factors that can potentially harm the skin. These factors consist of excessive pressure, shear and friction, and moisture.

Excessive Pressure

Blood is pumped out of the heart at a pressure that is close to the blood pressure that is measured in your arm. Blood flows down a pressure gradient from the left side of the heart to the arteries, capillaries, veins, and finally back to the right side of the heart. It is this pressure gradient that keeps the blood flowing. While a normal blood pressure in the artery of your arm is 120/70, the pressure in the capillaries is only 32 millimeters of mercury (mm Hg). Any pressure placed on the skin that exceeds the filling pressure of the capillaries 32 mm Hg will cut off blood flow to that part of the skin tissue. Bony points (tailbone, pelvis, hip, heels, scapula) are the areas that are most vulnerable to pressure-related injuries. Sitting up in bed on a standard hospital mattress can put up to 150 mm Hg of pressure on the area around your tailbone and bottom.[4]

We have seen many patients with a bedsore in the tailbone area who were also on a feeding tube. Standard protocols require that all patients who are receiving food through a feeding tube must have the head of the bed elevated at least 30 degrees during feeding. The idea here is that elevating the head of the bed will decrease the risk of getting pneumonia (but incidentally, there is no evidence that this works). Since feeding may take place for many hours during the day, either increased pressure will be put on the sacrum (tailbone and buttocks area) or the patient will be at increased risk for aspiration.

Sitting up in a chair is even worse, as it puts over 300 mm Hg of pressure on the coccyx area.[5] You must be asking yourself: "How come I don't get pressure ulcers when I go to the theater to watch a movie or sit down to read a book about aging?" One reason is that subconsciously we keep adjusting our weight as we sit in the chair. A combination of conditions suffered by many frail elderly patients may prevent them from doing this. Another reason we do not get bedsores is that we are generally much healthier than older adults who are in the hospital or nursing home.

Shear and Friction

Shear forces occur when the skin moves laterally relative to the underlying bone, muscles, and other tissues. Shearing forces can occur when bandages are not taken off carefully, when a person slouches in a chair, or when an area of skin is massaged. With friction the surface epithelium rubs off and can cause a friction burn. It can occur by dragging a patient across the bed sheet. It can also happen when a patient keeps sliding down in bed.

Moisture

Urine and diarrhea can act as chemical irritants and as sources of moisture for the skin on the buttocks and the tailbone area. This is the same area that is most vulnerable to pressure in people who are bed bound or confined to wheelchairs.

Acute Medical Illnesses

Acute illnesses, such as a serious infection or a hip fracture, often put the body in a state where the metabolism is markedly increased. Many other changes also occur, including a decrease in appetite and an increase in the breakdown of muscle tissue. We cannot overemphasize these points enough. They are a major reason why many frail elderly get bedsores when they are admitted to the hospital or transferred to a nursing home.

As we discussed in chapter 9, hospitals have a strong financial incentive to move patients from the hospital to a skilled nursing unit at a nursing home as soon as possible. The new nursing home resident often arrives from the hospital still in this high-metabolism/high–tissue breakdown state.

All this occurs at a time when patients have a decreased appetite. When you cut back on the food, the body prioritizes where the limited fuel will go. The brain and heart come first. Muscle and skin tissue are last. In fact, the body will use its own muscle tissue as an energy source to feed the other organs.

Patients with fractures and other illnesses can end up lying in the emergency room or on an operating table for hours, causing further damage to the skin. All of this damage may not become apparent until days or weeks later.

Chronic Illnesses

Many seniors suffer from multiple diseases for which there are no cures. For example, patients with cancer, end-stage heart failure, or emphysema are often in the high-metabolism state described above. Many also become bedridden. Strokes and severe arthritis can cause patients to have trouble shifting their weight to decrease pressure. Older adults with a decreased level of consciousness or dementia often do not shift their weight to relieve pressure and may be incontinent. Seniors with diabetes or who used tobacco may have poor blood flow in the arteries of the leg, which increases the risk of pressure ulcers to the heels.

Obesity is another risk factor. The excess weight of obese patients can lead to increased pressure on areas such as the tailbone or buttocks. The areas between the fat folds may also be areas where moisture accumulates. Many obese patients have diabetes, which puts them at further risk for skin infections.

HOW ARE PRESSURE ULCERS DOCUMENTED?

In the healthcare field, we break down pressure ulcers into one of four stages, as shown below:

Stage   Skin Changes

I   Redness of the skin that does not turn white when you press on it.

II	Shallow blister that goes partially through the skin.
III	Ulcer that penetrates through the skin and into the underlying tissue.
IV	Ulcer that penetrates into the muscle, tendons, and bones.

Rating the severity of pressure ulcers is difficult. It is based on visual inspection of the appearance and the depth of tissue damage, which can only be determined after all the dead tissue is removed. If there is scab tissue (*eschar*) in place, this, too, needs to be removed before the wound can be accurately assessed. With the eschar in place, we classify these wounds as *unstageable.*

In many cases, the damage does not progress in sequence with the above staging system. In other words, skin damage doesn't always occur in the expected top-down order. In fact, considerable damage may occur to the muscle tissue days or weeks before any skin changes are noticeable. What you see at the surface may only be the tip of the iceberg. This is called a *deep tissue injury* (DTI). This point cannot be overemphasized. In some cases you may see a stage I ulcer and think that it will easily go away. After a week or two, the wound may get worse, despite a good wound care plan.

It is not uncommon for two healthcare professionals to document the same wound somewhat differently. That is why many hospitals and other facilities will either photograph the wound or use tracing paper to outline its exact dimensions.

IS THE WOUND INFECTED?

Like any open wounds, pressure ulcers are at high risk for becoming infected. It is a good idea to be on the lookout for signs of infection. These can include the drainage of pus or painful reddened tissue that extends beyond the border of the wound. In more severe cases the person can get a fever, shaking chills, or even become delirious.

WHAT CAN WE DO TO TRY TO MINIMIZE THE RISK OF GETTING A BEDSORE?

- Inspect the skin frequently. Toileting, dressing, and bathing are good opportunities to inspect the skin.
- Minimize soiling from stool and urine.

- Make sure the person is receiving enough water, protein, and calories.
- Reduce excessive pressure for bedridden patients using proper positioning, turning techniques, and specialty mattresses.
- Proper positioning—pillows or special boots are often ordered to keep the heels off the mattress. Pillows may also be placed between the knees so that they do not rub against each other.
- Turning schedule—the standard protocol for residents is to turn patients in bed every two hours. Where did this standard come from? What scientific rationale is it based on? It is in fact not based on any hard scientific research studies. Rather, it comes from the recommendation made at a national meeting of experts on bedsores in 1994, which suggested that patients need to be repositioned more frequently while sitting.[6] The truth is that no one really knows whether we should be turning people more often or less often.[7] We also do not know how far to turn patients. Should we turn them 30 degrees, 45 degrees, or even 90 degrees? Many patients actually resist these turning efforts and insist on assuming the same position for many hours.[8] Is it ethical to forcibly turn these patients even if it causes much pain and discomfort?
- There are special mattresses for patients who are not able to change positions or have multiple bedsores. There are numerous brands out there, but they can be broadly grouped into several categories. Some are thick foam pads that are placed over a regular hospital mattress, and others are expensive devices that circulate small beads or air through the mattress.

Do These Expensive Mattresses Work Any Better?

No one really knows if the air mattresses work better than placing a six-inch foam pad over a standard hospital mattress. One problem is that there are too many different products out there to compare. Many of the studies looking at the effectiveness of these products did not involve frail older adults. Another concern is that the air/fluid mattresses often lose their effectiveness if the head of the bed is elevated.[9]

CAN YOU PREVENT BEDSORES IN FRAIL SENIORS?

As geriatricians, even we can't tell you for certain which patients are going to have skin breakdown and which ones aren't. While the steps we listed above may decrease the risk of bedsores to a degree, they cannot totally prevent skin break-down. There is a belief among many healthcare professionals that if a senior gets a bedsore, it is proof that he received poor care. To equate the formation of a bedsore with poor care is too simplistic. For patients who are seriously ill or who are dying, no one can guarantee that the skin will remain intact.

TREATING PRESSURE ULCERS IS NOT EASY

Knowing what to do is difficult because interventions that have been shown to be of benefit in the trauma or spinal cord injury population may be ineffective or poorly studied in the frail elderly. This distinction is important because the ninety-five-year-old has underlying skin changes, biochemical changes, and chronic medical illnesses that are not present in the younger patients.

Numerous ointments, dressings, and other products exist for treating pressure ulcers. There are so many different products that no one has enough experience using all of them. The best type of products to be used will depend on the location, size, depth, and drainage of the wound.

That being said, some basic principles apply: The treatment of stage I ulcers does not require any surgery or cutting. What is needed is to relieve the pressure from that area. The idea is to redistribute pressure over a larger surface area rather than have it all focused on one spot on the skin. This may require repositioning cushions or using padding when sitting. Careful positioning is also needed when lying in bed. If there are stage I ulcers on the heels, then elevating them and placing special pressure-relieving boots on the feet is essential.

In many cases, a pressure ulcer that is not infected and has adequate blood flow may show some improvement in two to four weeks. While the healthcare team may try their best, it is important to realize that the majority of stage III and stage IV deep pressure ulcers will NOT heal in frail elderly residents.[10]

The treatment of deep pressure ulcers involves the removal of infected and dead tissue from the wounds. Sometimes the scablike covering (*eschar*) needs to be removed in order to fully assess and treat the wound.

The process of removing tissue from the wound is often referred to as *debridement*. Debridement can be done in a variety of ways. There are creams that are placed on the wounds containing enzymes that slowly dissolve the dead tissue. Many types of special bandage dressings can also assist in the debridement process. For large wounds or for wounds with evidence of infection, the dead tissue may need to be removed surgically. Oftentimes, doctors are not able to remove all the dead tissue at one time and the person will need to go back for several treatment sessions.

For wounds that no longer have dead tissue and are not infected, platelet-derived growth factor (PDGF) gel may be ordered. Studies have shown that applying PDGF gel (Regranex) to diabetic ulcers of the foot can stimulate normal tissue to regrow and may help speed up the healing of the wound.[11]

HOW IMPORTANT IS GOOD NUTRITION?

Medical research has shown that addressing nutritional issues can lower the risk of bedsores forming in nursing home residents. It has also been shown among young paralyzed patients and critically ill hospitalized patients that increasing the amount of food and nutrition can increase the chances that a pressure ulcer will heal.

Unfortunately, the pressure ulcers that occur in the frail elderly often do not heal even with aggressive nutritional support. Recall in chapter 18 when we discussed the concept of *cachexia*: we stated that many sick patients are in a state of rapid protein and tissue breakdown. For many patients this poorly understood state cannot simply be reversed with some extra calories. Newer approaches to treat cachexia will hopefully be developed in the future.

Some healthcare professionals will recommend the use of vitamin C or zinc in order to improve wound healing. What limited data are available suggest that vitamin C and zinc have no benefit in healing the wounds of frail elderly patients.[12] Some people may advocate the use of special amino acid supplements to help promote wound healing. While there is some evidence that this may work in younger people, it is still too early to tell whether the amino acid arginine promotes wound healing in the frail elderly. Although these three supplements are generally very safe, you should talk to your doctor before using any of these products.

ARE THERE ANY PEOPLE WHO ARE EXPERTS IN DEALING WITH THESE WOUNDS?

In the hospital or nursing home, the patient will be seen by a certified wound care nurse who has special training in the management of pressure ulcers. The nurse will make recommendations to the doctor regarding the equipment needed to provide pressure relief and the types of dressings and treatments needed to treat this wound.

In some cases the doctor may refer the patient to a surgeon for further recommendations. The doctor may even refer the patient to an outpatient wound care center if there is one available in the community. This type of center focuses exclusively on difficult-to-heal wounds. It may be staffed by physicians with expertise in fields such as plastic surgery, vascular surgery, podiatry, and infectious disease.

WHAT IF THE ULCER IS NOT HEALING?

Some pressure ulcers may extend down to the bone, causing an infection known as *osteomyelitis*. The doctor will often order blood work, an x-ray, a bone scan, or even an MRI to help make that diagnosis. These bone infections are difficult to heal without the use of antibiotics for several months and/or surgical removal of the infected bone.

For severe ulcers on the sacral area, *diverting colostomies* are done in order to prevent stools from continuously contaminating a wound. In this procedure the fecal material in the colon is diverted to come out into a pouch in the abdomen rather than through the rectum.

Many families ask if a Foley catheter can be placed to help lower the potential for urine to contribute to the creation and growth of a bedsore. While this may seem to make sense, remember that Foley catheters greatly increase the risk of urinary tract infections. To minimize soiling from urine, most doctors recommend using a Foley catheter only if the patient has a stage III or IV bedsore on the buttocks or tailbone area.

In some cases, the doctor may order a *vacuum assisted closure* (VAC) *device* to help try to get the wound to close faster. With this device, special dressings are hooked up to a vacuum pump that applies negative pressure to the wound. This allows for the removal of harmful substances from the wound and for some patients it may promote faster wound healing.[13]

THINGS YOU CAN DO FOR A FAMILY MEMBER

- Ask if there is an outpatient wound care center in the community.
- Assist with turning or with reminding the patient to shift from side to side when sitting in a chair.
- Do not massage the skin over the tailbone and or buttocks.
- Do not bring any donut-shaped cushions for comfort when sitting.
- Encourage the patient to eat to maintain good nutrition.
- Make sure the patient is wearing the pressure-relieving boots.

Chapter 27

WHAT CAN BE DONE TO CONTROL PAIN?

Chronic pain is more common in the elderly than in any other age group. For example, 40 to 80 percent of nursing home residents have complaints of pain. The majority of these complaints are due to arthritis and lower back pain (*nociceptive pain*). Other seniors may suffer from what is known as *neuropathic pain*, which is a complex type of pain due to damage to the nerves. Neuropathic pain often presents as:

- burning in the feet of patients with long-standing diabetes
- burning in an area of skin due to shingles
- burning in the hands due to carpal tunnel syndrome

WHY IS IT SO IMPORTANT TO ASSESS PAIN?

Healthcare workers often get so busy taking care of the patient's numerous medical problems that they can forget to ask about pain. Many seniors will not complain of their pain, as they believe that this is part of the normal aging process. Others won't complain of pain because they are concerned that they will be put on potentially dangerous medications.

Failure to treat pain can have a serious impact on the quality of the person's life. Think about how hard it would be to do simple household chores if you were suffering from pain. Now try to think about how hard it would be to fall asleep at night if you were having severe hip, knee, or lower back pain. Social activities, such as walking in the mall or dancing, are also hard to do if you are in pain.

There is a strong association between chronic pain and depression. In many cases they are often greatly intertwined. People with chronic pain often become depressed. Those with depression may have a lower threshold for experiencing pain. It has been our experience that people who are depressed are less likely to comply with their physical therapy. Therefore, the recognition and treatment of depression becomes an important component of chronic pain therapy.

Pain in the legs and back may also lead to an increased risk of falls and deconditioning. As with many issues in geriatrics, pain is often due to a variety of complicated factors. Medication alone is often not enough to treat chronic pain. Other avenues exist as well.

ARE YOU IN PAIN?

All seniors should be assessed for pain. Doctors and nurses will often ask the patient, "Are you experiencing pain?" If the answer is yes, the next question is to quantify the pain on a scale of zero to ten. Zero is for no pain. Ten is for unbearable pain. If you are a caregiver, you can ask your loved one the same question.

For seniors with dementia, scales used to quantify the amount of pain may not be helpful. Some may not even be able to say, "Hey, I am having pain!" Others may be able to complain of pain but won't be able to remember how this pain compares to previous episodes of pain.

So how can we tell whether a person with dementia is having pain? The answer is that it is not easy. Some of the signs that we look for include:

- aggression (hitting, biting)
- crying or moaning
- facial wrinkling or grimacing
- guarding an area of the body
- irritability or greater confusion

WHAT CAUSES PAIN?

The sensation of pain is a complex process of our nervous system that allows us to sense danger in the environment. Our skin, muscles, and joints contain receptors that, when damaged, send signals via the nerves to sections of the spinal cord and then to specific parts of the brain. At certain points in the process, the brain sends back signals to the nerves that may change how the pain is being perceived. Understanding this pathway helps to highlight the most effective areas to target pain therapy. There are many treatment options available. We will discuss the use of medications first and then we will discuss other things that can be done to decrease pain.

SOME GENERAL PRINCIPLES ABOUT PAIN MEDICATIONS IN THE ELDERLY

- "Start low and go slow." What this means is that older adults are more sensitive to the effects of medication (see chapter 8). In order to minimize the risks of drug side effects, we try to start out at a low dose and increase the dose slowly.
- Taking medications on a specific schedule may be more effective than waiting for the pain to become severe.
- Using several medications at a low dose rather than high doses of a single drug may lower the potential risk of bad side effects.

Acetaminophen (Tylenol)

Acetaminophen is often the first drug ordered for the treatment of mild or moderate pain. Acetaminophen can be purchased over the counter. We are all familiar with Tylenol, which is one of the brand names for acetaminophen. Acetaminophen is also mixed with many narcotics, such as Lortab or Tylenol #3.

How does acetaminophen work? It is surprising that after all these years we are still not exactly sure how this drug works. We do know that it does **not** decrease inflammation.

Is it a good pain reliever? Many patients get angry when we suggest that they try acetaminophen because they claim that they already took it and it did not work. Upon further questioning, it turns out that they took only one or two pills. Several studies have shown that acetaminophen provides as much pain relief as the nonsteroidal anti-inflammatory drugs ibuprofen (Advil, Motrin)[1] and celecoxib (Celebrex).[2] In these studies, acetaminophen was taken at very high doses (1,300 mg three times daily). The standard Tylenol pill is 325 mg and the extra-strength pills are 500 or 650 mg. The package insert says not to exceed the 4-gram-per-day maximum dose, as Tylenol intoxication can severely damage the liver. We generally recommend that seniors not exceed 3 grams per day. If you have liver disease or hepatitis, or if you drink alcohol, you should talk to your doctor before you take any Tylenol.

Nonsteroidal Anti-inflammatory Drugs (NSAIDs)

Nonsteroidal anti-inflammatory drugs (NSAIDs) work by decreasing inflammation. Some NSAIDs are available over the counter and others require a prescription. Even those purchased over the counter can potentially cause some serious side effects. Table 27.1 lists the more commonly used NSAIDs.

TABLE 27.1. COMMONLY USED NSAIDS

- celecoxib (Celebrex)
- diclofenac (Voltaren, Arthrotec)
- etodolac (Lodine)
- ibuprofen (Advil, Motrin)
- indomethacin (Indocin)
- ketolac (Toradol)
- ketoprofen (Orudis, Oruvail)
- meloxicam (Mobic)
- nabumetone (Relafen)
- naproxen (Naprosyn, Aleve, Anaprox)
- oxaprozin (Daypro)
- piroxicam (Feldene)
- sulindac (Clinoril)

Even those purchased over the counter can cause some serious side effects:

- heart attacks
- increased high blood pressure
- kidney damage
- stomach bleeding
- stomach ulcers

The increased risk of stomach ulcers is quite serious. Twenty percent of patients who use NSAIDs long term will develop ulcers.[3] The patients at the highest risk for serious bleeding from NSAIDs are those over the age of seventy and those with a prior history of stomach ulcers. The higher the dose and the longer this medication is used, the greater the risk. These medications should be used with extreme caution if you are on blood thinners such as war-farin (Coumadin), aspirin/dipyridamole (Aggrenox), clopidogrel (Plavix), or enoxaparin (Lovenox).

If you are going to use one of these over-the-counter medications, make sure you tell your doctor. You may be told to take a pill such as omeprazole (Prilosec) or famotidine (Pepcid) to help lower your risk of ulcers from the NSAID.

All NSAIDs are not equal. Some pose a much higher risk of causing bleeding ulcers. Table 27.2 compares the risk among the different NSAIDs.[4]

TABLE 27.2. RISK OF GASTROINTESTINAL BLEEDING IN OLDER ADULTS WHO USE NSAIDS

NSAID	Increase in Risk (compared to ibuprofen)
ibuprofen (Motrin, Advil)	Baseline of 100 percent
diclofenac (Voltaren)	180 percent
naproxen (Naprosyn)	220 percent
indomethacin (Indocin)	240 percent
piroxicam (Feldene)	380 percent

NSAIDs can also potentially injure the kidneys. The kidneys can be dam-aged through a variety of complicated mechanisms. The kidneys are espe-cially at risk of being damaged when a person becomes dehydrated due to diarrhea, fever, vomiting, or a very poor appetite. If you suffer from hyper-tension, don't forget that NSAIDs can also raise your blood pressure.

Is Celecoxib (Celebrex) Safer?

The main benefit of Celebrex is that it causes fewer ulcers compared to the other NSAIDs.[5] The pain relief is equal between Celebrex and older drugs, such as ibuprofen. However, the dosage of ibuprofen used in these studies was quite high (for example, 800 mg of ibuprofen was taken three times a day). This is a large dose when you consider that an Advil tablet contains 200 mg of ibuprofen.

Celebrex is no safer but no worse for your kidneys than other NSAIDs. While safer than Vioxx, the FDA determined that the long-term use of prob-ably **all** NSAIDs is associated with a higher risk of heart attacks when they are compared to a placebo.[6] For these reasons, Celebrex is a good, safe option for short-term pain management in older adults.

What Happened with Vioxx?

In the late 1990s, Celebrex and Vioxx were developed as safer alternatives to traditional NSAIDs. Research showed that these medications had a lower risk of stomach ulcers and gastrointestinal bleeding as compared to other NSAIDs.[7]

When people looked more closely at the results of these studies, however, they found that patients who received Vioxx had a higher rate of heart attacks than those who took Naprosyn. Vioxx was then pulled from the market several years later after a study showed that patients who took Vioxx had a higher risk of heart attacks compared to those who took a placebo agent (see chapter 4 for an explanation on the use of a placebo in drug research studies).

What about Meloxicam (Mobic)?

Meloxicam is another NSAID said to have a similar benefit as Celebrex with regard to the prevention of stomach ulcers. At the dose of 7.5 mg, there is a lower risk of ulcers, but at 15 mg, the risk is similar to other NSAIDs.[8]

Don't Use Indomethacin (Indocin)!

Indomethacin is a commonly used NSAID that should not be used in the elderly. It has a higher risk of causing stomach ulcers when compared to ibuprofen. In addition, indomethacin can actually cause some older adults to become delirious.[9]

NSAIDs Can Be Applied to the Skin

While we usually think of NSAIDs as pills, they can also be made into creams and lotions. Many studies have shown that these topical medications are effective for use in people who have acute and chronic pain. Topical creams and lotions using ketoprofen, ibuprofen, and piroxicam have been shown to work.[10] These medications seem to work in the joints and barely get absorbed into the blood, where they can damage the kidneys and stomach.[11] These creams are not available at your standard pharmacies. You need to go to what's called a *specialty pharmacy*. The specialty pharmacy will make this cream for you. They will often mix it with lidocaine, which helps numb the skin. The cream can be applied directly to the skin or through an ultrasound machine that delivers the medication to the deeper tissue layers.[12] Another option your doctor has is to prescribe the diclofenac patch (Flector). This patch is FDA approved for the treatment of pain due to minor strains, sprains, and contusions.

There is also a lidocaine patch (Lidoderm) that is applied to the skin daily. This patch is used to treat nerve pains, such as those that occur with herniated discs in the lower back.

What about Glucosamine?

Glucosamine is a compound that is found in many arthritis nutritional supplements. At the beginning of the decade there were several major studies showing that glucosamine could improve the pain symptoms and decrease the damage that arthritis can do to the knees. More recent studies have shown no benefit.[13]

If you look closely at the labels for glucosamine products, you will see that chondroitin sulfate is also added. Research does not show any benefit from chondroitin.[14] Fortunately, both glucosamine and chondroitin sulfate seem to be very safe.

What about Fish Oil?

If you go on the Internet you will see numerous Web sites describing the benefits of fish oil in treating arthritis pain. At the present time it appears that fish oil may have some anti-inflammatory properties at high doses.[15] If you are taking this medication for your arthritis, it may take up to four weeks to notice an effect. If you are taking an NSAID or aspirin, do not expect the fish oil to work. Taking an NSAID on the same days you are taking omega-3 fatty acids may block the anti-inflammatory effects of the omega-3 fatty acids.

WHEN SHOULD A NARCOTIC BE PRESCRIBED?

Narcotic medications are often prescribed for severe pain. There are many different narcotic medications on the market. They can be broken down into two general categories. The short-acting ones begin to take effect quickly and last for several hours. These medications are prescribed for the new onset of pain. Examples of short-acting agents include Percocet, Tylenol #3, oxycodone, and Lortab.

For patients who require chronic pain relief, a long-acting agent is used. These medications act for twelve to twenty-four hours to provide a more stable control of the pain symptoms, but they take longer to begin working. Examples of long-acting narcotics include OxyContin, MS Contin, Kadian, Roxanol, and methadone. Even while the patient is taking a long-acting narcotic, he should always have a short-acting narcotic ordered in case pain should arise at some point during the day or night.

WHAT IF THE PATIENT CAN'T SWALLOW A PILL?

Many seniors are unable to swallow pills when they become very ill. Some people with dementia will adamantly refuse to swallow pills. We already discussed the use of NSAID creams and the lidocaine patch (Lidoderm). There is also a narcotic patch that can be applied every seventy-two hours for long-acting pain control. This patch goes by the name of fentanyl (Duragesic). It can take anywhere from six to twelve hours to begin working. After the patch is removed, it may take up to twenty-four hours for the drug to work its way out of the body.

There are preparations of morphine that can be placed under the tongue or on the lining of the cheek. Both of these areas are moist mucous membranes that allow drugs to be easily absorbed into the bloodstream.

Many doctors who work with hospice patients have found that inhaling morphine as a vapor is also effective. Like the lining of your mouth, the lining of the lungs is a great way for certain medications to be absorbed into the bloodstream. Remember that the function of the lungs is to absorb oxygen and transfer it to the bloodstream.

The inhalation of morphine is not something that we recommend for the chronic treatment of pain. Its two most common uses are in the emergency setting for trauma-related pain and in the care of the dying patient.

ARE NARCOTICS ADDICTIVE?

Many physicians are reluctant to order narcotics due to a fear that the senior will become addicted to the medication. The prescribing of narcotics and benzodiazepines is monitored by the DEA. Physicians can get in trouble for prescribing these medications inappropriately.

In some cases, people suffering from drug addiction come to the office asking or even demanding a prescription for narcotics. However, studies have shown that it is very rare for people with serious pain to become addicted to narcotics if they are using the medication correctly.

SIDE EFFECTS OF NARCOTICS

Older adults need to be careful when taking narcotics. Morphine, for example, may have more of an effect in the elderly than in younger patients. It also takes 50 percent longer for the elderly body to metabolize the narcotic. Narcotics may make patients appear more lethargic (i.e., stoned). They are also associated with constipation in the elderly. There is an increase in the number of opiate receptors in the cells of the wall of the colon. Therefore, narcotic (opioid) medications will have a greater effect at slowing down the movement of an older person's colon. Seniors who are prescribed narcotic medications should be given a medication that will help with their bowel movements. Additional side effects of narcotics include:

- decreased drive to breathe
- decreased blood pressure
- difficulty urinating
- itching
- nausea

> Any of these side effects may have a major impact on the ability to provide rehab (chapter 16). In some cases, your doctor may add other pain medications, such as an NSAID, in order to help reduce the amount of narcotic needed.

In theory, you may want to avoid long-acting morphine in patients with bad kidneys, as morphine is broken down by the kidneys.[16] Another subtle danger is the potential for acetaminophen liver damage. Many narcotics pills listed in table 27.3 are mixed with acetaminophen (Tylenol).

TABLE 27.3. NARCOTICS CONTAINING ACETAMINOPHEN

- Darvocet (propoxyphene and acetaminophen)
- Lortab, Lorcet, Vicodin, Zydone (hydrocodone and acetaminophen)
- Percocet, Roxicet, Tylox (oxycodone and acetaminophen)
- Ultracet (tramadol and acetaminophen)

The medications in table 27.3 contain acetominophen. Too much acetominophen can cause liver damage. Avoid taking over-the-counter acetominophen if you take these drugs.

WHAT IS A PCA PUMP?

For patients with severe pain, the use of *patient-controlled analgesia* (PCA) *pump* has increased in popularity. PCA pumps are very commonly used in the hospital to treat patients following surgery or with cancer pain. The PCA pump utilizes an IV form of either morphine, fentanyl, or hydromorphone. The IV medication will be set so that there is often a low, continuous infusion rate. If the patient is still having pain, all he has to do is press a button and he will receive a set amount of medication from the IV. The patient-controlled dose and the rate at which he can push the button can be adjusted to prevent the administration of excessive medication. Compared with the standard practice of taking narcotic pills, patients who use a PCA pump use less of the drug, have less sedation, and experience fewer of the complications associated with narcotics.[17]

WHAT IS TRAMADOL (ULTRAM, ULTRAM ER)?

Tramadol is a medication that binds to the same receptors in the nervous system as narcotics. Technically this medication is not addictive, but it should be avoided in patients with a history of drug abuse. In addition, this drug does not cause the decreased drive to breathe that we see with narcotic pain medications.[18] Some seniors report feeling nauseous or dizzy when they take this medication.[19]

In theory, this medication should not be taken if you are taking an antidepressant such as fluoxetine (Prozac), paroxetine (Paxil), sertraline (Zoloft), citalopram (Celexa), escitalopram (Lexapro), venlafaxine (Effexor), or duloxetine (Cymbalta). The medication is available in an extended-release form (Ultram ER).

WHAT ABOUT MUSCLE RELAXERS?

Many cases of musculoskeletal pain involve small areas of muscle spasms known as *trigger points*. There are medicines out there for these conditions that are referred to as *muscle relaxers*. On the surface this sounds great: a muscle relaxer for a muscle spasm. The truth is that some of these medications, such as methocarbamol (Robaxin) and cyclobenzaprine (Flexeril), do not appear to have any benefit in the treatment of localized muscle spasms. These medications can cause a variety of side effects, including dry mouth, constipation, a drop in blood pressure upon standing, and increased confusion.[20]

ANTIDEPRESSANT DRUGS USED FOR PAIN?

Antidepressants are sometimes used to treat pain that is due to damage of the nerves. Seniors with long-standing diabetes may get a burning sensation in their legs. Herpes zoster (shingles) may lead to a similar burning sensation at an affected skin area. Examples of the types of antidepressants used in these cases include amitriptyline (Elavil), doxepin (Sinequan), and nortriptyline (Pamelor). These medications are virtually never used to treat seniors with depression any more because they have some very severe side effects. Even at low doses, these drugs can cause side effects. The dose used for pain relief is only a small fraction of the dose used to treat depression. So if the person is also depressed, another antidepressant will be needed.

Two of the newer antidepressants—venlafaxine (Effexor) and duloxetine (Cymbalta)—have been shown to be effective for the treatment of pain associated with diabetic peripheral neuropathy. Both drugs are commonly used to treat depression in the elderly.

Fluoxetine (Prozac), sertraline (Zoloft), paroxetine (Paxil), citalopram (Celexa), escitalopram (Lexapro), bupropion (Wellbutrin), mirtazapine (Remeron), and buspirone (Buspar) are other antidepressants drugs. They do not have a role in pain relief. However, many seniors with chronic pain may become depressed. Addressing symptoms of depression is an important component in the treatment of chronic pain issues.

SEIZURE MEDICATIONS USED FOR PAIN?

The doctor may recommend a seizure medication to help with the pain. The most commonly used seizure medications are gabapentin (Neurontin), pregabalin (Lyrica), and tegretol. These medications are generally not helpful for arthritis pain, however. Where they are most effective is in the treatment of pain due to nerve damage, for example, from long-standing diabetes. The idea here is that the seizure medications may help to slow down the transmission of nerve impulses from the peripheral nerves to the brain.

WHAT ELSE CAN BE USED TO TREAT PAIN BESIDES MEDICATIONS?

We live in a society where people generally have no patience. People want immediate results. It does not matter that it took many years for their arthritis to form. Many people like pain pills because they work so quickly. Doctors and patients must always remember that nearly all medications have potential side effects. For pain medications to have their best chance of working, it is important to utilize them in conjunction with nondrug treatments.

A variety of nondrug treatments are available:

- physical therapy
- assistive devices such as canes, walkers, braces, and even shoe insoles
- biofeedback
- cognitive behavior therapy
- electrical stimulation
- heating pads
- hydrotherapy
- massage therapy
- surgical intervention (not based on x-rays)
- weight loss

Do I Really Need to See a Physical Therapist?

Physical therapy has helped many seniors regain their mobility by improving muscle strength, flexibility, and strength (chapter 16). Physical therapists also use a variety of modalities, such as ultrasound, heat, and localized deep tissue massage to provide pain relief.[21] A good physical therapist will also provide an opportunity to address the poor body mechanics that continue to aggravate the pain. They can show the patient what needs to be done to minimize the stress on the body when sleeping, sitting, driving, exercising, and so on.

Canes and Walkers

In chapter 17, we discussed that when used properly, a cane can take some of the weight off a bad hip or knee. Walkers can provide a similar benefit.

Shoe Insoles

We see many elderly people with arthritis of their hips or knees who have a variety of foot problems. In many cases fallen arches shift the angle of the knees and hips. Properly fitting shoes with arch support may help provide more support for the hip, knee, and lower back.

Why Does My Doctor Keep Nagging Me to Lose Weight?

We cannot overemphasize how important it is for obese patients to lose weight. We see many obese patients complaining of hip, knee, and lower back pain. Many get upset when you tell them that they need to lose some weight. But as doctors we have to be honest and tell patients the truth. The extra weight is more of a load for the hips and knees to carry. A big belly puts added stress on the lower back. Many obese patients are limited in their ability to exercise due to their weight, arthritis, and chronic illnesses.

WHAT ABOUT ALTERNATIVE MEDICINE?

Many patients with pain are drawn to alternative medicine therapies out of a fear or distrust of the traditional medical system. For young adults this attitude usually does not lead to any problems as most young and middle-aged adults are generally healthy. For the elderly who may suffer from many illnesses, the rejection of modern healthcare can be dangerous. You need to be cautious when considering treatment by alternative medicine providers who claim to have cured illnesses that doctors and hospitals couldn't.

While some of these alternative therapies may have a beneficial role in treating people, we prefer to use the term *complementary medicine* instead. The term *alternative medicine* implies that the therapy is used in place of conventional treatment. Complementary medicine therapy should be used to supplement conventional treatment, not replace it, in order for you to have the best chance at treatment and recovery.

Does Acupuncture Work?

About 1 million US consumers use acupuncture each year. Many studies have tried to determine whether acupuncture is helpful in treating chronic pain. Some have shown a benefit, but just as many have shown no difference.

One large recent study looked at the use of acupuncture in patients with fibromyalgia.[22] Fibromyalgia is a disorder where patients complain of severe pain in many different parts of the body. It is different from arthritis, which is a destructive process of the joints. No one is really sure what causes fibromyalgia or how to treat it. In this study, patients were randomized to receive acupuncture versus "sham acupuncture" (randomly placing acupuncture needles under the skin). Acupuncture was no better than sham acupuncture at relieving fibromyalgia pain.

Two recent studies compared traditional Chinese acupuncture versus sham acupuncture versus doctor visits without any acupuncture.[23] Pain relief was equal in both the acupuncture and the sham acupuncture groups. The pain relief was better for both of these groups compared to the group that only had the doctor visits. The authors concluded that the benefit seen in the acupuncture group could be due to the placebo effect or from some unknown beneficial effect of needling.

Can a Chiropractor Help?

Chiropractic care is based on the principle that good health results from a spine that is well aligned. If the bones of the spine are not well aligned, a variety of illnesses may result. It is unclear whether spinal manipulation will improve back pain in the elderly. While chiropractic adjustments are generally safe in younger and middle-aged patients, there are several things that the elderly patient needs to be beware of:

- The spine of an older adult may be more fragile due to osteoporosis.
- The spine of an older adult is also more difficult to adjust. Many will have spinal conditions, such as a hunched back.
- Inappropriate neck movements in patients with atherosclerosis of the carotid artery (the arteries that travel through the neck to supply the brain with blood) can in theory cause a stroke.[24]
- Chiropractors have expertise treating muscles and bones but not in the care of patients with multiple chronic medical illnesses. Remember, even medical doctors are often not knowledgeable about all the complexities of healthcare of the elderly. Do not rely solely on a chiropractor for medical diagnoses and treatments.

AM I TOO OLD FOR SURGERY?

Each year, many elderly people have their hips and knees replaced. For the large majority, there are no significant problems after the surgery. With advances in anesthesiology and surgical technique, doctors are now able to operate on older adults who would have been labeled as "too weak" years ago.

With that said, we must remember that we are talking about elective surgery here. If you have a fracture or dislocation, that is a completely different topic (chapter 15). The decision to undergo surgery should never be taken lightly. Surgery of the hip or knee should not be done just because your x-ray looks terrible or your knee looks bad. It should be a last resort for people whose lives have been severely impaired by their arthritis. Many of these people can neither tolerate nor get significant benefit from pain medications. Many have already tried the other nondrug treatments listed above.

One should always be aware of the risks prior to undergoing any operation. If you have questions about the surgery, do not be embarrassed about asking.

THINGS YOU CAN DO TO HELP!

- Discuss with your loved one the importance of telling the hospital or nursing home staff if he or she is experiencing pain.
- Make sure to tell the doctor:
    - what makes the pain better or worse.
    - what times of the day it is better or worse.
- If the pain is not being controlled, then ask to see a pain specialist.
- Discuss with the doctor any alternatives to drugs that may help in treating pain.

Part 4

PLANNING AHEAD
BEFORE IT'S TOO LATE

Chapter 28

GROWING OLD IS EXPENSIVE

"I will be eighty-three years old on December 12 and I've decided to retire while I'm still young."
Bob Barker, on announcing his retirement from
The Price Is Right

When most people think about retiring, they often have visions of the fun things they will do in their free time. Retirement offers more time to play golf and tennis. Or maybe it is finally time to plan a vacation to the Fiji Islands or to Greece.

For many seniors, such dreams are interrupted by the economic realities of growing old in the twenty-first century. As we discussed in the previous chapters, people are living longer now with more medical problems than ever before in human history. The **real truth** is that the longer you live, the more money you will need to get you through your later years. In this chapter, we will tell you what to expect and how to prepare for this financial challenge.

BEFORE YOU BEGIN SAVING, YOU NEED TO THINK ABOUT A FEW THINGS

In the 1960s if a man retired from work at age sixty-five, he had an average life expectancy of four years.[1] Today's retirees, many of whom are women, can expect to live an average of almost twenty years after their sixty-fifth birthday. This means that you are going to have to do some very careful long-term planning. So before you can try to figure out how much money you need to save, you need to think about a few things:

- At what age do you want to stop working?
  - Will you become ill or forced to retire early?
  - Are you going to work part-time after you retire?
- What type of lifestyle do you want to lead during retirement?
  - Are you going to live in a small one-bedroom condominium, or are you going to need a summer home as well?
  - Do you plan on eating out a lot?
  - Are you going to do a lot of traveling?
- How much money have you saved?
- How long do you plan to live?

SO HOW MUCH MONEY WILL YOU NEED?

The conventional wisdom is that you need to save enough money so that your investments will bring in the equivalent of 70 to 80 percent of your preretirement income. So how much does a person need to save? It depends on how early you start. People in their twenties need to save only about 10 percent of their incomes while those who have waited until their forties may need about 30 percent.[2]

If you are able to save only 25 percent instead of 30 percent, you may still be doing much better than many of your friends. Many people have almost nothing saved. Studies have shown that nearly 60 percent of American workers have less than fifty thousand dollars—excluding the value of their home and IRA/401(k)—set aside for their retirement.[3] The key is to start saving right now! There is no government tooth fairy that will provide this money for you.

WARNING! EVEN THE BEST PLANS CAN SOMETIMES FALL APART

Almost all financial planning assumes that over the long haul, investments will increase in value. It is further assumed that the financial markets will not take a nose dive and inflation will not skyrocket at the time you are ready to retire.

Unfortunately, in 2007 both the housing market and the stock market began to tank. Many companies have either stopped or cut back on their stock dividends. Bank and CD interest rates have fallen as well. If that wasn't bad enough, seniors have more high-inflation expenses (property taxes, insurance premiums, healthcare, and long-term care costs) than younger adults.[4]

For baby boomers looking to retire and for retirees on fixed incomes, this spells trouble. What they face is a world in which their assets are decreasing while their expenses are skyrocketing. For the time being, the overall inflation rate is low. Should the inflation rate increase like it did in the 1970s, retirees will find themselves in even bigger trouble.

To make matters even more complicated, there is no guarantee of how long someone will live once he reaches retirement. There are tables that can tell you a person's average life expectancy when he turns sixty-five. The problem with an average number is that most people either live longer or shorter than it. If you guess wrong you could spend all your money and then be broke for ten to twenty years. On the flip side, you could live like a cheapskate and die early with a lot of money in the bank.

HEALTHCARE COSTS ARE INCREASING

For decades, healthcare costs have been increasing much faster than the general inflation rate. Studies have been conducted to estimate the amount of money that a sixty-five-year-old couple will need in order to pay the healthcare expenses not covered by Medicare. Fidelity estimates that a sixty-five-year-old couple will need about $225,000 to pay for the medical costs not covered by Medicare.[5]

Does $225,000 seem too high? Actually, it may be low. This figure does not include the cost of nursing home care. It also assumes that there are no future Medicare cuts. Medicare may start running deficits in the near future and some say it is slated for bankruptcy in the year 2019.[6] Rest assured that the government will be scaling back benefits to seniors. As the cost of this program to taxpayers continues to skyrocket, seniors will almost certainly be asked to pay for a larger share of the costs.

CAN YOU AFFORD LONG-TERM CARE?

In chapter 12 we tried to provide you with advice about how to choose a nursing home. Before you go out and start looking at facilities, you need to know how much this would cost.

For the 50 percent of residents who are not poor enough to qualify for Medicaid, long-term care can be an enormous expense. The average cost for nursing home care in 2007 was $68,985 per year.[7] This is for a semiprivate room. Would you like a roommate who screams all night long and stinks up the room? If that's not the case, then you need to know that the average private room will cost $77,745 per year. The nicer facilities will likely cost more. If you assume a 6 percent increase per year (which is a fairly conservative estimate), the cost of that semiprivate room will be about $102,000 in 2015.

WHAT ABOUT LONG-TERM CARE INSURANCE?

Long-term care insurance is a policy that you can buy to cover the high cost of nursing home care should you need such services. Not all policies are the same. Below are some helpful questions to ask before choosing a long-term care insurance policy:

- *Is the insurer a high-quality company?* The policy you buy today is one that you may not call on to collect for decades. Therefore, you want to choose from among the most stable companies. You want to look for companies that have a rating of A– or better.
- *Does it have inflation protection?* As time goes on, the cost of long-term care will increase. Similarly, your other expenses will be increasing as well.
- *Is there a sufficient benefit period?* The benefit period is the amount of time that the insurance company will pay your long-term care expenses. We generally recommend that you purchase a policy that will cover you for two to five years.
- *Is home care included?* You want to make sure that the policy you purchase will cover you for home health aides and assistance should you wish to stay at home rather than go to a nursing home.
- *What is the elimination period?* The *elimination period* is the amount of time that you will be expected to pay for your long-term care expenses before the policy kicks in. You can lower your premiums by increasing the length of the elimination period.

WILL SOCIAL SECURITY AND MEDICARE COME TO YOUR RESCUE?

The people who designed Social Security never expected that there would be so many elderly living for so long. As a result there are increasingly more people collecting Social Security and fewer people contributing.[8] In the 1950s there were 16 working-age people contributing to Social Security for every 1 person receiving this benefit. Now the ratio has dropped to 3.3 to 1. By 2030 the ratio will be approaching 2 to 1. An ever-increasing financial burden will therefore be placed on a smaller percentage of workers to pay for Social Security and Medicare.

Where's the Money?

Since it began in 1935, Social Security has taken in more money than what was paid out to recipients. The same applies to Medicare, which started in 1965. All that is about to change, however.

As of 2009 Medicare will likely start paying out more than it takes in. The same will apply for Social Security around 2018. You may be saying to yourself: What about all those surpluses that accumulated over all the years? The truth is that there were trillions of extra dollars collected by Social Security and Medicare over the decades. Unfortunately, all of that money was "borrowed" over the years by the government for the general federal budget.

So how is the federal government going to pay back all the money it borrowed? Money will have to be pumped into Social Security and Medicare from the general budget, which is already running a massive deficit. In order to keep Medicare and Social Security from going bankrupt, some tough decisions are going to have to be made.

So What Do the Experts Say?

In order to pay for entitlements for an ever-increasing older population, the government will have no choice other than to do one or more of the following:

- decrease funding for entitlement programs
- decrease nonentitlement spending
- increase taxes
- increase the budget deficit

Former treasury secretary Henry Paulson has remarked that delaying changes to Social Security will decrease the number of people who will have to bear the burden of reform. Faster economic growth will not solve Social Security's money problems.[9]

WHAT ABOUT PENSIONS?

In a global competitive market, fewer and fewer American companies are offering pension plans.[10] What seemed like a nice thing to do decades ago has become a major financial burden that can affect the profitability and long-term survival of many companies. Many companies and local governments simply cannot afford to pay pensions for tens of thousands of retired employees. In the global marketplace, American companies that are offering pensions are at a major economic disadvantage when they compete against third world companies that offer no such benefits.

Just because you currently work for a company that offers a pension plan does not mean that you can ignore careful financial planning. Think about the things that can go wrong:

- You may leave your job or get fired before your benefits kick in.
- The company may go out of business or declare bankruptcy.
- The pension may be too small to cover your retirement expenses.

WHAT ABOUT INHERITANCE?

People are living so long that you may be old yourself by the time your parents die. Increased life expectancy along with the high rate of senior inflation means that older adults will need more money to retire. If you are relying on an inheritance, beware that your parents will need more of this money for themselves and may therefore have less to leave to you.

WHAT CAN A SENIOR CITIZEN DO?

Younger workers have time to reassess their spending habits and investment strategies. For some seniors it is already too late. With few options to make money, many seniors have been forced to:

- cash in a life insurance policy
- delay retirement
- look for a new job
- lower their standard of living
- run up credit card debt
- sell personal belongings

- try to sell their homes
- take out a reverse mortgage

What Is a Reverse Mortgage?

Reverse mortgages have become a popular alternative for older adults who want to live in their home but lack the income to pay their monthly bills. The requirements for a reverse mortgage are that you:

- own the home outright
- are age sixty-two or over
- live in the home

Advantages of a reverse mortgage over the traditional mortgage:

- No need to make monthly payments.
- No need to show that you have the income to qualify.

The disadvantages of a reverse mortgage are:

- Over time your debt will increase and your equity in the home will decrease. If the interest rate rises, the equity will decrease at an even faster rate.
- With a reverse mortgage, a longer life means less equity to pass on to heirs.

It goes beyond the scope of this book to discuss all the many nuances of reverse mortgages. The US Department of Housing and Urban Development offers free counseling and a list of government-approved lenders. We recommend that you call their toll free number at 1-800-569-4287 if you are considering a reverse mortgage.

It may seem that we have presented a bunch of problems with few solutions. Preparing for retirement is very complicated and must take into account unknown variables, such as how long you will live and what will the economy look like in the decades to come. Rather than tell you what to do or where to invest your money, our goal is to open your eyes to the financial complexities of growing old in the twenty-first century. Once again, beware of those who claim to have the simple answer for you.

Chapter 29

WHEN IS IT TIME TO GIVE UP DRIVING?

On July 16, 2003, Russell Weller, eighty-six, was driving through Santa Monica, California. Unfortunately, he did not realize that the streets were closed to traffic for a twice-a-week farmers market. Instead of hitting the brakes, Mr. Weller hit the gas. Reaching speeds of 70 mph, he hit fifty people, killing ten.

For most people, driving is something that can be done with little thought or effort. However, for many older adults, driving can be a difficult and potentially dangerous task. Drivers over the age of eighty-five are at a higher risk for car accidents than any other age group.[1] One of the reasons you do not see more accidents involving the elderly is that many seniors have already cut back on the amount of driving they do. Many avoid driving at night and in heavy traffic. However, per mile driven, the elderly are at the highest risk for automobile accidents.

AGING AND THE DANGERS OF GETTING BEHIND THE WHEEL

The Eyes Change as You Get Older

In addition to generally worsening eyesight (chapter 2), the ability of the eyes to adapt to changes in the amount of light in the environment is delayed. On a dark road, where headlights may appear suddenly, the ability of the pupils to adjust to sudden changes in lighting is impaired.

Older adults also have a harder time discriminating between different surfaces. This could be a problem if you are unable to see the puddle on the road or the gravel on the shoulder of a highway.

Many older adults also suffer from cataracts. Cataracts develop in 95 percent of people over the age of eighty-five. Cataracts result in a clouding of the lens of the eye, which decreases vision and increases glare, making driving at night even more difficult. Age-related macular degeneration is another eye disorder that affects many elderly people. Some patients may complain of decreased vision when they try to focus on a particular object.

Changes in Brain Function

Driving in traffic requires more than just the ability to see the road and other cars. When you drive, you are seeing many things at the same time. Some are moving and some are not. You will see the road, the trees, the clouds, other cars, people walking, and so on. You need to be able to follow all these objects simultaneously to determine which ones are potential problems or dangers.

With aging there is a decrease in coordination and reaction time. People with dementia have even greater difficulty following directions, judging the distance between objects, and processing new information. Think about how dangerous it would be if you could not react to a child running out into the street from the sidewalk or a truck running through a stop sign to your right. This is one of the many reasons why people with dementia should not be driving at all.

The Eyes Are Connected to the Body

A stiff neck may make it difficult for an older driver to see what's going on in the periphery. If the driver cannot turn to look around, it will be hard to see a car in the driver's blind spot or behind the car to see a child playing or a bicycle approaching.

What if Grandpa can't hear too well? Having bad hearing certainly doesn't help with driving, but it is not a major factor that leads to unsafe driving.

Medical Problems

Many medical problems can make it harder for a senior to drive because it increases the risk of getting into a serious car accident. Seizures, poorly controlled diabetes, abnormal heart rhythms, and arthritis of the neck and shoulders may all be problems for the older adult driver.

Warning! Talk to the patient's doctor about whether it is safe for a loved one to drive after any of the following:

- hypoglycemic events (low blood sugar)
- narcolepsy (sleep attacks)
- recent myocardial infarction (heart attack)
- recent stroke
- seizures
- syncope (passing out)

WHAT ARE THE WARNING SIGNS THAT A LOVED ONE HAS A PROBLEM WITH DRIVING?

- near accident
- recent accident
- warning or ticket for a moving violation
- gets lost in department stores, supermarkets, and other familiar places
- gets lost while driving
- others are scared to get in the car with him

EVALUATING YOUR ABILITY TO DRIVE

Families often go to the doctor with concerns about whether their loved one can still safely drive. In many cases, what the doctor faces is a patient who is adamant about driving and a family who is desperately pleading the person to turn in the keys to the car. Trying to assess a patient's ability to drive is very difficult for a doctor in the hospital or office setting. Many doctors don't really know how to evaluate a senior's driving ability. Some do not know the process for reporting a potentially dangerous driver to the state. Others will not have the time or resources available. Even the experts do not agree as to the best way to evaluate driving safety in seniors.[2]

Most states do not require that the doctor report to the state's department of motor vehicles a patient who may pose a threat while driving. Many states, nonetheless, do allow doctors the option to report patients without fear of legal action.[3] In a few states, doctors may be responsible if one of their patients is involved in a motor vehicle accident that was due to a medical condition that wasn't reported.

Elderly people with poor vision and dementia urgently need to be identified as they are at an increased risk of auto accidents and accident-related injuries to themselves and others. Florida requires seniors over the age of eighty to take a vision test before renewing their license. We believe that the simple vision test performed at most DMVs is insufficient to identify many who are potentially dangerous drivers.

In 2000 the American Academy of Neurology published guidelines for the risk of driving in patients with Alzheimer's disease.[4] They recommended that patients with even mild dementia should not drive. They also recommend that patients with pre-Alzheimer's disease or mild cognitive impairment (chapter 22) should be referred for a driving evaluation every six months.

WHAT ABOUT A DRIVING EVALUATION?

Driving safety can be tested in a number of ways. There are computer programs that can test a person's ability to see a variety of images. There are even simulation machines that resemble video games. However, the best way to evaluate driving is in an actual car.

See if there are any driver rehabilitation specialists in your community. These specialists are usually occupational therapists who can perform detailed evaluations of a senior's driving ability. They will assess the older driver's vision, cognition, muscle strength, and range of motion. The assessment may also involve actual testing of the person's driving ability. AARP offers driver safety courses for older adults. They also have a CD-ROM that can test the person's ability to correctly perceive images.

Medicare will not pay for driving evaluations. Medicare does not consider testing a person's ability to drive to be a medically necessary activity. Therefore, you and your family will be expected to pay between $150 to $300 for any evaluation involving a driving rehabilitation specialist. That may seem like a lot of money, but these tests are labor intensive for the specialist. In fact, many rehabilitation departments do not offer these driving evaluations because they are not profitable.

Passing a driving test does not guarantee safe driving. If memory loss gets worse, for example, driving must stop. An acute illness may make the patient too frail to drive.

WHAT CAN A SENIOR DO TO BE A SAFER DRIVER?

First, get vision checkups. Cataracts can be removed and new lenses implanted. Medications, such as benzodiazepines, that can make one groggy need to be stopped (chapter 8). The seats and mirrors can be adjusted to help compensate for limitations of movement in the neck. An occupational therapist can often be of assistance with these adjustments. By avoiding driving at night, in bad weather, or on busy roads, seniors can further minimize their risk of an accident.

DON'T BE SO EAGER TO TAKE AWAY SOMEONE'S DRIVING PRIVILEGES!

The decision to stop driving is an issue of paramount importance in the lives of many older adults. While the states define driving as a privilege, we all know that it is a very important privilege. Many older people are already trying to adjust to the changes that occur with retirement and increased frailty. Many are no longer working and do not live near family and friends. Without the ability to drive, seniors can lose their independence, dignity, and autonomy. Without a car, they may have less access to healthcare, food, social activities, and so on. Some seniors have even told us that they don't want to stop driving since they are afraid of becoming a "bigger burden" on their families.

THE TIME TO HAVE THE CONVERSATION ABOUT DRIVING IS NOW!

Many families dread the thought of discussing this difficult topic with their loved ones. People can get hurt or even killed by an unsafe driver. The Hartford and MIT Age Lab has an excellent online booklet that gives suggestions on how to discuss this difficult topic with a loved one.[5] The booklet also discusses alternative transportation options as well.

There is a time when many seniors need to stop driving and consider their safety and the safety of others. Regular reassessment of driving ability is very important. Consider both sides of the situation, including the isolation if the senior cannot connect with friends. Affordable alternative transportation options may be available. Discuss this important topic openly and consult publications such as the booklet provided by the Hartford and MIT Age Lab, which gives pointers on how to comfortably discuss this topic with the older adult in your life.

Chapter 30

WHAT YOU NEED TO KNOW BEFORE YOU TRAVEL!

"I will never give in to old age until I become old. And I'm not old yet!"

Tina Turner (1939–)

Each year, millions of seniors are traveling via our nation's roads and airports. While many people may find traveling to be somewhat inconvenient, for seniors with health problems it can be quite a challenge. Traveling long distances often involves changes in a person's normal sleep pattern, urinary pattern, and diet. The person may also be traveling to a location where the weather, pollution, or altitude may vary greatly from what they are used to.

As a retired colonel in the US Army Reserve, Dr. Silverman has extensive experience dealing with travel-related medical problems. While some issues may arise unexpectedly, there are important steps seniors can take while planning that dream vacation:

- Don't forget to bring all of your medications. Always bring an extra few days' worth in case your trip runs a little longer than you expected.
- Your medications should stay with you in your carry-on luggage. Do not put them with your check-in luggage.
- If you use syringes for insulin or narcotic medications for pain, bring documentation from your doctor or pharmacist. You don't want to have problems with security personnel in a domestic or foreign airport.

- Many third world countries do not have the medical facilities that we have grown accustomed to here in the United States. If you get injured abroad, you may be in big trouble. So don't take any chances doing risky activities, such as climbing ladders, swimming after drinking alcohol, and so on.
- Get travel insurance if you are going to be in a foreign country. Medicare does not cover the costs incurred in other countries. In some places the healthcare is so poor that you will want to get out of there as soon as possible in the event of a medical emergency. If you need to be airlifted, it can cost anywhere from thirty thousand to a hundred thousand dollars, depending on where you are. Make sure you know the restrictions and clauses that address preexisting conditions.
- Since heart attacks can happen overseas, it is a good idea to bring a copy of your most recent EKG. In many cases one of the fastest ways to tell if there is a problem with your heart is to check an EKG and compare it with an old one.
- Consider how you will be traveling. You may want to hire a town car or taxi rather than using congested public transportation or driving on unfamiliar roads.
- If you are going to be traveling outside the United States, check to make sure you don't need any additional immunizations. You can find out which immunizations are recommended by the Centers for Disease Control and Prevention by going to www.cdc.gov. Additional vaccines may include one or more of the following:
  - ° hepatitis A
  - ° hepatitis B
  - ° tetanus booster (every ten years)
  - ° typhoid fever
  - ° yellow fever
- Don't wait until the day or the week before your trip to get your vaccinations. Some vaccines may take weeks before they can protect you from an infection. Most likely your primary care doctor will not have these immunizations available. You may need to go to a travel medicine clinic or your local health department. Medicare will not cover the cost of any immunizations other than influenza, tetanus, and Pneumovax (for pneumonia).
- Be careful to follow all recommendations regarding the local food and water. Older adults are more vulnerable to becoming dehydrated from traveler's diarrhea. We often recommend that people they take a five-

day course of an antibiotic, such as ciprofloxacin (Cipro), with them and probably some Immodium for diarrhea. Be sure to check with the person's doctor before making medication changes.

- Make sure you leave a copy of your travel itinerary with family or friends. In case of an emergency, you want to make sure that someone can contact you.
- Because of the disruption that occurs with traveling (change in sleep schedule, diet, etc.), diabetics need to be more careful about checking their blood sugar.
- Bring an extra set of eyeglasses.
- Bring comfortable footwear.
- Bring an alcohol-based hand wash.
- At higher altitudes, the air has less oxygen. If you have congestive heart failure, heart disease, anemia, or COPD/emphysema, check with your doctor before traveling to a place that is at a high altitude. This decrease in oxygen can even be a problem during the airplane trip itself. Ask your doctor about whether supplemental oxygen will be of any benefit for you.
- If you are going to a third world country, avoid wearing perfume, as this can attract flying insects that carry diseases. You may want to consider using an insect repellant as well.

CAN GRANDMA TRAVEL ALONE ON AN AIRPLANE?

The airlines are not required to transfer passengers from wheelchair to wheelchair, wheelchair to aircraft seat, or wheelchair to lavatory seat. Furthermore, airline personnel are not obliged to assist with feeding, bodily functions, or providing medication to travelers. Disabled passengers who cannot transfer themselves or care for themselves should travel with a companion or an attendant.

Some Extra Tips for Traveling with a Frail Senior

- Bring an extra set of underwear and pants for your loved one. You never know if and when an accident may occur.
- You can bring cards to hand to staff and other passengers that tell people your loved one has dementia.
- If you are traveling with someone with dementia, remember that the greater the disruption to their normal schedule for sleeping, eating, and activities, the higher the risk that the person will become delirious.

Preventing Blood Clots in Your Legs while Traveling

For many years, doctors have known that seniors are at particular risk for developing blood clots in their legs after traveling long distances by plane, car, train, or bus.[1]

- When traveling by car, stop every hour or two to stretch and walk around. Failure to do so increases the risk of lower back pain, and more importantly, of developing a blood clot in the leg known as *deep vein thrombosis* (DVT). The risk of dangerous blood clots increases dramatically with sitting for more than five hours.
- When traveling by plane, train, or bus, get up and walk around every hour or two.
- Take a low-dose (81 mg) aspirin daily.
- Wear compression hose.
- Use foot stretches to flex the calf muscles and leg stretches to flex the thigh muscles.
- Stay well hydrated while traveling. Avoid drinks with caffeine or alcohol.

FIGHTING JET LAG

Jet lag has been found to be a problem whenever travel involves crossing three or more time zones. The severity of jet lag is worse among older adults compared to younger travelers. Jet lag is different from the travel fatigue that occurs due to difficulty sleeping, changes in diet, and other difficulties associated with traveling.[2] While travel fatigue is relieved with a good night's sleep, people suffering from jet lag may need several days to adjust to their new environment.

Traveling Eastbound

If you are traveling eastward you will need to adjust your body to awaking one hour later and going to bed one hour earlier each night for three nights before your trip. When you get to Italy, for example, the clock on the nightstand says 11 PM, but your body still thinks it is only 3 PM. Some suggestions to prevent eastbound jet lag:

- Wake up an hour earlier each day before your trip.
- Light therapy—turn on bright lights upon awakening.

- Melatonin—doses of 0.5 mg have been shown to be as effective as those of 3 mg. However, most studies that analyzed whether melatonin was helpful for jet lag involved only younger patients.

Studies have shown that people who use all three of these interventions can decrease their jet lag symptoms.

Traveling Westbound

If you are traveling from New York to Hawaii, your body will think that it is nighttime when it is actually the afternoon. Some things that you should do to minimize westbound jet lag:

- When you arrive, try to stay awake while it is daylight and to go to sleep when it gets dark.
- Avoid caffeine and alcohol.
- Eat at the times the locals eat...unless the custom is to eat at one in the morning!

AM I TRAVELING TO A DANGEROUS PLACE?

There are no guarantees in life. However, you should take some basic steps and be aware of your new surroundings:

- The US Department of State has a Web site that lists all the travel warnings for Americans traveling abroad. The Web site is www.travel.state.gov.
- Stay out of the "bad" parts of town.
- Talk to the staff at the hotel to get an idea about which neighborhoods are safe to walk around at night.
- Do not wear any jewelry.

DON'T LEAVE YOUR COMMON SENSE AT HOME!

Just because you are on vacation does not mean that your brain should go on vacation, too. There are some commonsense things you need to remember:

- Wear sunscreen when you are outside.
- Wear seatbelts.
- Don't get too drunk.
- Be extra careful riding a motorbike.
- Stay out of dangerous neighborhoods.

MEDICAL TOURISM

In recent years, many people have traveled to other countries for the purpose of receiving medical care at just a fraction of what it costs in the United States. With major Medicare cutbacks planned in the near future, more seniors will likely be going overseas for healthcare.

You may find that you can save money this way, but you need to be aware of the following issues:

- What if you have a complication and get very sick in another country?
- What if you have a complication from your surgery when you return?
- Where will you find a doctor to fix the problem once you return?

ARE YOU A SNOWBIRD?

As geriatricians in the state of Florida, Dr. Silverman and Dr. Golden have taken care of many snowbird patients. Snowbirds are people who live in Florida, Arizona, and California in the fall and winter, and in the Northeast or Midwest during the summer.

If you are a snowbird, it is a good idea for you to have a doctor in both locations. When you head down south for the winter, make sure to bring a copy of your recent blood work and radiology reports. If you have been admitted to a hospital while up north, get a copy of your discharge summary for your doctor down south.

TIPS FOR PURCHASING/LEASING A VACATION HOME

- Make sure that the house or townhouse has at least one bedroom and bathroom on the first floor. You may have no problems with your knees and hips now, but you never know what the future holds. Millions of seniors will become ill, develop severe arthritis, or fracture their hips. When this happens those stairs will seem like Mt. Everest.

- Find an area that is in walking distance to stores, restaurants, the post office, and so on. Many people dream of retiring to a remote beach, farmhouse, or maybe an exclusive golf resort. The problem with all three options is that once you are unable to drive, you will lose much of your independence. Or even worse you may continue to drive, even when you know it is not safe to do so. By walking to do your errands you will remain more active and less of a burden on your family and friends. By being able to get out of the house on your own, you will be able to preserve more of your social contacts.
- Retire to an area that has good public transportation for seniors.
- Find a place that is near a good medical center. Before you move into your dream log cabin out to the country, you need to ask yourself: Am I too far from a good hospital? What are you going to do if and when you have a heart attack, stroke, pneumonia, or hip fracture? The key word here is not *if*, but *when*. Everyone at some point will get sick and need help.

When an elderly person decides to travel or to buy a retirement home, there are important issues to consider. Don't just impulsively act. Think carefully and plan ahead! Travel and vacations are supposed to be fun; planning ahead can keep the experience positive.

Chapter 31

ARE YOU PREPARED FOR
A HURRICANE OR
OTHER DISASTER?

HURRICANES

As geriatricians in the state of Florida, Dr. Golden and Dr. Silverman have extensive experience dealing with problems associated with hurricanes. While the media gives a lot of advice about how to prepare homes and apartments for wind and rain damage, they often neglect providing advice to seniors.

Do You Have Everything You Need?

When a storm approaches you will hear on the news that everyone should stock up on emergency supplies. These supplies consist of water, nonperishable food, and batteries. Most sources say to have at least a seventy-two-hour supply. Based on our experience, seniors need to prepare themselves in many more ways.

The Essentials

Information—Keep all important documents in a waterproof container

- Healthcare policy numbers
- Identification documents (passport, Social Security card, driver's license)

- List of medical illnesses, medications, allergies
- Names and contact information of relatives, power of attorney, health-care providers
- Insurance documents, bank statements

Supplies

- Assistive devices (wheelchair, cane, walker, etc.)
- Battery-powered radio
- Cash—banks and ATM machines may not be working
- Credit cards
- Eyeglasses, dentures, hearing aids
- Flashlight
- A generous amount of incontinence supplies, if needed (chapter 21)
- One-week supply of clothing
- One-week supply of food and water
- Pet food
- Plenty of batteries
- A three-week supply of medications—your pharmacy or doctor's office may be out of commission after the storm

In addition, make sure the gas tank in your car is full. With no electricity, the pumps at many gas stations may not be working.

Having a Plan Is Not Enough

You need to have a hurricane plan that suits your needs, *and* you must institute that plan early. Don't wait or it may be too late. The roads will be jammed and the hotels in neighboring towns will all be booked. Trying to leave town on the last day possible will certainly leave you in bumper-to-bumper traffic. For the older adult with special needs, getting stuck in a ten-hour traffic jam is not such a great idea.

What about Emergency Shelters?

Local governments and the media make an emphatic plea to seniors that they seek emergency shelter when a storm approaches. The danger from the storm itself is only part of the problem. After the storm, seniors will have to cope with the loss of electricity, loss of running water, and poor sanitary conditions.

Remaining in a hurricane-damaged zone in the heat of summer is difficult for even the strongest of people. What about for a frail older person? Without air-conditioning and adequate drinking water, seniors are at a higher risk of becoming dehydrated.

When you look back at the damage caused by hurricanes Andrew, Katrina, Rita, Wilma, and others, you may wonder: why on earth would elderly people not evacuate when they are told to do so? Dr. Golden and Dr. Silverman have spoken to many elderly people who adamantly refused to leave when a hurricane approached. Many were more fearful of going to a shelter than they were of the potential danger of riding the storm out. While we do not recommend that people ignore orders to evacuate, we can understand why many remain reluctant to leave their homes.

Emergency shelters have trouble providing for the special needs of the frail elderly. Even ones that claim to be special-needs shelters usually have limited personnel trained to deal with the special issues of this vulnerable population. If nursing homes and hospitals are having trouble finding trained staff during the best of times, it is unlikely that a rescue shelter is going to have this level of expertise in a crisis.

For the millions of older adults with urinary problems, the two to three bathrooms in the corner of a high school hallway will not suffice. Lying on a mattress on the floor may be difficult as well. Also, during times of environmental change, patients with dementia are more likely to suffer from delirium and behavioral problems, such as agitation (chapter 24).

We have heard many elderly people complain that they were shipped off to shelters in unfamiliar neighborhoods where they were terrified they would be robbed or attacked. Many seniors live alone and the only companionship they have is with their pets. Parting with their dog or cat was simply not an option.

What about Nursing Homes?

After Hurricane Katrina, there were many news reports about several nursing homes where everyone died in the storm. There are many variables that have an impact on how well a nursing home will fare in the event of a hurricane. The path and strength of the storm, as well as the construction of the building, will play roles in determining how much physical damage the facility suffers.

Even if the building remains structurally intact, the facility may lose electrical power and running water. Delivery of supplies may be delayed.[1]

Don't forget the staffing issues, too. Even in the best of circumstances, most nursing homes struggle to maintain enough staff to meet all the needs of their residents. In the event of a natural disaster, maintaing adequate staffing will be a major problem since employees will be dealing with their own personal property losses and transportation issues. The employees who do remain will certainly be working harder as they may have to move residents and supplies without the use of elevators and other conveniences.[2] Water may need to be carried for drinking, bathing, and for flushing toilets.

Without air-conditioning, room temperatures will likely be above 90 degrees with a humidity in the 90-percent range as well. Body fluid losses can increase substantially under these conditions.[3] As we discussed earlier, the elderly are at a higher risk for dehydration. Keeping up with this increased loss of fluids would likely be too much for the limited nursing home staff.

The knee-jerk reaction of sending patients to the nearest hospital emergency room may not even be an option. The roads may be closed and access to hospitals may be limited.

Remember, while all people should have a plan in the case of a natural disaster, seniors need to be extra prepared. Taking some time to make some basic preparations and to think about a disaster plan can save a tremendous amount of pain and suffering for you and your family.

Chapter 32

THE TIME TO DISCUSS
END-OF-LIFE ISSUES IS NOW!

*"On the plus side, death is one of the few things that can
be done just as easily lying down."*

Woody Allen (1935–)

OLD PEOPLE GET SICK

Advances in medicine have led to a dramatic increase in life expectancy. Defibrillators and medications can be used to restart a heart after it has stopped beating. Ventilators can move air in and out of lungs that have failed. Feeding tubes can provide nutrition when the patient is unable to swallow. Dialysis machines can remove fluid and toxins from the body when the kidneys have failed. The relatively easy access to these life-prolonging devices raises many ethical concerns when they are used on frail elderly patients with terminal illnesses.

WHAT ARE ADVANCED DIRECTIVES?

At some point, many seniors become so ill that they are unconscious, delirious, or unable to talk. Others may also have dementia. It is almost impossible for patients in these states to make tough decisions regarding their medical treatment.

So how are doctors supposed to know what the patient would like the healthcare team to do? In theory, the person's wishes or needs are recorded in documents known as *advanced directives*. Advanced directives can take several forms:

1. *Living will.* This document outlines what medical procedures and interventions a person would want if he were too sick to make those decisions for himself.
2. *Durable power of attorney for healthcare (healthcare surrogate).* This document names someone to make healthcare decisions in the event a person is too sick to make those decisions himself. We recommend that people also appoint an alternate healthcare surrogate in case the primary surrogate is unavailable, incapacitated, or dead. Many people have both a living will and a durable power of attorney for healthcare.
3. *Guardianship.* For those who do not have someone who can act as a surrogate, the court can appoint a legal guardian to make decisions in cases in which the person is no longer able to do so himself.

All hospitals, long-term care facilities, home health agencies, hospice programs, and HMOs that receive federal funds are required to ask if the patient has an AD at the time of admission. The hospital or nursing home must provide information about the AD if the person wants to learn more about how to fill out these forms.

TALK TO YOUR FAMILY

Although no one enjoys talking about end-of-life issues, it is something that everyone should do. Even if you trust your family to carry out your wishes, it is still a good idea to talk about these issues and make a plan to follow. Such a discussion will allow you to express your thoughts and wishes with people who know you well. They may bring up good points or questions that you may want to discuss with a doctor. For the family, it may be an opportunity to learn what a patient's actual wishes are on a particular issue.

You may be surprised at what these conversations may reveal. In a study with an outcome that resembled the old *Newlywed Game Show*, families incorrectly predicted the patients' end-of-life preferences in a third of the cases.[1]

While family discussions can be helpful, the family still needs to make one person the decision maker. The need for one decision maker is critical, as many decisions will need to be made quickly. When making these decisions it is important to put yourself in the shoes of the patient and try to determine how the person, if he were aware of what was going on, would decide.

By agreeing to be the healthcare surrogate or the durable power of attorney for someone, you are not obligating yourself to manage the person's finances. Nor will you be responsible for any debts that this person has or incurs.

As geriatricians we are always surprised by the fact that anywhere from 30 to 40 percent of nursing home residents and frail homebound seniors have no advanced directives.[2] Many patients with severe dementia, emphysema, and/or heart disease do not have a written advance care plan that addresses resuscitation and ventilator use. What happens then is that these patients are needlessly poked and prodded by the medical system despite having a limited life expectancy.

AND NOW THE **REAL TRUTH** ABOUT ADVANCED DIRECTIVES!

Just because you or your family member has an advanced directive does not mean that you are out of the woods. An advanced directive provides a general overview of the person's wishes, but the **real truth** is that no one document can cover all of the potential scenarios and gray medical areas that can arise.

Because there are many potential ambiguities that may occur, there is no guarantee that the doctor will totally understand, let alone follow, your true intentions. In some cases the technology has changed or progressed, which for instance makes a living will even harder to interpret. In other cases, the patient's family situation may have changed, making the listed healthcare surrogate outdated. Over time, the patient's or surrogate's outlook on life may change. If advanced directives are not updated, the healthcare staff may not know the patient's current wishes.

WHAT IS A DO NOT RESUSCITATE (DNR) FORM?

When a patient stops breathing or her heart stops beating, healthcare professionals will try to resuscitate her. *Cardiopulmonary resuscitation* (CPR) refers to the chest compressions that are done when the heart stops beating. The purpose of the chest compressions is to keep blood pumping out of the heart to other parts of the body. A defibrillator is used to provide electrical shock that will hopefully reset the heart rhythm. The patient may also be given powerful drugs to try to fix the abnormal heart rhythm. If the lungs fail, we can stick a tube down the person's throat and hook the tube up to a mechanical ventilation machine.

In the hospital setting, these interventions are enacted immediately. Most emergency medical personnel arriving at the scene of an emergency will also initiate these lifesaving procedures. For seniors at the end stages of underlying diseases, such as cancer, heart disease, Alzheimer's disease, or renal failure, these interventions offer very little chance for the patient to fully recover after the heart stops or the lungs fail.

We have found that the decision to sign a DNR form is often based on how it is presented. If you are asked if you want doctors to keep you alive in the event that your heart stops beating or your lungs stop working, most people would say, "Of course!" If you were instead asked if you wanted to be shocked and have a tube rammed down your throat, many people would respond differently. As geriatricians, we emphasize to our elderly patients and their families that in many cases, aggressive medical care does not always lead to better outcomes. In some cases it may actually increase suffering.

The DNR form applies only to CPR, shocking the heart, administering advanced cardiac drugs, and intubation for mechanical ventilation. We have seen cases where patients with a Do Not Resuscitate form were not transferred to an intensive care unit or did not receive IV antibiotics because it was assumed that they would not want to be treated "aggressively." The American Medical Association's Council on Ethical and Judicial Affairs stated that a signed Do Not Resuscitate form "should not influence other therapeutic interventions that may be appropriate."[3] A less aggressive treatment plan should not be simply inferred because the resident has a DNR order. DNR stands for *do not resuscitate*, not *comfort care measures only*.

DOES CPR WORK FOR THE FRAIL ELDERLY?

While you will see CPR commonly done on younger patients without a problem on TV, for the frail elderly it can be quite traumatic. Many times, the chest compressions lead to fractures of the sternum (breastbone) and ribs. On TV you will see many patients recover with CPR or defibrillation. The **real truth** is that the survival rate for frail seniors who require CPR at home or at a nursing home has been measured to be between 0 and 3 percent.[4]

REFUSING LIFE-SUSTAINING CARE

For many seniors there may come a point when they do not want to proceed with medical treatment. It is often hard for doctors and family to accept that an elderly patient has the right to refuse treatment for one or more illnesses. A patient has a right to refuse medical care even if it means that he will die sooner.

That being said, we as doctors need to make sure that patients understand all the facts before making any decisions. Maybe the patient has misunderstood something the doctors told him?

DECISION-MAKING CAPACITY (DMC)

When assessing seniors for their insight and ability to make decisions regarding medical treatment and other healthcare matters, we ask ourselves several important questions:

- Can the person express personal preferences?
- Can she give reasons for the alternative selected?
- Are the supporting reasons rational?
- Can she comprehend the risks and benefits of the various choices being presented?

DMC may fluctuate depending on the patient's medical illnesses, medications, and so on. If you remember the case involving Anna Nicole Smith and her husband, J. Howard Marshall, the whole legal issue centered on whether her eighty-eight-year-old husband had decision-making capacity for his financial affairs at the time he married her. She claims he did and his son claimed he did not.

Legally, doctors cannot deem a person to be incompetent. Competency is a legal term. Doctors can assess a person's capacity to make decisions, but only a court can determine if someone is actually competent.

WHEN SHOULD A PERSON SET UP HIS ADVANCED DIRECTIVE?

The answer is *now*, not later! This is one of the few issues in geriatrics that has a simple answer. Even if you feel great and your doctor just gave you a clean bill of health, there is still no excuse to procrastinate. No one is immortal.

If your family member has just been diagnosed with mild cognitive impairment or mild dementia, you had better hurry up! Remember that the person has to have the mental capacity to understand what she is agreeing to when she signs her advanced directive form. When the dementia has progressed or the patient is acutely ill, it will be too late for the person to have the decision-making capacity needed to sign an advanced directive.

THINGS YOU CAN DO TO HELP!

- Talk with your loved one about CPR, mechanical intubation, tube feeding, and so on, so choices can be made. Although no one enjoys talking about this, it is better than the 3 AM phone call from the hospital to get your consent for an emergency procedure or surgery for your loved one. Under those circumstances, you need to know what your loved one wants rather than living with the guilt that you made the wrong decision.
- Frail elderly patients with severe or terminal illnesses should always ask their doctors whether recommended medical procedures will improve their comfort or their long-term prognosis.
- If you have an advanced directive, make sure your doctor, family, and long-term care facility have a copy on file.

Some advice for caregivers: Not only do we recommend having an advanced directive prepared for your loved one, but we also recommend that you get one for yourself. We have seen many cases where the patient is left without a decision maker due to illness or death.

THE FIVE WISHES DOCUMENT

We recommend the Five Wishes Document, which combines the essential elements of a healthcare surrogate and a living will. It also addresses the patient's emotional and spiritual concerns. This document does not require a lawyer and is recognized in thirty-eight states as well as the District of Columbia. Copies of this form can be ordered at a very low price through www.agingwithdignity.com (1-888-594-7437).

DO I NEED AN ATTORNEY TO HELP WITH
THE ADVANCED DIRECTIVE?

Technically, you do not need an attorney to set up a durable power of attorney, a living will, or a DNR. Standard forms exist for these types of advanced directives, but they may vary depending upon the state in which you live. If you agree with the wording in these forms and you have a designated family member or friend to be the decision maker, then you will likely be fine. Don't forget that you need two witnesses in order for this document to be legal.

We do suggest that you contact an attorney under the following circumstances:

- *Family complexity*—this involves situations where the family does not agree or does not get along.
- *Financial complexity*—the estate has significant assets. The more assets, the more likely someone may contest the advanced directive.
- *Wording complexity*—this involves situations where the forms need to be customized.

WHAT DO YOU DO WHEN THE OLDER ADULT
NEGLECTS HIMSELF?

We have taken care of many patients who do not want to take any medications and do not want any laboratory or other testing. These patients may refuse hospitalization when they are ill or may leave against medical advice when they are admitted. Oftentimes families are extremely upset at the patient's stubbornness.

In some cases the patient may be stubborn. In other cases, the patient may be severely depressed or demented. If you are concerned that there may be an issue of self-neglect, be on the lookout for some of the other signs:

- The bills are not being paid.
- The house is filthy.
- There is no food in the kitchen.

When the patient adamantly refuses to take care of the basic healthcare and household needs, the family becomes caught in a difficult situation. Balancing a person's independence with personal safety is tricky. By law, patients are considered competent to make their own decisions until the courts have determined they are incompetent. This determination must therefore be made by the courts. To make matters even more complicated, with the recent changes in medical privacy law—foremost, the Health Insurance Portability and Accountability Act (HIPPA)—the doctor will need to get the patient's permission before discussing the patient's healthcare issues with friends or family.

TIPS FOR FAMILIES WITH OLDER ADULTS
WHO REFUSE TO TAKE CARE OF THEMSELVES

- If the patient will go to the doctor, ask the doctor to assess the patient's decision-making capacity.
- If you are concerned that the patient is a danger to self or others, contact the state department that deals with elder affairs. They can send out a case manager or social worker to do an emergency evaluation.
- Contact an elder law attorney as soon as possible. This is especially important if you are concerned that other family members or friends may be exploiting your elderly family member.

Chapter 33
THE DYING PROCESS

"Old age isn't so bad when you consider the alternatives."
Maurice Chevalier (1888–1972)

Death is an inevitable fact of life. Even though modern medicine has allowed people to live longer, at a certain point even the best doctors and the best hospitals will not be able to make the person healthier or live any longer. There comes a point for many patients when more medical testing and procedures will not lead to a better quality of life.

Studies have shown that healthcare at the end of life can be expensive. Almost 20 percent of all Medicare costs occur during the last six months of life.[1] In many of these cases, expensive healthcare does not mean better healthcare. A significant amount of the Medicare budget is spent providing medical treatment that in the big picture will not help patients.

WHAT IS PALLIATIVE CARE?

Palliative care is an approach that involves addressing the symptoms of a disease rather than trying to halt or cure it. The goal of palliative care is the achievement of the best possible quality of life for patients and their families. Many hospitals and nursing homes have palliative care units that can provide this kind of focused healthcare. In addition to providing medical care, these units also help the patients and families come to terms with many of the difficult decisions that need to be addressed.

WHAT IS HOSPICE?

An important component of the palliative care approach has been the development of hospice programs. Hospice is a philosophy that emphasizes pain and symptom management for patients whose life expectancy is limited. For example, a hospice will treat the pain and distress associated with a terminal breast cancer rather than trying to treat the cancer itself.

The dying process is often difficult for patients to deal with. Depression, guilt, and anxiety are issues that need to be discussed and addressed through a combination of professional counseling and medication. Many dying older adults are afraid that no one will listen to their complaints and that they will die in severe pain. The goal of hospice care is to maximize physical and psychological comfort for the patient. Hospice agencies also strive to provide support for the family before and after the patient dies.

In 2006, 1.3 million Americans received hospice care.[2] Medicare will provide coverage of hospice services for enrollees who agree to hospice services and forego "curative treatments" for their illnesses. Both the patient's doctor and the hospice medical director must certify that the person has a life expectancy of six months or less. You may be asking yourself, how are the doctors able to make such a prediction? The **real truth** is that it is very hard to predict if a person will have six months or less to live. (We will discuss this in more detail later in the chapter.)

Patients must also have specific diseases that Medicare recognizes as qualifying for hospice services. These diagnoses include end-stage:

- cancer
- dementia
- heart disease
- HIV
- kidney disease
- liver disease
- stroke/coma

Although many patients wish to die at home, in some cases, the patient and family find it too distressing to have the person dying there. Many hospice agencies make arrangements with nursing homes or hospitals in order to get the patient out of the home.

HOSPICE FOR END-STAGE DEMENTIA

About one in ten patients with end-stage dementia will receive hospice care. One of the problems that many healthcare professionals face is that the criteria used to classify end-stage dementia for hospice has been shown not to accurately predict six-month survival.[3] Rather than treat end-stage dementia as a terminal illness, many of these people receive aggressive care that involves multiple hospitalizations and procedures that do not improve the patient's quality of life.

WHO PAYS FOR HOSPICE?

Seniors are covered for hospice under Medicare Part A. Medicare pays the hospice agency a set fee per patient enrolled per day. The patient does not need to make any copayments. All medications, supplies, and equipment related to the hospice diagnosis are covered. Hospice offers some additional services that are not covered by home healthcare under Medicare. Hospice can provide for home health aides who help with basic chores, such as house cleaning and bathing. Counseling and bereavement services are available for the caregiver. What about expensive treatments, such as dialysis, blood transfusions, or radiation therapy? Medicare does not regulate what treatments hospice agencies have to provide. Some hospice agencies may be able to afford the expensive treatments while others may not.[4]

HOSPICE MYTHS THAT NEED TO BE DISPELLED

- You can enroll in hospice only if you have a caregiver.
- You must sign a do not resuscitate form in order to enroll.
- Care can only be provided in the home.
- All medical treatments are discontinued.
- All invasive interventions, such as dialysis or radiation therapy, are stopped.
- After six months patients are kicked out of the program.

BUT WHAT IF THE PATIENT LIVES LONGER THAN SIX MONTHS?

In some cases hospice patients live past the six-month period. In these situations, hospice services can be renewed if the patient is still suffering from the same terminal diagnosis.

REVOKING THE HOSPICE BENEFIT

Patients can choose to quit the hospice at any time. When they do so, the Medicare benefits are restarted immediately.

HOW MUCH TIME DO THEY HAVE LEFT?

Families often ask how much longer a dying patient has. As physicians, we always feel uncomfortable when we are asked this question. For patients who are not responsive, not drinking, and having trouble breathing, we usually say that they have hours or days to live. For patients with advanced cancer, congestive heart failure, or Alzheimer's disease, giving a specific time frame becomes more difficult to answer. Even with many years of experience of taking care of thousands of dying patients, it is sometimes difficult for us to predict much longer a dying patient has. We have seen cases where we wrongly thought the person was going to die very soon. Some lived for only a few months while others lived for several years. In most cases the intuition of the doctor, however, is relatively accurate in predicting which patients have less than six months to live.

DO YOU HAVE TO FORGO ALL TREATMENTS IF YOU SIGN UP WITH HOSPICE?

The general focus with hospice care is to provide pain control, psychological support, and spiritual support. The active treatment of medical illnesses is not the focus. That being said, some treatments may still be provided while under hospice care. Dialysis may continue and you may receive radiation therapy for cancer if it can help relieve pain that you are having. You may also receive medical treatments that are unrelated to your hospice diagnosis. Let's say you are in hospice for lung cancer and you accidentally step on a nail. You will still get your foot fixed.

THE **REAL TRUTH** IS THAT MANY PEOPLE WON'T SIGN UP FOR HOSPICE CARE!

The average length of stay in hospice is seventy-two days.[5] Some patients are enrolled only hours or days before they die. This suggests that many of these people are signing up too late and are receiving aggressive care up until the end.

I JUST DON'T WANT TO GIVE UP HOPE!

The dying process is difficult for most families to deal with. Part of the reason is that people in our society have very high expectations that our medical system will be able to cure nearly any health problem. Many families do not want to consider a hospice. The word *hospice* may have a strong negative connotation that conveys a sense of hopelessness. By agreeing to hospice care, they are giving up hope for recovery. It has been our experience that many families would feel guilty if they were to give up trying to help a family member. In most cases, everything has already been tried by the time the hospice is offered. We often tell families that the guilt of not doing enough needs to be weighed against the guilt of doing too much.

As doctors, it is very easy for us to keep sending a patient back to the hospital for more tests, treatments, and procedures. We can always poke a patient for more blood or send him for one more CT scan. We have seen many patients continue to receive chemotherapy even though there was no hope that the cancer would be cured. In many cases, this aggressive approach does little to make the patient feel better. In fact, all this extra poking and sticking can make the patient feel even worse.

OFTENTIMES DOCTORS DON'T HELP THE SITUATION

We have discussed how end-of-life issues are often difficult for patients and their families to deal with. We should not forget that many doctors and other healthcare professionals are also uncomfortable discussing death-related issues with their patients. As doctors we are trained to do whatever it takes to make our patients better. Many of us work in large state-of-the-art hospitals that are filled with lifesaving technology. Doctors sometimes feel subconsciously that they may be giving up too soon.

Many specialists get so focused on their specific organ system that they fail to see the big picture with regard to the long-term and overall health of the patient. As the specialist explains the specific treatments, families often get a false sense of hope. We have heard many of these talented specialists say things such as, "If we can fix the kidneys with dialysis, then we can fix the clogged arteries of the heart. After that we will be able to try to operate on the patient's cancer."

As geriatricians who see frail ill patients every day, we realize the importance of treating the entire patient. In the big picture it is essential to ask if a medical treatment will allow the patient to live longer or improve his or her quality of life.

BE SURE YOU HAVE A DIAGNOSIS

It is very common for frail elderly patients to exhibit symptoms that may be due to a cancer. These include rectal bleeding, severe weight loss, or coughing up blood. In these cases we may inadvertently find a mass that is suspicious for cancer on a chest x-ray or CT scan. Other times, we may find a mass by accident when we order tests for another reason.

There is an old saying that if it looks like a duck and quacks like a duck, then it is likely a duck. This logic works well when you are duck hunting but can be quite dangerous when you are diagnosing people with terminal cancers. In order to make a more definitive diagnosis, further testing is often needed. This may involve a surgeon, gastroenterologist, or radiologist taking a biopsy.

You may be saying to yourself, why not just treat it like a cancer and save the person the agony of having a needle stuck into his lung or abdomen to get a tissue sample? We can't begin to tell you how many times we have seen cases where the senior or the family refuses a diagnostic biopsy because it would be "too difficult." Instead, the patient ends up getting sent to the ER on multiple occasions for a variety of symptoms, such as fever, cough, dehydration, and so on. Without a clear diagnosis it is hard to give patients and families a clear plan for what to expect in the coming weeks to months.

WHAT ABOUT WITHDRAWING FEEDINGS AND FLUIDS?

During the dying process, medical care that is seen as futile and not helping to relieve discomfort is often withdrawn. The courts have determined that artificial nutrition and hydration are not different from other forms of medical treatment that can be withdrawn or withheld.

WHAT CAN I EXPECT TO SEE DURING THE DYING PROCESS?

In the weeks preceding death, patients may withdraw from the activities and the company they used to enjoy. As a caregiver, do not take it personally if your loved one shows little interest in the activities you have planned. The person will also spend more time in bed. Other changes that you may notice include:

- decreased appetite
- decrease in blood pressure
- decreased energy
- eyes will generally remain closed
- increased breathing rate
- increased paleness

In the last few minutes or hours of life, you may notice the patient gasping for air.

No Thirst or Appetite

Most will lose the interest or the ability to eat or drink. Despite the position of the courts and the American Medical Association that artificial nutrition and hydration is a "life-prolonging medical treatment," many doctors and nurses may still think that withdrawing nutrition and hydration amounts to killing the patient. While these healthcare providers are entitled to their moral beliefs, they should realize that they may be imposing their personal beliefs upon frail and ailing seniors or their families.

While dehydration and malnutrition are generally thought of as horrible things, many experts in geriatrics make the point that for patients with dementia who are within hours or days of dying, this may be the preferred natural course.

It is important to remember that the effects of dehydration are different in the dying patient than in a younger, healthier person. Foregoing food and water in dying patients with end-stage dementia does not appear to increase patient discomfort.[6]

The few studies that have been done have shown that those without hunger or thirst have experienced increased pain when tube fed. An important study once asked the question, Do terminally ill cancer patients experience hunger or thirst? What they found was that 63 percent never experienced any hunger, 34 percent had hunger only initially, and 63 percent had thirst only initially or not at all. All hunger or thirst was relieved with very small amounts of fluid, food, or ice chips.[7]

The lack of water and food leads to decreased saliva, which makes it easier for the patient to breathe without gurgling. It also decreases the need to urinate, which further increases the comfort of the dying patient.

Skin Breakdown

Some people, even many doctors, will say out of ignorance that ailing bed-bound people are being neglected if they have bedsores (pressure ulcers). As noted earlier, the **real truth** is that no one can guarantee that if the body is dying that the body's largest organ, the skin, can be kept intact. As a patient becomes weaker, she will at some point become unable to get out of bed. In many cases, turning the patient may cause as much discomfort as the formation of a bedsore. The patient may become so weak that he or she can't even get up to use the bathroom. Adult diapers are frequently needed. All of these factors increase the already high risk of developing pressure ulcers.

Gurgling Noises

Laymen sometimes refer to gurgling noises as the *death rattle*. As the person becomes more lethargic, the ability to swallow effectively and cough up secretions is lost. Saliva is then pooled in the back of the throat. At the same time, the lips become quite dry and chapped. Good mouth care is quite helpful. Medications such as a scopolamine patch can be given to decrease the amount of mouth secretions. Other alternatives to scopolamine are hyoscyamine or atropine drops.

Difficulty Breathing

Many times you will see the person gasping for air. This can be quite distressing to watch. It can also cause much anxiety for the patient, especially if she is alert. Very low doses of morphine are often helpful. In other cases oxygen therapy may help. The goal here is to minimize suffering. If the patient is very anxious, low doses of Ativan or Xanax can be used.

Pain

Pain is the symptom that patients fear most about dying. Many patients with cancer have severe pain as the tumor invades organs, bones, and other tissues. Other patients may have pain as a result of being confined to a bed. While hospitals are great at delivering the latest medical care, their mattresses are often not that comfortable.

Nevertheless, we treat pain very aggressively for the dying patient. Nonsteroidal anti-inflammatory drugs are often helpful in cases that involve bone pain. Narcotics are commonly used to treat the pain that dying patients are facing. We do not worry about the problem of addiction at this stage of the game.

Even if the patient is too weak to swallow pills, we have several effective alternatives:

- inhaled morphine vapor
- morphine rectal suppositories
- morphine that can be applied under the tongue
- narcotic skin patches

Nausea

Many things can cause a person to become nauseous. Medications, such as chemotherapy agents and narcotics, are common causes of nausea. Fortunately, this can be treated with a variety of medications:

- metoclopramide (Reglan)
- ondansetron (Zofran)
- promethazine (Phenergan)

Delirium

Many patients become quite confused during this stage. Low-dose antipsychotics or benzodiazepines are often used to help relax the patient.

COPING WITH THE LOSS OF A LOVED ONE

You may have heard people say that when a person dies, the surviving spouse is at a higher risk of dying within the following months. The **real truth** is that something like this is hard to measure scientifically. However, it would be naive of us not to acknowledge that the death of a spouse is one of the most painful experiences that a person will ever face. This is one of the main reasons why hospice services provide psychological support to loved ones even after the death of a loved one.

SOME PARTING THOUGHTS

When regulators are assessing nursing homes, they often focus on the facility's ability to restore the health of the individual. Some overlook the fact that many nursing home residents have incurable diseases that will progress in severity. Many would easily qualify for hospice services. In other words, the nursing homes are expected to stabilize or even fix up patients who will die no matter what is done. Instead of letting nature take its course, the homes often become quite aggressive with the use of tube feeding, intravenous fluids, and hospitalization. The nursing homes must do this in order to document that they have "tried to prevent" bedsores, malnutrition, dehydration, falls, and so on.

THINGS YOU CAN DO TO HELP!

- Be willing to spend time listening to your loved one.
- Help the healthcare provider understand what the patient would define as an "acceptable" or "unacceptable" quality of life.
- Encourage good communication with the healthcare team.
- Be willing to talk to the healthcare provider about dying and the patient's expressed wishes.

The point of this chapter is not to scare you or frighten you. Rather, our goal is to provide you with an understanding of what to expect and what can be done to try to make the dying process more comfortable. Remember that there are many highly trained healthcare professionals who will be able to help guide you and your family through this difficult journey.

Afterword
MOVING ON

"Life is a dash between two numbers on a tombstone. It takes 250 million sperms to fertilize an egg. We are all winning sperms. We won the lottery. If one other sperm or egg joined together, we would not experience this wonderful journey on earth . . . so enjoy the dash."

Neil Shulman, MD

There are many beliefs about the afterlife—religious, spiritual, and individual. We all are entitled to our own answers or non-answers. Psychologists, philosophers, and preachers have all described the various mental states one experiences when dying. They have also offered many ways to approach the various stages of mourning the loss of a loved one. One thing is obvious: our ancestors and forebears want us to make the best of our dash. They wouldn't want our lives to end just because theirs have. Whether we or our loved ones have a short dash or a long dash, all dashes are gifts. If you are ever having a difficult day, stop in your tracks, pat yourself on the back, and say, "I'm a winning egg and sperm!"

If you can find some way to be creative, help others, and laugh at yourself, it will go a long way in helping you enjoy the gift of life. When we're feeling weighed down by the uncontrollable, we all need to find ways to feel empowered in our own lives. Creativity is one valuable tool for this. We all need to let new creativity rise from the ashes of our grieving. The dash of life is too short for you to be confined by the fear of rejection or failure. Instead, focus on the challenge of creating an eternal piece of yourself to leave for those who follow in your footsteps, whether it be a work of art, a collection of poems, a novel, a new dance step, a therapeutic technique, an invention or discovery, or a belief system.

In addition to creative self-expression, it is infinitely rewarding to feel you can have a positive impact in others' lives. It's relatively easy to help other people, whether matching up a couple, feeding the homeless, assisting an elderly person, or comforting someone during a psychological crisis. Not only is it easy to do, but it makes life easier for you in times of suffering. Getting your mind off of your own suffering by helping someone else is something you DO have control over, which makes you feel less overwhelmed by your own problems. Taking on personal challenges like playing a sport or playing chess can also help you feel better, whether physically or mentally. Again, you're diverting your attention elsewhere, to positive ends.

When you can't avoid the circumstances that upset you, look for ways of seeing the humor in the situation. It's a fact that if you can laugh about something, you're going to feel much more comfortable about it.

Of course, most of us also need to focus on work so we can have resources to live, but the process of thinking about money all day can narrow our minds, making us forget about our time and good deeds. If the focus on money becomes an unnecessary extreme, then the joys of life are needlessly tossed aside. The self-esteem that is tied to accumulating wealth is precarious, at best. On the other hand, a life rich with meaningful experiences gives one an unshakeable sense of well-being and self-confidence.

We hope that as you or your loved ones approach your later years, you will continue to value your dash and move through suffering and sorrow with your creativity and sense of purpose intact. One of the most remarkable traits of the human species is our ability to adapt. When confronted with great adversity, we often feel we will not be able to survive it . . . but somehow, most of the time, we do. Throughout the ages people have again and again lost loved ones who meant the world to them and then ultimately bounced back, found their world again, and went on living. We encourage you to remember this wonderful human legacy of which we are all a part.

We have written this book with one goal in mind. We want to help elders to be as healthy as possible and to be empowered to deal with the aging process. We are aging ourselves. The opportunity to research the literature and share the lessons we have learned from our own patients has improved our dashes. We thank our readers for passing on the advice in this book to others.

We hope that by demystifying the process of aging, and by providing practical advice, we have had an impact on many dashes. Hail to keeping those dashes as healthy and upbeat as possible.

ENDNOTES

CHAPTER 1

1. *Merriam-Webster's Online Dictionary*, http://www.merriam-webster.com/dictionary/aging (accessed July 1, 2008).

2. Bruce R. Troen, "The Biology of Aging," *Mount Sinai Journal of Medicine* 79, no. 1 (January 2003): 3–21.

3. Pier G. Pelicci, "Do Tumor-Suppressive Mechanisms Contribute to Organism Aging by Inducing Stem Cell Senescence?" *Journal of Clinical Investigation* 113, no. 1 (January 1, 2004): 4–7.

4. Maris Kuningas et al., "Genes Encoding Longevity: From Model Organisms to Humans," *Aging Cell* 7, no. 2 (April 2008): 270–80.

5. Bruce R. Troen and Donald A. Jurivich, "Biology," *Geriatric Review Syllabus*, 6th ed., ed. Peter Pompei and John B. Murphy (New York: American Geriatric Society, 2006), pp. 8–16.

6. Steven Austad, "Advances in Vertebrate Aging Research 2007," *Aging Cell* 7, no. 2 (April 2008): 119–24.

7. Madlyn I. Frisard et al., "Aging, Resting Metabolic Rate and Oxidative Damage: Results from the Louisiana Healthy Aging Study," *Journal of Gerontology: Medical Sciences* 62A, no. 7 (2007): 752–59.

8. Troen and Jurivich, *Geriatric Review Syllabus*.

9. Mark H. Beers et al., "Age-Old Questions," *Merck Manual for Health and Aging* (Whitehouse Station, NJ: Merck Research Laboratories, 2004), pp. 1–6.

10. Robert L. Kane et al., "Clinical Implications of the Aging Process," *Essentials of Clinical Geriatrics*, 5th ed. (New York: McGraw-Hill, 2004), pp. 3–16.

CHAPTER 2

1. Robert L. Kane et al., "Clinical Implications of the Aging Process," *Essentials of Clinical Geriatrics*, 5th ed. (New York: McGraw-Hill, 2004), pp. 3–16.

2. J. D. Pearson et al., "Age-Associated Changes in Blood Pressure in a Longitudinal Study of Healthy Men and Women," *Journal of Gerontology* 52A, no. 3 (May 1997): M177–M183.

3. T. Peter Stein and Douglas R. Bolster, "Insights into Muscle Atrophy and Recovery Pathway Based on Genetic Models," *Current Opinion in Clinical Nutrition and Metabolic Care* 9, no. 4 (July 2006): 395–402.

4. Ali A. Rizvi, "Management of Diabetes in Older Adults," *American Journal of the Medical Sciences* 333, no. 1 (January 2007): 35–47.

5. Alan J. Sinclair and Simon C. M. Croxson, "Diabetes Mellitus," in *Brocklehurst's Textbook of Geriatric Medicine and Gerontology*, 6th ed., ed. Raymond C. Tallis and Howard M. Fillit (London: Churchill Livingstone, 2003), pp. 1193–1218.

6. Raul Raz and Walter E. Stamm, "A Controlled Trial of Intravaginal Estriol in Postmenopausal Women with Recurrent Urinary Tract Infections," *New England Journal of Medicine* 329, no. 11 (September 9, 1993): 753–56.

7. Bruce R. Troen and Donald A. Jurivich, "Biology," *Geriatric Review Syllabus*, 6th ed., ed. Peter Pompei and John B. Murphy (New York: American Geriatric Society, 2006), pp. 8–16.

8. Joëlle Nafziger et al., "Decreased Erythropoietin Responsiveness to Iron Deficiency Anemia in the Elderly," *American Journal of Hematology* 43, no. 3 (July 1993): 172–76.

9. David Sarraf and Anne L. Coleman, "Visual Impairment," in *Geriatric Review Syllabus*, 6th ed., ed. Peter Pompei and John B. Murphy (New York: American Geriatric Society, 2006), pp. 149–55.

10. Ibid.

11. Ibid.

12. Akshay Bagai, Paaladinesh Thavendiranathan, and Allan S. Dentsky, "Does This Patient Have Hearing Impairment?" *Journal of the American Medical Association* 295, no. 4 (January 25, 2006): 416–28.

13. Ibid.

14. Ibid.

15. Ibid.

16. Ibid.

CHAPTER 3

1. Kim T. B. Knoops et al., "Mediterranean Diet, Lifestyle Factors, and 10-Year Mortality in Elderly European Men and Women," *Journal of the American Medical Association* 292, no. 12 (September 22/29, 2004): 1433–39.

2. American Cancer Society, "Can Prostate Cancer Be Found Early?" June 14, 2007, http://www.cancer.org/docroot/CRI/content/CRI_2_4_3X_Can_prostate _cancer_be_found_early_36.asp?sitearea (accessed August 4, 2008).

3. US Preventive Services Task Force, "Screening for Prostate Cancer: US Preventive Services Task Force Recommendation Statement," *Annals of Internal Medicine* 149, no. 3 (August 5, 2008): 185–99.

4. Sylvia K. Oboler et al., "Public Expectations and Attitudes for Annual Physical Examinations and Testing," *Annals of Internal Medicine* 136, no. 9 (May 2002): 652–59.

5. Fredric C. Blow, "Substance Abuse among Older Adults. Treatment Improvement Protocol (TIP) Series 26," DHHS pub. no. (SMA) 98–3179, US Department of Abuse and Mental Health Services Administration, Center for Substance Abuse Treatment, 1998.

6. Kristin L. Nichol et al., "Influenza Vaccination and Reduction in Hospitalizations for Cardiac Disease and Stroke among the Elderly," *New England Journal of Medicine* 348, no. 14 (April 3, 2003): 1322–32.

7. US Preventive Services Task Force, "Screening for Breast Cancer," http:// www.ahrq.gov/clinic/uspstf/uspsbrca.htm (accessed July 2, 2008).

8. Brian D. Badgwell et al., "Mammography before Diagnosis among Women Age 80 Years and Older with Breast Cancer," *Journal of Clinical Oncology* 26, no. 15 (May 10, 2008): 1–8.

9. Christiane K. Kuhl et al., "MRI for Diagnosis of Pure Ductal Carcinoma In Situ: A Prospective Observational Study," *Lancet* 370, no. 9586 (August 11, 2007): 485–92.

10. Louise C. Walter et al., "PSA Screening among Elderly Men with Limited Life Expectancies," *Journal of the American Medical Association* 296, no. 19 (November 15, 2006): 2336–42.

11. US Preventive Services Task Force, *Annals of Internal Medicine* 149, no. 3 (August 5, 2008): 185–99.

12. Walter et al., "PSA Screening among Elderly Men with Limited Life Expectancies."

13. Theodore R. Levin et al., "Complications of Colonoscopy in an Integrated Health Care Delivery System," *Annals of Internal Medicine* 145, no. 12 (December 19, 2006): 880–86.

14. US Preventive Services Task Force, "Screening for Lung Cancer," http://www.ahrq.gov/clinic/us[stfis[s;img/htm (accessed July 2, 2008).

15. International Early Lung Cancer Action Program Investigators, "Survival of Patients with Stage-1 Lung Cancer Detected on CT Screening," *New England Journal of Medicine* 355, no. 17 (October 26, 2006): 1763–71.

16. Radiology Info, "Is Whole-Body CT Screening Worthwhile?" http://www .radiolgyinfo.org/en/news/newdetarget.cfm?id=5 (accessed July 10, 2008).

17. David J. Brenner and Eric J. Hall, "Computed Tomography—An Increasing Source of Radiation Exposure," *New England Journal of Medicine* 357, no. 22 (November 29, 2007): 2277–84.

CHAPTER 4

1. Eugenia Chan, "Quality of Efficacy Research in Complementary and Alternative Medicine," *New England Journal of Medicine* 299, no. 2 (June 11, 2008): 2685–88.

2. National Center for Biotechnology Information, "PubMed," www.pubmed .gov (accessed August 18, 2008).

CHAPTER 5

1. Thomas H. Perls, Neal R. Reisman, and S. Jay Olshansky, "Provision or Distribution of Growth Hormone for 'Anti-aging,'" *Journal of the American Medical Association* 294, no. 16 (October 26, 2005): 2086–90; S. Jay Olshansky and Thomas T. Perls, "New Developments in the Illegal Provision of Growth Hormone for 'Anti-aging' and Bodybuilding," *Journal of the American Medical Association* 299, no. 23 (June 18, 2008): 2792–94.

2. US Food and Drug Administration, "Warning Letter from FDA to Genentech," August 23, 2003, http://www.fda.gov/cder/warn/2003/11522.pdf (accessed May 4, 2008).

3. Daniel Rudman et al., "Effects of Human Growth Hormone in Men over 60 Years Old," *New England Journal of Medicine* 323, no. 1 (July 5, 1990): 1–6.

4. Marc R. Blackman et al., "Growth Hormone and Sex Steroid Administration in Healthy Aged Women and Men," *Journal of the American Medical Association* 288, no. 18 (November 13, 2002): 2282–92.

5. Ibid.

6. Patrick Maison et al., "Growth Hormone as Risk for Premature Mortality in Healthy Subjects: Data from the Paris Prospective Study," *British Medical Journal* 316, no. 7138 (April 11, 1998): 1132–33.

7. Giuseppe Paolisso et al., "Serum Levels of Insulin-Like Growth Factor-I (IGF-I) and IGF—Binding Protein-3 in Healthy Centenarians: Relationship with Plasma Leptin and Lipid Concentrations, Insulin Action, and Cognitive Function," *Journal of Clinical Endocrinology and Metabolism* 82, no. 7 (July 1997): 2204–2209.

8. Yousin Suh et al., "Functionally Significant Insulin-Like Growth Factor 1 Receptor Mutations in Centenarians," *Proceedings of the National Academy of Sciences* 105, no. 9 (March 4, 2008): 3438–42.

9. Jukka Takala et al., "Increased Mortality Associated with Growth Hormone Treatment in Critically Ill Adults," *New England Journal of Medicine* 341, no. 11 (September 9, 1999): 785–92.

10. Mohammed Kazi, Stephen A. Geraci, and Christian A. Koch, "Considerations for the Diagnosis and Treatment of Testosterone Deficiency in Elderly Men," *American Journal of Medicine* 120, no. 10 (October 2007): 835–40.

11. K. Sreekumarn Nair et al., "DHEA in Elderly Women and DHEA or Testos-

terone in Elderly Men," *New England Journal of Medicine* 355, no. 16 (October 19, 2006): 1647–49.

12. Lise Mazat et al., "Prospective Measurement of Dehydroepiandrosterone Sulfate in a Cohort of Elderly Subjects: Relationship to Gender, Subjective Health, Smoking Habits and 10-Year Mortality," *Proceedings of the National Academy of Sciences* 98, no. 14 (July 3, 2001): 8145–50.

13. Nair et al., "DHEA in Elderly Women and DHEA or Testosterone in Elderly Men."

14. Donna Kritz-Silverstein et al., "Effects of Dehyroepiandrosterone Supplementation on Cognitive Function and Quality of Life: The DHEA and Well-Ness (DAWN) Trial," *Journal of the American Geriatric Society* 56, no. 7 (July 2008): 1292–98.

CHAPTER 6

1. NIH State-of-the-Science Panel, "National Institutes of Health State-of-the-Science Conference Statement: Multivitamin/Mineral Supplements and Chronic Disease Prevention," *Annals of Internal Medicine* 145, no. 5 (September 5, 2006): 364–71.

2. Ibid.

3. Goran Bjelakovic et al., "Antioxidant Supplements for Prevention of Mortality in Healthy Participants and Patients with Various Diseases," *Cochrane Database of Systemic Reviews* 2 (2008).

4. Brian D. Lawenda et al., "Should Supplemental Antioxidant Administration Be Avoided during Chemotherapy and Radiation Therapy?" *Journal of the National Cancer Institute* 100, no. 11 (May 27, 2008): 773–83.

5. NIH State-of-the-Science Panel, "National Institutes of Health State-of-the-Science Conference Statement."

6. Lydia A. Bazzano et al., "Effect of Folic Acid Supplementation on Risk of Cardiovascular Diseases: A Meta-analysis of Randomized Controlled Trials," *Journal of the American Medical Association* 296, no. 22 (December 13, 2006): 2720–26.

7. F. Michael Gloth, "The ABD's of Long-Term Care: A Review of the Use of Some Vitamin Supplements in the LTC Setting," *Annals of Long-Term Care* 16, no. 2 (February 2008): 28–32.

8. Stephen Sander et al., "The Impact of Coenzyme Q10 on Systolic Function in Patients with Chronic Heart Failure," *Journal of Cardiac Failure* 12, no. 6 (August 2006): 464–72.

9. Cynthia A. Weber and Michael E. Ernst, "Antioxidants, Supplements, and Parkinson's Disease," *Annals of Pharmacotherapy* 40, no. 5 (May 2006): 935–38.

10. Joanna M. Young et al., "Effect of Coenzyme Q10 Supplementation on Simvastatin-Induced Myalgia," *American Journal of Cardiology* 100, no. 9 (November 1, 2007): 1400–1403.

11. Larry C. Clark et al., "Nutritional Prevention of Cancer Study Group. Effects

of Selenium Supplementation for Cancer Prevention in Patients with Carcinoma of the Skin. A Randomized Controlled Trial," *Journal of the American Medical Association* 276, no. 24 (December 25, 1996): 1957–63.

12. Saverio Stranges et al., "Effects of Long-Term Selenium Supplementation on the Incidence of Type 2 Diabetes," *Annals of Internal Medicine* 147, no. 4 (August 21, 2007): 217–23.

13. Scott M. Lippman et al., "Effect of Selenium and Vitamin E on Risk of Prostate Cancer and Other Cancers Selenium and Vitamin E Cancer Prevention Trial (SELECT)," *Journal of the American Medical Association* 301, no. 1 (January 7, 2009): 39–51.

14. E. Paul Cherniak, Hermes J. Florez, and Bruce R. Troen, "Emerging Therapies to Treat Frailty Syndrome in the Elderly," *Alternative Medicine Review* 12, no. 3 (September 2007): 246–58.

15. Phillippe Autier and Sara Gandini, "Vitamin D Supplementation Decreases All-Cause Mortality in Adults and Older Individuals," *Archives of Internal Medicine* 167, no. 16 (September 10, 2007): 1730–37.

16. Joel A. Simon, *ACP Journal Club* 148, no. 2 (March/April 2008): 30.

17. Age-Related Eye Disease Study Group, "A Randomized, Placebo-Controlled, Clinical Trial of High-Dose Supplementation with Vitamins C, and E, Beta Carotene, and Zinc for Age-Related Macular Degeneration and Vision Loss: AREDS Report no. 8," *Archives of Ophthalmology* 119, no. 10 (October 2001): 1417–36.

18. Bruce Arroll, "Non-antibiotic Treatments for Upper-Respiratory Tract Infections (Common Cold)," *Respiratory Medicine* 99, no. 12 (December 2005): 1477–84.

19. Jacqueline Birks and J. Evans Grimley, "Ginkgo Biloba for Cognitive Impairment and Dementia," *Cochrane Database of Systematic Reviews* 2 (2008).

20. Benjamin W. Beckert, "The Effect of Herbal Medicines on Platelet Function: An In Vivo Experiment and Review of the Literature," *Plastic and Reconstructive Surgery* 120, no. 7 (December 2007): 2044–50.

21. Naghma Khan and Hasan Mukhtar, "Tea Polyphenols for Health Promotion," *Life Sciences* 81, no. 7 (July 26, 2007): 519–33.

22. Shinichi Kuriyama et al., "Green Tea Consumption and Mortality Due to Cardiovascular Disease, Cancer, and All Causes in Japan: The Ohsaki Study," *Journal of the American Medical Association* 296, no. 10 (September 13, 2006): 1255–65.

23. John H. Lee et al., "Omega-3 Fatty Acids for Cardioprotection," *Mayo Clinic Proceedings* 83, no. 3 (March 2008): 324–32.

24. Ibid.

25. Daniel O. Clegg et al., "Glucosamine, Chondroitin Sulfate, and the Two in Combination for Painful Knee Osteoarthritis," *New England Journal of Medicine* 354, no. 8 (February 23, 2006): 795–808.

26. Ibid.

27. National Osteoporosis Foundation, "National Osteoporosis Foundation's Updated Recommendations for Calcium and Vitamin D Intake," July 26, 2007, http://www.nof.org/prevention/calcium_and_VitaminD.htm (accessed August 19, 2008).

28. Ramon Estruch et al., "Effects of a Mediterranean-Style Diet on Cardiovascular Risk Factors," *Annals of Internal Medicine* 145, no. 1 (July 4, 2006): 1–11.

29. I. Dilova, E. Easlon, and S. J. Lin, "Calorie Restriction and the Nutrient Sensing Signaling Pathways," *Cellular and Molecular Life Sciences* 64, no. 6 (March 2007): 752–67.

30. Leonard Guarente, "Mitochondria—A Nexus for Aging, Calorie Restriction, and Sirtuins?" *Cell* 132, no. 2 (January 25, 2008): 171–75.

31. George S. Roth et al., "Aging in Rhesus Monkeys: Relevance to Human Health Interventions," *Science* 305, no. 5689 (September 3, 2004): 1423–26.

32. Arthur V. Everitt and David G. LeCouteur, "Life Extension by Calorie Restriction in Humans," *Annals of the New York Academy of Science* 1114 (2007): 428–33.

33. Joseph A. Baur and David Sinclair, "Therapeutic Potential of Resveratrol: The In Vivo Evidence," *Nature Reviews* 5 (June 2006): 493–506.

34. Jamie L. Barger et al., "A Low Dose of Dietary Resveratrol Partially Mimics Caloric Restriction and Retards Aging Parameters in Mice," *PLoS ONE* 3, no. 6 (June 2008): e2264.

CHAPTER 7

1. National Institute on Aging, *Exercise: A Guide from the National Institute on Aging*, NIH pub. no. 01-4258 (2008), http://www.nia.nih.gov/HealthInformation/Publications/ExerciseGuide (accessed March 23, 2008).

2. Nancy K. Latham et al., "Systematic Review of Progressive Resistance Strength Training in Older Adults," *Journal of Gerontology* 59A, no. 1 (2004): 48–61.

3. Alexander Voukelatos et al., "A Randomized, Controlled Trial of Tai Chi for the Prevention of Falls: The Central Sydney Tai Chi Trial," *Journal of the American Geriatrics Society* 55, no. 8 (August 2007): 1185–91.

CHAPTER 8

1. US Department of Health and Human Services, "Medicare Prescription Drug Plan Finder," http://www.medicare.gov/MPDPF (accessed August 1, 2008).

2. Social Security Online, "What You Should Know about the Medicare Prescription Drug Plans," http://www.ssa.gov/pubs/10126.html (accessed July 10, 2008).

3. John Hsu et al., "Medicare Beneficiaries' Knowledge of Part D Prescription Drug Program Benefits and Responses to Drug Costs," *Journal of the American Medical Association* 299, no. 16 (April 23/30, 2008): 1929–36.

4. Board of Trustees of the Federal Hospital Insurance and Federal Supplementary Medical Insurance Trust Funds, "2008 Annual Report," March, 25, 2008, www.cms.hhs.gov/ReportsTrustFunds/downloads/tr2008.pdf (accessed August 21, 2008).

5. Center for Drug Evaluation and Research, "Preventable Adverse Drug Reactions: A Focus on Drug Interactions," July 31, 2002, http://www.fda.gov/CDER/DRUG/drugReactions/default.htm (accessed August 19, 2008).

6. S. L. Gray et al., "Adverse Drug Events in Hospitalized Elderly," *Journal of Gerontology: Biological Sciences* 53A, no. 1 (January 1998): M59–M63.

7. Donna M. Fick et al., "Updating the Beers Criteria for Potentially Inappropriate Medication Use in Older Adults," *Archives of Internal Medicine* 163, no. 18 (October 13, 2003): 2716–24.

8. Ibid.

9. Nabil S. Kamel and Julie K. Gammack, "Insomnia in the Elderly: Cause, Approach, and Treatment," *American Journal of Medicine* 119, no. 6 (June 2006): 463–69.

10. David J. Greenblatt, Jerold S. Harmatz, and Richard I. Shader, "Clinical Pharmacokinetics of Anxiolytics and Hypnotics in the Elderly," *Clinical Pharmacokinetics* 21, no. 3 (1991): 165–77.

11. David J. Greenblatt, Jerold S. Harmatz, Richard I. Shader, "Clinical Pharmacokinetics of Anxiolytics and Hypnotics in the Elderly," *Clinical Pharmacokinetics* 21, no. 4 (1991): 262–73.

12. Melinda J. Barker et al., "Persistence of Cognitive Effects after Withdrawal from Long-Term Benzodiazepine Use: A Meta-analysis," *Archives of Clinical Neuropsychology* 19, no. 3 (April 2004): 437–54.

13. Adam G. Golden et al., "Inappropriate Medication Prescribing in Homebound Older Adults," *Journal of the American Geriatrics Society* 47, no. 8 (August 1999): 948–53.

14. Fick et al., "Updating the Beers Criteria for Potentially Inappropriate Medication Use in Older Adults."

15. T. Sunderland et al., "Anticholinergic Sensitivity in Patients with Dementia of the Alzheimer Type and Age-Matched Controls. A Dose-Response Study," *Archives of General Psychiatry* 44, no. 5 (May 1987): 418–26.

16. Fick et al., "Updating the Beers Criteria for Potentially Inappropriate Medication Use in Older Adults."

17. Ibid.

18. Dima M. Qato et al., "Use of Prescription and Over-the-Counter Medications and Dietary Supplements among Older Adults in the United States," *Journal of the American Medical Association* 300, no. 24 (December 24/31, 2008) 2867–78.

19. Fick et al., "Updating the Beers Criteria for Potentially Inappropriate Medication Use in Older Adults."

20. Saunjoo L. Yoon and Susan D. Schaffer, "Herbal, Prescribed, and Over-the-Counter Drug Use in Older Women: Prevalence of Drug Interactions," *Geriatric Nursing* 27, no. 2 (March/April 2006): 118–29.

21. American Association of Retired People, "Complementary and Alternative Medicine: What People 50 and Older Are Using and Discussing with Their Physicians," http://assets.aarp.org/rgcenter/health/cam_2007.pdf (accessed June 28, 2008).

CHAPTER 9

1. National Center for Healthcare Statistics, "Life Expectancy," http://209.217 .72.34/aging/Reportfolders/Reportfolders.aspx?IFActivePathName=PTLife %expectancy (accessed August 19, 2008).

2. Ibid.

3. US Census Bureau, "Table 1. Annual Estimates of the Population by Sex and Five-Year Age Groups for the United States: April 1, 2000 to July 1, 2007," NC-EST2007-01, http://www.census.gov/popest/national/asrh/NC-EST2007-sa.html (accessed April 18, 2008).

4. US Census Bureau, "National Population Projections," 2008, www.census.gov/ population/www/projections/files/nation/summary/np2008-t12.xls (accessed August 19, 2008).

5. US Census Bureau, "Table 1. Annual Estimates of the Population by Sex and Five-Year Age Groups for the United States."

6. US Census Bureau, "National Population Projections."

7. US Census Bureau, "Table 1. Annual Estimates of the Population by Sex and Five-Year Age Groups for the United States."

8. US Census Bureau, "National Population Projections."

9. Kevin Kinsella and David R. Phillips, "Global Aging: The Challenge of Success," *Population Bulletin* 60, no. 1 (Washington, DC: Population Reference Bureau, 2005), http://www.prb.org/pdf05/60.1GlobalAging.pdf (accessed June 14, 2008).

10. Joseph H. Flaherty et al., "China: The Aging Giant," *Journal of the American Geriatrics Society* 55, no. 8 (August 2007): 1295–1300.

11. Kinsella and Phillips, "Global Aging."

12. Ibid.

13. Ibid.

14. Ibid.

15. Paul S. Mueller, Christopher Hook, and Kevin C. Fleming, "Ethical Issues in Geriatrics: A Guide for Clinicians," *Mayo Clinic Proceedings* 79 (April 2004): 554–62.

16. Joseph S. Alpert and Pamela J. Powers, "Who Will Care for the Frail Elderly?" *American Journal of Medicine* 120, no. 6 (June 2007): 469–71.

17. Agency for Healthcare Research and Quality, *2007 National Healthcare Disparities Report*, AHRQ pub. no. 08-0041.P67 (Rockville, MD: US Department of Health and Human Services, Agency for Healthcare Research and Quality, February 2008).

18. Mark H. Beers et al., "The Aging of America," in *Merck Manual for Health and Aging* (Whitehouse Station, NJ: Merck Research Laboratories, 2004), pp. 1–6.

19. US Department of Health and Human Services, "Table 99. Discharges and Average Length of Stay in Non-Federal Short-Stay Hospitals, according to Sex, Age, and Selected First-Listed Diagnoses: United States, Selected Years 1990–2003," http://www.ncbi.nlm.nih.gov/books/bv.fcgi?indexed=google&rid=healthus05.table.44 7 (accessed July 15, 2008).

20. Centers for Medicare and Medicaid Services, "Medicare Coverage of Skilled Nursing Facility Care," pub. no. CMS 10153, April 2002, http://www.medicare .gov/publications/pubs/pdf/snf.pdf (accessed June 23, 2008).

21. Centers for Medicare and Medicaid Services, "Fact Sheets—CMS Announces Medicare Premiums, Deductibles for 2008," October 1, 2007, http:// www.cms.hhs.gov/pf/printpage.asp?ref (accessed August 21, 2008).

22. Agency for Health Care Administration, "Florida Medicaid Nursing Homes, July 2008 Rate Semester Initial Per Diems," http://www.fdhc.state.fl.us/ Medicaid/cost_reim/pdf/2008_07_initial_rates.pdf (accessed August 20, 2008).

23. Jack M. Colwill, James M Cultice, and Robin L. Kruse, "Will Generalist Physician Supply Meet Demands of an Increasing and Aging Population?" *Health Affairs* 27, no. 3 (April 2008): W232–W241.

24. National Institute on Aging, "Talking with Your Doctor," http:// www.niapublications.org/pubs/talking/Talking_with_your_Doctor.pdf (accessed May 18, 2008).

25. American Board of Internal Medicine, "Candidates Certified," http:// www.abim.org/about/examInfo/data-candidates-certified.asp (accessed July 21, 2008).

26. Ibid.

27. Thomas Bodenheimer, "Coordinating Care: A Major (Unreimbursed) Task of Primary Care," *Annals of Internal Medicine* 147, no. 10 (November 2007): 730–31.

CHAPTER 10

1. Jennifer L. Wolff and Debra L. Roter, "Hidden in Plain Sight—Medical Visit Companions as a Resource for Vulnerable Older Adults," *Archives of Internal Medicine* 168, no. 13 (July 14, 2008): 1409–15.

2. National Institute on Aging, "Talking with Your Doctor," http://www.nia publications.org/pubs/talking/Talking_with_your_Doctor.pdf (accessed May 18, 2008).

CHAPTER 11

1. Charlene Harrington, "Nursing Home Staffing Standards," Henry J. Kaiser Family Foundation, June 2002, www.kff.org (accessed June 4, 2008).

2. Sally C. Stearns and Laura P. D'Arcy, "Staying the Course: Facility and Profession Retention among Nursing Home Assistants in Nursing Homes," *Journal of Gerontology* 63B, no. 3 (May 2008): S113–S121.

3. Donna Gates, Evelyn Fitzwater, and Paul Succop, "Reducing Assaults against Nursing Home Caregivers," *Nursing Research* 53, no. 2, (March/April 2005): 119–27.

CHAPTER 12

1. Henry J. Kaiser Family Foundation, "Views about the Quality of Long-Term Care Services in the United States," pub. no. 7719, December 2007, www.kff.org (accessed July 21, 2008).

2. Consumer Reports, "Nursing Homes: Business as Usual," September 2006, http://www.consumerreports.org/cro/health-fitness/health-care/nursing-homes-9-06/overview/0609_nursing-homes_ov.htm?EXTKEY=SP72F00&CMP=KNC-CROYPIHEALTH&HBX_OU=51&HBX_PK=pi (accessed July 14, 2008).

3. Charlene Harrington, "Nursing Home Staffing Standards," Kaiser Commission on Medicaid and the Uninsured, June 2002, http://www.kff.org/medicaid/loader .cfm?url=/commonspot/security/getfile.cfm&PageID=14106 (accessed June 30, 2008).

4. Mercedes Bern-Klug and Sarah Forbes-Thompson, "Family Member's Responsibilities to Nursing Home Residents," *Journal of Gerontological Nursing* 34, no. 2 (February 2008): 43–52.

5. Agency for Health Care Administration, "Florida Medicaid Nursing Homes, July 2008 Rate Semester Initial Per Diems," http://www.fdhc.state.fl.us/Medicaid/cost_reim/pdf/2008_07_initial_rates.pdf (accessed August 20, 2008).

6. Robert L. Kane, "Assuring Quality in Nursing Home Care," *Journal of the American Geriatric Society* 46, no. 2 (February 1998): 232–37.

7. Medicare, "Nursing Home Compare," www.medicare.gov/nhcompare/home.asp (accessed June 1, 2008).

8. "Nursing Home Guide," www.consumerreports.org/nursinghomes (accessed March 18, 2008).

CHAPTER 13

1. Leslie A. Wei et al., "The Confusion Assessment Method: A Systematic Review of Current Usage," *Journal of the American Geriatrics Society* 56, no. 5 (May 2008): 823–30.

2. Mark H. Beers et al., "Delirium," in *Merck Manual for Health and Aging* (Whitehouse Station, NJ: Merck Research Laboratories, 2004), pp. 300–306.

3. Donna M. Fick and Lorraine C. Milon, "Delirium Superimposed on Dementia," *American Journal of Nursing* 108, no. 1 (January 2008): 52–60.

4. Dylan Harris, "Delirium in Advanced Disease," *Postgraduate Medicine Journal* 83 (2007): 525–28.

5. John G. Canto et al., "Atypical Presentations among Medicare Beneficiaries with Unstable Angina Pectoris," *American Journal of Cardiology* 90, no. 3 (August 1, 2002): 248–53.

6. Wilbert S. Aronow et al., "Prevalence of and Association between Silent

Myocardial Ischemia and New Coronary Events in Older Men and Women with and without Cardiovascular Disease," *Journal of the American Geriatric Society* 50, no. 6 (June 2002): 1075–78.

7. Frédéric Aubrun and Frédéric Marmion, "The Elderly Patient and Postoperative Pain Treatment," *Best Practice & Research Clinical Anaesthesiology* 21, no. 1 (2006): 109–27.

8. Donald P. Kotler, "Cachexia," *Annals of Internal Medicine* 133, no. 8 (October 17, 2000): 622–34.

CHAPTER 14

1. David A. Ganz et al., "Will My Patient Fall?" *Journal of the American Medical Association* 297, no. 1 (January 3, 2007): 77–86.

2. Ibid.

3. Ray Freeman, "Neurogenic Orthostatic Hypotension," *New England Journal of Medicine* 358, no. 6 (February 7, 2008): 615–24.

4. Sirpa Hartikainen, Eija Lönnroos, and Kirsti Louhivuori, "Medication as a Risk Factor for Falls: Critical Systematic Review," *Journal of Gerontology* 62A, no. 10 (October 2007): 1172–81.

5. Ibid.

6. Allan F. Tencer, "Biomechanical Properties of Shoes and Risk of Falls in Older Adults," *Journal of the American Geriatrics Society* 52, no. 11 (November 2004): 1840–46.

7. Alexander Voukelatos et al., "A Randomized, Controlled Trial of Tai Chi for the Prevention of Falls: The Central Sydney Tai Chi Trial," *Journal of the American Geriatrics Society* 55, no. 8 (August 2007): 1185–91.

8. Wayne A. Ray et al., "A Randomized Trial of a Consultation Service to Reduce Falls in Nursing Homes," *Journal of the American Medical Association* 278, no. 7 (August 20, 1997): 557–62; Jane Jensen et al., "Fall and Injury Prevention in Older People Living in Residential Care Facilities: A Cluster Randomized Trial," *Annals of Internal Medicine* 136, no. 10 (May 21, 2002): 733–41; Kimberly Rask et al., "Implementation and Evaluation of a Nursing Home Fall Management Program," *Journal of the American Geriatric Society* 55, no. 3 (2007): 342–49.

9. Pekka Kannus and Jari Parkkari, "Hip Protectors for Preventing Hip Fracture," *Journal of the American Medical Association* 298, no. 4 (July 25, 2007): 454–55.

CHAPTER 15

1. B. Lawrence Riggs and L. Joseph Melton, "Involutional Osteoporosis," *New England Journal of Medicine* 314, no. 26 (June 26, 1986): 1676–86.

2. Angela M. Cheung and Allan S. Detsky, "Osteoporosis and Fractures: Missing

the Bridge?" *Journal of the American Medical Association* 299, no. 12 (March 26, 2008): 1468–70.

3. Ibid.

4. Consuelo H. Wilkins and Stanley J. Birge, "Prevention of Osteoporotic Fractures in the Elderly," *American Journal of Medicine* 118, no. 11 (November 2005): 1190–95; Hosam K. Kamel, "Update on Osteoporosis Management in Long-Term Care: Focus on Bisphosphonates," *Journal of the American Medical Directors Association* 8, no. 7 (September 2007): 434–40.

5. Susan M. Ott, "Osteoporosis and Osteomalacia," in *Principles of Geriatric Medicine and Gerontology*, 4th ed., ed. William R. Hazzard et al. (New York: McGraw-Hill, 1999) pp. 1057–84.

6. Deborah M. Kado, Katherine Prenovost, and Carolyn Crandall, "Narrative Review: Hyperkyphosis in Older Persons," *Annals of Internal Medicine* 147, no. 5 (September 4, 2007): 330–38.

7. Robert G. W. Lambert, "Vertebroplasty for Osteoporotic Vertebral Fracture," *British Medical Journal* 336 (June 7, 2008): 1261–62.

8. Mark H. Beers, "Fractures," in *Merck Manual of Health and Aging* (Whitehouse Station, NJ: Merck Research Laboratories, 2004), pp. 268–84; Richard Keen, "Osteoporosis: Strategies for Prevention and Management," *Best Practice & Research Clinical Rheumatology* 21, no. 1 (2007): 109–22.

9. Keen, "Osteoporosis."

10. Edward R. Marcantonio et al., "Reducing Delirium after Hip Fracture: A Randomized Trial," *Journal of the American Geriatric Society* 49, no. 5 (May 2001): 516–22.

11. National Osteoporosis Foundation, "Osteoporosis Medications," http://www.nof.org/patientinfo/medications.htm (accessed August 18, 2008).

12. Ibid.

13. Ibid.

14. Keen, "Osteoporosis."

15. Ibid.

16. Eli Lilly, "Evista Prescribing Information," http://pi.lilly.com/us/evista-pi-pdf (accessed August 18, 2008).

17. National Osteoporosis Foundation, "Osteoporosis Medications."

18. Ibid.

19. Ibid.

20. Ibid.

21. Benjamin M. Tang et al., "Use of Calcium or Calcium in Combination with Vitamin D Supplementation to Prevent Fractures and Bone Loss in People Age 50 Years and Older: A Meta-analysis," *Lancet* 370, no. 9588 (August 25/31, 2007): 657–66.

CHAPTER 16

1. Allie J. Turton and Elizabeth Britton, "A Pilot Randomized Controlled Trial of a Daily Muscle Stretch Regime to Prevent Contractures in the Arm after a Stroke," *Clinical Rehabilitation* 19 (2005): 600–12.

2. Scott E. Rand et al., "The Physical Therapy Prescription," *American Family Physician* 76, no. 11 (December 1, 2007): 1661–66.

3. Kathleen Kline Mangione et al., "Interventions Used by Physical Therapists in Home Care for People after Hip Fracture," *Physical Therapy* 88, no. 2 (February 2008): 199–210.

4. Mark H. Beers, "Fractures," in *Merck Manual of Health and Aging* (Whitehouse Station, NJ: Merck Research Laboratories, 2004), pp. 268–84.

5. Ellen F. Binder et al., "Effects of Extended Outpatient Rehabilitation after Hip Fracture," *Journal of the American Medical Association* 292, no. 7 (August 18, 2004): 837–46.

CHAPTER 17

1. Helen Hoenig, "Assistive Technology and Mobility Aids for the Older Patient with Disability," *Annals of Long-Term Care* 12, no. 9 (2004): 12–19.

2. Ibid.

3. Ibid.

4. Ibid

5. ABLEDATA, "Products," http://www.abledata.com/abledata.cfm?pageid =19327&ksectionid=19327 (accessed August 17, 2008).

CHAPTER 18

1. Thomas T. Yoshikawa, "Antimicrobial Resistance and Aging: Beginning of the End of the Antibiotic Era?" *Journal of the American Geriatric Society* 50, no. S6 (January 2002): S206–S209.

2. Kevin P. High, "Infection in the Elderly," *Principles of Geriatric Medicine and Gerontology*, 4th ed., ed. William R. Hazzard et al. (New York: McGraw-Hill, 1999), pp. 1443–54.

3. Irving H. Gomolin, Paula Lester, and Simcha Pollack, "Older Is Colder: Observations on Body Temperature among Nursing Home Subjects," *Journal of the American Medical Directors Association* 8, no. 5 (June 2007): 335–37.

4. High, "Infection in the Elderly."

5. Jane Siegel et al., "Guideline for Isolation Precautions: Preventing Transmission of Infectious Agents in Healthcare Settings," June 2007, http://www.cdc.gov/ ncidod/dhqp/pdf/isolation2007.pdf (accessed April 8, 2008).

6. Priya Sampathkumar, "Methicillin-Resistant Staphylococcus Aureus: The Latest Health Scare," *Mayo Clinic Proceedings* 82, no. 12 (December 2007): 1463–67.

7. Sanjay Saint et al., "Condom versus Indwelling Urinary Catheters: A Randomized Trial," *Journal of the American Geriatric Society* 54, no. 7 (July 2006): 1055–61.

8. Jen-Hau Chen, "Occurrence and Treatment of Suspected Pneumonia in Long-Term Care Residents Dying with Advanced Dementia," *Journal of the American Geriatrics Society* 54, no. 2 (February 2006): 290–95.

9. Takeyoshi Yoneyama et al., "Oral Care Reduces Pneumonia in Older Patients in Nursing Homes," *Journal of the American Geriatric Society* 50, no. 3 (March 2002): 430–33.

10. Anne Moscona, "Neuraminidase Inhibitors for Influenza," *New England Journal of Medicine* 353, no. 13 (September 29, 2005): 1363–73.

11. Ibid.

12. Warren R. Heymann, "The Herpes Zoster Vaccine," *Journal of the American Academy of Dermatology* 58, no. 5 (2008): 872–73.

13. M. N. Oxman, "A Vaccine to Prevent Herpes Zoster and Postherpetic Neuralgia in Older Adults," *New England Journal of Medicine* 352, no. 22 (June 2, 2005): 2271–84.

14. Advisory Committee on Immunization Practices, "Recommended Adult Immunization Schedule: United States, October 2007–September 2008," *Annals of Internal Medicine* 147, no. 10 (November 2007): 725–29.

15. Maxwell M. Chait, "The New Era of *C. difficile*–Associated Diarrhea," *Annals of Long-Term Care* 16, no. 7 (July 2008): 25–31.

16. Ibid.

17. Mary C. Vritis, "The *Clostridium difficile* Epidemic: A Potential Disaster for Long-Term Care," *Annals of Long-Term Care* 16, no. 7 (July 2008): 19–24.

18. Ibid.

CHAPTER 19

1. Mark H. Beers et al., "Nutritional Disorders," in *Merck Manual for Health and Aging* (Whitehouse Station, NJ: Merck Research Laboratories, 2004), pp. 199–213.

2. Claire Murphy et al., "Prevalence of Olfactory Impairment in Older Adults," *Journal of the American Medical Association* 288, no. 18 (November 13, 2002): 2307–12.

3. Donald P. Kotler, "Cachexia," *Annals of Internal Medicine* 133, no. 8 (October 17, 2000): 622–34.

4. Adam G. Golden et al., "University of Miami Division of Clinical Pharmacology Therapeutic Rounds: Medications Used to Treat Anorexia in the Frail Elderly," *American Journal of Therapeutics* 10, no. 4 (July/August 2003): 292–98.

5. Alan Shenkin, "Serum Prealbumin: Is It a Marker of Nutritional Status or of Risk of Malnutrition?" *Clinical Chemistry* 52, no. 12 (December 2006): 2177–79.

6. Cathy Gaillard et al., "Are Elderly Hospitalized Patients Getting Enough Protein?" *Journal of the American Geriatrics Society* 56, no. 6 (June 2008): 1045–49.

7. Sandra F. Simmons, Dan Osterweil, and John F. Schnelle, "Improving Food Intake in Nursing Home Residents with Feeding Assistance: A Staffing Analysis," *Journal of Gerontology: Medical Sciences* 56A, no. 12 (2001): M790–M794; Sanda F. Simmons and John F. Schnelle, "Feeding Assistance Needs of Long-Stay Nursing Home Residents and Staff Time to Provide Care," *Journal of the American Geriatrics Society* 54, no. 6 (June 2006): 919–24.

8. David R. Thomas et al., "Understanding Clinical Dehydration and Its Treatment," *Journal of the American Medical Directors Association* 9, no. 5 (June 2008): 292–301.

9. Maria A. Fiatarone et al., "Exercise Training and Nutritional Supplementation for Physical Frailty in Very Elderly People," *New England Journal of Medicine* 330, no. 25 (June 23, 1994): 1769–75.

10. Rajesambhaji Borade et al., "Nutritional Supplements Do Not Always Work," *Long-Term Care Interface* 8, no. 1 (January/February 2007): 26–30.

11. Matthew D. Parrott, Karen W. H. Young, and Carol E. Greenwood, "Energy-Containing Nutritional Supplements Can Affect Usual Energy Intake Postsupplementation in Institutionalized Seniors with Probable Alzheimer's Disease," *Journal of the American Geriatric Society* 54, no. 9 (September 2006): 1382–87.

12. Donna A. Fick, "Updating the Beers Criteria for Potentially Inappropriate Medication Use in Older Adults," *Archives of Internal Medicine* 163, no. 22 (December 8/22, 2003): 2716–24.

13. Shing-Shing Yeh, Sherri Lovitt, and Michael W. Schuster, "Pharmacological Treatment of Geriatric Cachexia: Evidence and Safety in Perspective," *Journal of the American Medical Directors Association* 8, no. 6 (July 2007): 363–77.

14. Shing-Shing Yeh et al., "Improvement in Quality-of-Life Measures and Stimulation of Weight Gain after Treatment with Megestrol Acetate Oral Suspension in Geriatric Cachexia: Results of a Double-Blind, Placebo-Controlled Study," *Journal of the American Geriatrics Society* 48, no. 5 (May 2000): 485–92; David B. Reuben et al., "The Effects of Megestrol Acetate Suspension for Elderly Patients with Reduced Appetite after Hospitalization: A Phase II Randomized Clinical Trial," *Journal of the American Geriatrics Society* 53, no. 6 (June 2005): 970–75.

15. Dennis H. Sullivan et al., "Effects of Muscle Strength Training and Megestrol Acetate on Strength, Muscle Mass and Function in Frail Older People," *Journal of the American Geriatrics Society* 55, no. 1 (January 2007): 20–28.

16. Shing-Shing Yeh et al., "Improvement in Quality-of-Life Measures and Stimulation of Weight Gain after Treatment with Megestrol Acetate Oral Suspension in Geriatric Cachexia."

17. Ibid.

18. Dennis H. Sullivan et al., "Effects of Muscle Strength Training and Megestrol Acetate on Strength, Muscle Mass and Function in Frail Older People."

19. Adam G. Golden et al., "University of Miami Division of Clinical Pharmacology Therapeutic Rounds."

CHAPTER 20

1. Donald Garrow et al., "Feeding Alternatives in Patients with Dementia: Examining the Evidence," *Clinical Gastroenterology and Hepatology* 5, no. 12 (December 2007): 1372–78.

2. American Medical Association, *Policy E-2.20: Withholding or Withdrawing Life-Sustaining Medical Treatment*, http://www.ama-assn.org/apps/pf_new/pf_online (accessed May 30, 2008).

3. Donald Garrow et al., "Feeding Alternatives in Patients with Dementia: Examining the Evidence"; Thomas E. Finucane, Colleen Christmas, and Kathy Travis, "Tube Feeding in Patients with Advanced Dementia," *Journal of the American Medical Association* 282, no. 14 (October 13, 1999): 1365–70.

4. Joseph W. Shega et al., "Barriers to Limiting the Practice of Feeding Tube Placement in Advanced Dementia," *Journal of Palliative Medicine* 6, no. 6 (December 2003): 885–93.

5. Garrow et al., "Feeding Alternatives in Patients with Dementia: Examining the Evidence."

6. Shai Gavi et al., "Management of Feeding Tube Complications in the Long-Term Care Resident," *Annals of Long-Term Care* 16, no. 4 (April 2008): 28–32.

CHAPTER 21

1. Rebecca G. Rogers, "Urinary Stress Incontinence in Women," *New England Journal of Medicine* 358, no. 10 (March 6, 2008): 1029–36.

2. Ibid.

3. Tatyana A. Shamliyan et al., "Systemic Review: Randomized, Controlled Trials of Nonsurgical Treatments for Urinary Incontinence in Women," *Annals of Internal Medicine* 148, no. 6 (March 18, 2008): 459–73.

4. Rogers, "Urinary Stress Incontinence in Women."

5. Charlotte Kelly, "Estrogen and Its Effect on Vaginal Atrophy in Postmenopausal Women," *Urologic Nursing* 27, no. 1 (February 2007): 40–46.

6. Shamliyan et al., "Systemic Review."

7. Nancy Krieger et al., "Hormone Replacement Therapy, Cancer, Controversies, and Women's Health: Historical Epidemiological, Biological, Clinical, and Advocacy Perspectives," *Journal of Epidemiology and Community Health* 59 (September 2005): 740–48.

8. John D. McConnell et al., "The Long-Term Effect of Doxazosin, Finasteride, and Combination Therapy on the Clinical Progression of Benign Prostatic Hyperplasia," *New England Journal of Medicine* 349, no. 25 (December 18, 2003): 2387–98.

9. S. Bent, C. Kane, K. Shinohara et al., "Saw Palmetto for Benign Prostatic Hyperplasia," *New England Journal of Medicine* 354 (2006): 557–66.

10. Mary H. Wilde and Kathyrn Getliffe, "Urinary Catheter Care for Older Adults," *Annals of Long-Term Care* 14, no. 8 (August 2006): 38–42.

11. Sanjay Saint et al., "Condom versus Indwelling Urinary Catheters: A Randomized Trial," *Journal of the American Geriatric Society* 54, no. 7 (July 2006): 1055–61.

CHAPTER 22

1. Jürgen Untüzer, "Late Life Depression," *New England Journal of Medicine* 357, no. 22 (November 29, 2007): 2269–76.

2. Wayne Katon et al., "Impact of Antidepressant Drug Adherence on Comorbid Medication Use and Resource Utilization," *Archives of Internal Medicine* 165, no. 21 (November 28, 2005): 2497–2503.

3. Mugdha Thakur and Dan G. Blazer, "Depression in Long-Term Care," *Journal of the American Medical Directors Association* 9, no. 2 (February 2008): 82–87.

4. Untüzer, "Late Life Depression."

5. Wan He et. al., "Social and Other Characteristics, '65+ in the United States,'" in *Current Population Reports* (Washington, DC: US Government Printing Office, 2005), pp. 145–82.

6. Sheldon H. Preskorn, "Reproducibility of the In Vivo Effect of the Selective Serotonin Reuptake Inhibitors on the In Vivo Function of Cytochrome P450 2D6: An Update (part II)," *Journal of Psychiatric Practice* 9, no. 3 (May 2003): 228–35.

7. Untüzer, "Late Life Depression"; Thakur and Blazer, "Depression in Long-Term Care."

8. Ibid.

9. Untüzer, "Late Life Depression."

10. Ibid.

11. Ibid.

12. Ibid.

CHAPTER 23

1. Mark H. Beers et al., "Dementia," *Merck Manual for Health and Aging* (Whitehouse Station, NJ: Merck Research Laboratories, 2004), pp. 306–25.

2. Susan L. Mitchell, "A 93-Year-Old Man with Advanced Dementia and Eating Problems," *Journal of the American Medical Association* 298, no. 21 (December 5, 2007): 2527–36.

3. Ibid.

4. Thomas D. Bird, "Genetic Aspects of Alzheimer's Disease," *Genetic Medicine* 10, no. 4 (April 2008): 231–39.

5. Ibid.

6. Ibid.

7. Daniel Weintraub and Howard I. Hurtig, "Presentation and Management of Psychosis in Parkinson's Disease and Dementia with Lewy Bodies," *American Journal of Psychiatry* 164, no. 10 (October 2007): 1491–98.

8. Kenneth M. Langa, Norman L. Foster, and Eric B. Larson, "Mixed Dementia-Emerging Concepts and Therapeutic Implications," *Journal of the American Medical Association* 292, no. 23 (December 15, 2004): 2901–2908.

9. Marvin Bergsneider, "Surgical Management of Idiopathic Normal-Pressure Hydrocephalus," *Neurosurgery* 57, no. 3 (September 2005): S2-29–S2-39.

10. Cynthia Barton et al., "Dementia," in *Geriatric Review Syllabus*, 6th ed., ed. Peter Pompei and John B. Murphy (New York: American Geriatrics Society, 2006), pp. 221–30.

11. Michele L Ries et al., "Magnetic Resonance Imaging Characterization of Brain Structure and Function in Mild Cognitive Impairment: A Review," *Journal of the American Geriatrics Society* 56, no. 5 (May 2008): 920–34.

12. Amir Qaseem et al., "Current Pharmacologic Treatment of Dementia: A Clinical Practice Guideline from the American College of Physicians and the American Academy of Family Physicians," *Annals of Internal Medicine* 148, no. 5 (March 4, 2008): 370–78.

13. Hanna Kaduszkiewicz et al., "Cholinesterase Inhibitors for Patients with Alzheimer's Disease: Systemic Review of Randomized Clinical Trials," *British Medical Journal* 331, no. 7512 (August 6, 2005): 321–27.

14. Parminder Raina et al., "Effectiveness of Cholinesterase Inhibitors and Memantine for Treating Dementia: Evidence Review for a Clinical Practice Guideline," *Annals of Internal Medicine* 148, no. 5 (March 4, 2008): 379–97.

15. Pierre N. Tariot et al., "Memantine Treatment in Patients with Moderate to Severe Alzheimer Disease Already Receiving Donepezil: A Randomized Controlled Trial," *Journal of the American Medical Association* 291, no. 3 (January 21, 2004): 317–24.

16. Parminder Raina, et al., "Effectiveness of Cholinesterase Inhibitors and Memantine for Treating Dementia."

17. Jacqueline Birks and J. Evans Grimley, "Ginkgo Biloba for Cognitive Impairment and Dementia," *Cochrane Database of Systematic Reviews* 2 (2008).

18. Benjamin W. Beckert, "The Effect of Herbal Medicines on Platelet Function: An In Vivo Experiment and Review of the Literature," *Plastic and Reconstructive Surgery* 120, no. 7 (December 2007): 2044–50.

19. Antonio Cheubini et al., "Low Plasma N-3 Fatty Acids and Dementia in Older Persons: The InCHIANTI Study," *Journal of Gerontology* 62A, no. 10 (October 2007): 1120–26.

20. Shelly L. Gray et al., "Antioxidant Vitamin Supplement Use and Risk of Dementia or Alzheimer's Disease in Older Adults," *Journal of the American Geriatrics Society* 56, no. 2 (February 2008): 291–96.

21. NIH State-of-the-Science Panel, "National Institutes of Health State-of-the-

Science Conference Statement: Multivitamin/Mineral Supplements and Chronic Disease Prevention," *Annals of Internal Medicine* 145, no. 5 (September 5, 2006): 364–71.

22. Sally A. Shumaker et al., "Conjugated Equine Estrogens and Incidence of Probable Dementia and Mild Cognitive Impairment in Postmenopausal Women," *Journal of the American Medical Association* 291, no. 4 (June 23/30, 2004): 2947–58; Ruth A. Mulnard et al., "Estrogen Replacement Therapy for Treatment of Mild to Moderate Alzheimer Disease: A Randomized Controlled Trial," *Journal of the American Medical Association* 283, no. 8 (February 23, 2000): 1007–15.

23. C. Cramer et al., "Use of Statins and Incidence of Dementia and Cognitive Impairment without Dementia in a Cohort Study," *Neurology* 71, no. 5 (July 29, 2008): 344–50.

24. Z. Arvanitakis et al., "Statins, Incident Alzheimer Disease, Change in Cognitive Function, and Neuropathology," *Neurology* 70, no. 19 (May 6, 2008): 1795–1802.

25. Amarilis Acevedo and David A. Lowenstein, "Nonpharmacological Cognitive Interventions in Aging and Dementia," *Journal of Geriatric Psychiatry and Neurology* 20, no. 4 (December 2007): 239–49.

26. James Butcher, "Mind Games—Do They Work?" *British Journal of Medicine* 336 (February 2, 2008): 246–48.

27. Acevedo and Lowenstein, "Nonpharmacological Cognitive Interventions in Aging and Dementia."

28. Mitchell, "A 93-Year-Old Man with Advanced Dementia and Eating Problems."

CHAPTER 24

1. Clive Ballard et al., "Atypical Antipsychotics for Aggression and Psychosis in Alzheimer's Disease," *Cochrane Database of Systematic Reviews* 2 (2008).

2. American Psychiatric Association, "Practice Guideline for the Treatment of Patients with Alzheimer's Disease and Other Dementias, Second Edition," *American Journal of Psychiatry* 164, no. 12 (December 2007).

3. US Department of Health and Human Services, *Alzheimer's Disease: Unraveling the Mystery*, NIH pub. no. 02-3782 (Washington, DC: US Department of Health and Human Services, 2002).

4. Pierre N. Tariot et al., "Divalproex Sodium in Nursing Home Residents with Possible or Probable Alzheimer Disease Complicated by Agitation: A Randomized, Controlled Trial," *American Journal of Geriatric Psychiatry* 13, no. 11 (November 2005): 942–49.

5. Robert J. Howard et al., "Donepezil for the Treatment of Agitation in Alzheimer's Disease," *New England Journal of Medicine* 357, no. 14 (October 4, 2007): 1382–92.

6. Dilip V. Jeste et al., "Atypical Antipsychotics in Elderly Patients with Dementia

or Schizophrenia: Review of Recent Literature," *Harvard Review Psychiatry* 13, no. 6 (November/December 2005): 340–51.

7. Ibid.

8. Lori S. Schneider et al., "Effectiveness of Atypical Antipsychotic Drugs in Patients with Alzheimer's Disease," *New England Journal of Medicine* 355, no. 15 (October 12, 2006): 1525–38.

9. Dilip V. Jeste et al., "Atypical Antipsychotics in Elderly Patients with Dementia or Schizophrenia."

10. Ibid.; US Food and Drug Administration, "Risperdal (Risperidone)," http://www.fda.gov/medwatch/safety/2005/aug_PI/Risperdal_Oral_PI.pdf (accessed August 15, 2008).

11. Dilip V. Jeste et al., "Atypical Antipsychotics in Elderly Patients with Dementia or Schizophrenia."

12. Patricia R. Recupero and Samara E. Rainey, "Managing Risk when Considering the Use of Atypical Antipsychotics for Elderly Patients with Dementia-Related Psychosis," *Journal of Psychiatric Practice* 13, no. 3 (May 2007): 143–52.

13. Dilip V. Jeste et al., "Atypical Antipsychotics in Elderly Patients with Dementia or Schizophrenia"; Donna A. Fick, "Updating the Beers Criteria for Potentially Inappropriate Medication Use in Older Adults," *Archives of Internal Medicine* 163, no. 22 (December 8/22, 2003): 2716–24.

14. Recupero and Rainey, "Managing Risk when Considering the Use of Atypical Antipsychotics for Elderly Patients with Dementia-Related Psychosis."

15. Ann Kolanowski et al., "Spouses of Persons with Dementia: Their Healthcare Problems, Utilization, and Costs," *Research in Nursing & Health* 27 (2004): 296–306.

CHAPTER 25

1. J. Brandon Birath and Jennifer L. Martin, "Common Sleep Problems Affecting Older Adults," *Annals of Long-Term Care* 15, no. 2 (December 2007): 20–26.

2. Ibid.

3. Ibid.

4. Carlos A. Vaz Fragoso and Thomas M. Gill, "Sleep Complaints in Community-Living Older Persons: A Multifactorial Geriatric Syndrome," *Journal of the American Geriatric Society* 55, no. 11 (November 2007): 1853–66.

5. Eric Ball and Christine K. Caivano, "Internal Medicine: Guidance to the Diagnosis and Management of Restless Legs Syndrome," *Southern Medical Journal* 101, no. 6 (June 2008): 631–34.

6. Scott S. Campbell, Patricia J. Murphy, and Thomas N. Stauble, "Effects of a Nap on Nighttime Sleep and Waking Function in Older Subjects," *Journal of the American Geriatrics Society* 53, no. 1 (January 2005): 48–53.

7. Phillip D. Sloane, Mariana Figueiro, and Lauren Cohen, "Light as Therapy for

Sleep Disorders and Depression in Older Adults," *Clinical Geriatrics* 16, no. 3 (March 2008): 25–32.

8. Melinda J. Barker et al., "Cognitive Effects of Long-Term Benzodiazepine Use: A Meta-analysis," *CNS Drugs* 18, no. 1 (January 2004): 37–48.

9. David J. Greenblatt, Jerold S. Harmatz, and Richard I. Shader, "Clinical Pharmacokinetics of Anxiolytics and Hypnotics in the Elderly," *Clinical Pharmacokinetics* 21, no. 3 (1991): 165–77.

10. Nabil S. Kamel and Julie K. Gammack, "Insomnia in the Elderly: Cause, Approach, and Treatment," *American Journal of Medicine* 119, no. 6 (June 2006): 463–69.

11. Esa R. Korpi, Gerhard Gründer, and Hartmut Lüddens, "Drug Interactions at GABA$_A$ Receptors," *Progress in Neurobiology* 67, no. 2 (June 2002): 113–59.

12. Kamel and Gammack, "Insomnia in the Elderly: Cause, Approach, and Treatment."

13. James K. Walsh, Christina Soubrane, and Thomas Roth, "Efficacy and Safety of Zolpidem Extended Release in Elderly Primary Insomnia Patients," *American Journal of Geriatric Psychiatry* 16, no. 1 (January 2008): 44–57.

14. Kamel and Gammack, "Insomnia in the Elderly: Cause, Approach, and Treatment."

15. Ibid.

16. Altun and B. Uger-Altun, "Melatonin: Therapeutic and Clinical Utilization," *Clinical Practice* 61, no. 5 (May 2007): 835–45.

17. Nina Buscemi et al., "Efficacy and Safety of Exogenous Melatonin for Secondary Sleep Disorders and Sleep Disorders Accompanying Sleep Restriction: Meta-analysis," *BMJ* 332, no. 7538 (February 18, 2006): 385–93.

18. Barbara J. Messinger-Rapport et al., "Intensive Session: New Approaches to Medical Issues in Long-Term Care," *Journal of the American Medical Directors Association* 8, no. 7 (September 2007): 421–33.

19. US Drug Enforcement Administration, "Drug Scheduling," http://www.usdoj.gov/dea/pubs/scheduling.html (accessed on August 14, 2008).

CHAPTER 26

1. Department of Health and Human Services (DHHS) Centers for Medicare and Medicaid Services, "CMS Manual System, State Operations Provider Certification," pub. no. 100-07, October 20, 2006, www.cms.hhs.gov/transmittals/downloads/R21SOMA.pdf (accessed August 19, 2008).

2. Jeffrey M. Levine, "Preparing for the New Medicare Reimbursement Guidelines: Part 1—When Are Pressure Ulcers in the Hospital Avoidable?" *Clinical Geriatrics* 16, no. 6 (June 2008): 19–24.

3. Robert A. Norman, "Common Skin Conditions in Geriatric Dermatology," *Annals of Long-Term Care* 16, no. 6 (June 2008): 40–45.

4. Richard Allman, "Pressure Ulcers," in *Principles of Geriatric Medicine and Gerontology*, 4th ed., ed. William R. Hazzard et al. (New York: McGraw-Hill, 1999), pp. 1577–84.

5. Ibid.

6. Ibid.; Agency for Health Care Policy and Research, *Treatment of Pressure Ulcers: Clinical Guideline Number 15* (Washington, DC: US Department of Health and Human Services, 1994).

7. Madhuri Reddy, Sudeep S. Gill, and Paula A. Rochon, "Preventing Pressure Ulcers: A Systemic Review," *Journal of the American Medical Association* 296, no. 8 (August 23/30, 2007): 974–84.

8. T. Young, "The 30 Degree Tilt Position vs. the 90 Degree Lateral and Supine Positions in Reducing the Incidence of Non-blanching Erythema in a Hospital Inpatient Population: A Randomized Controlled Trial," *Journal of Tissue Viability* 14, no. 3 (2004): 88, 90, 92–96.

9. Reddy, Gill, and Rochon, "Preventing Pressure Ulcers: A Systemic Review."

10. Katherine R. Jones and Kristopher Fennie, "Factors Influencing Pressure Ulcer Healing in Adults over 50: An Exploratory Study," *Journal of the American Medical Directors Association* 8, no. 6 (July 2007): 378–87.

11. David L. Steed, "Clinical Evaluation of Recombinant Human Platelet-Derived Growth Factor for the Treatment of Lower Extremity Ulcers," *Plastic and Reconstructive Surgery* 117, no. 7 (2006): 143S–149S.

12. Katherine J. Desneves et al., "Treatment with Supplementary Arginine, Vitamin C, and Zinc in Patients with Pressure Ulcers: A Randomized Controlled Trial," *Clinical Nutrition* 24, no. 6 (December 2005): 979–87.

13. Paul Takahashi et al., "Wound Care Technologies: Emerging Evidence for Appropriate Use in Long-Term Care," *Annals of Long-Term Care* 15, no. 11 (November 2007): 35–40.

CHAPTER 27

1. J. D. Bradley et al., "Comparison of an Anti-inflammatory Dose of Ibuprofen, an Analgesic Dose of Ibuprofen, and Acetaminophen in the Treatment of Patients with Osteoarthritis of the Knee," *New England Journal of Medicine* 325, no. 2 (July 11, 1991): 87–91.

2. M. J. Yelland et al., "Celecoxib Compared with Sustained-Release Paracetamol for Osteoarthritis: A Series of N-of-1 Trials," *Rheumatology* 46, no. 1 (January 2007): 135–40.

3. Lucina M. Jackson and Christopher J. Hawkey, "COX-2 Selective Nonsteroidal Anti-inflammatory Drugs," *Drugs* 59, no. 6 (June 2000): 1207–16.

4. Luis Alberto García Rodríguez et al., "Risk of Hospitalization for Upper Gastrointestinal Tract Bleeding Associated with Ketorolac, Other Nonsteroidal Anti-

inflammatory Drugs, Calcium Antagonists, and Other Antihypertensive Drugs," *Archives of Internal Medicine* 158, no. 1 (January 12, 1998): 33–39.

5. Claire Bombardier et al., "Comparison of Upper Gastrointestinal Toxicity of Rofecoxib and Naproxen in Patients with Rheumatoid Arthritis," *New England Journal of Medicine* 343, no. 21 (November 23, 2000): 1520–28.

6. John K. Jenkins, "Analysis and Recommendations for Agency Action regarding Non-steroidal Anti-inflammatory Drugs and Cardiovascular Risk," US Food and Drug Administration, Office of New Drugs, April 6, 2005.

7. Bombardier et al., "Comparison of Upper Gastrointestinal Toxicity of Rofe-coxib and Naproxen in Patients with Rheumatoid Arthritis."

8. Jackson and Hawkey, "COX-2 Selective Nonsteroidal Anti-inflammatory Drugs."

9. Donna M. Fick et al., "Updating the Beers Criteria for Potentially Inappropriate Medication Use in Older Adults," *Archives of Internal Medicine* 163, no. 22 (December 8/22, 2003): 2716–24.

10. R. A. Moore et al., "Quantitive Systematic Review of Topically Applied Nonsteroidal Anti-inflammatory Drugs," *BMJ* 316, no. 7 (January 31, 1998): 333–38.

11. Josef Zacher et al., "Topical Diclofenac and Its Role in Pain and Inflammation: An Evidence-Based Review," *Current Medical Research and Opinion* 24, no. 4 (April 2008): 925–50.

12. Scott E. Rand et al., "The Physical Therapy Prescription," *American Family Physician* 76, no. 11 (December 1, 2007): 1661–66.

13. Daniel O. Clegg et al., "Glucosamine, Chondroitin Sulfate, and the Two in Combination for Painful Knee Osteoarthritis," *New England Journal of Medicine* 354, no. 8 (February 23, 2006): 795–808.

14. John Distler and Amanda Anguelouch, "Evidence-Based Practice: Review of Clinical Evidence on the Efficacy of Glucosamine and Chondroitin in the Treatment of Osteoarthritis," *Journal of the American Academy of Nurse Practitioners* 18, no. 10 (October 2006): 487–93.

15. Robert J. Goldberg and Joel Katz, "A Meta-analysis of the Analgesic Effects of Omega-3 Polyunsaturated Fatty Acid Supplementation for Inflammatory Joint Pain," *Pain* 129, nos. 1–2 (May 2007): 210–23.

16. Frederic Aubrun and Frederic Marmion, "The Elderly Patient and Postoperative Pain Treatment," *Best Practices & Research Clinical Anaesthesiology* 21, no. 1 (March 2007): 109–27.

17. Ibid.

18. Robert Barkin, "Extended-Release Tramadol (Ultram ER): A Pharmacotherapeutic, Pharmacokinetic, and Pharmacodynamic Focus on Effectiveness and Safety in Patients with Chronic/Persistent Pain," *American Journal of Therapeutics* 15, no. 2 (March/April 2008): 157–68.

19. Ibid.

20. Fick et al., "Updating the Beers Criteria for Potentially Inappropriate Medication Use in Older Adults."

21. Rand et al., "The Physical Therapy Prescription."

22. Nassim P. Assefi et al., "A Randomized Clinical Trial of Acupuncture Compared with Sham Acupuncture in Fibromyalgia," *Annals of Internal Medicine* 143, no. 1 (July 5, 2005): 10–19.

23. Michael Haake et al., "German Acupuncture Trials (GERAC) for Chronic Low Back Pain: Randomized, Multicenter, Blinded, Parallel-Group Trial with 3 Groups," *Archives of Internal Medicine* 167, no. 17 (September 24, 2007): 1892–98; Hanns-Peter Schaff et al., "Acupuncture and Knee Osteoarthritis: A Three-Armed Randomized Trial," *Annals of Internal Medicine* 145, no. 1 (July 4, 2006): 12–20.

24. Michael T. Haneline and Gary Lewkowvich, "Identification of Internal Carotid Artery Dissection in Chiropractic Practice," *Journal of the Canadian Chiropractic Association* 48, no. 3 (September 2004): 206–10.

CHAPTER 28

1. Centers for Disease Control and Prevention, "United States Life Tables, 2003," *National Vital Statistics Reports* 15, no. 14, April 19, 2006, http://www.cdc.gov/nchs/data/nvsr/nvsr54/nvsr54_14.pdf (accessed July 7, 2008).

2. Scott Reeves, "Saving for Retirement at Any Age," Forbes.com, September 28, 2004, http://www.forbes.com/retirement/2004/09/28/cx_sr_0928retirement_2.html (accessed July 15, 2008).

3. "Falling Short," *Economist* 387, no. 8584 (June 14, 2008): 93–94.

4. Brett Arends, "The Danger in Senior Inflation," *Wall Street Journal*, March 6, 2008, http://finance.yahoo.com/focus-retirement/article/104562/The-danger-in-senior-inflation?mod=retirement-post-spending (accessed March 7, 2008).

5. Fidelity, "Fidelity Investments Estimates $225,000 Needed to Cover Retiree Health Care Costs," March 5, 2008, http://personal.fidelity.com/myfidelity/Inside Fidelity/index_NewsCenter.shtml?refhp=pr&ut=B65 (accessed March 6, 2008).

6. Henry Paulson, "Statement on the Social Security and Medicare Trust Fund Reports," US Department of the Treasury press release, March 25, 2008, www.ustreas.gov/press/releases/hp886.htm (accessed March 26, 2008).

7. MetLife Market Survey of Nursing Home & Assisted Living Costs, October 30, 2007, www.maturemarketinstitute.com (accessed August 19, 2008).

8. OASDI Trustees, "The 2008 Annual Report of the Board of Trustees of the Federal Old-Age and Survivors Insurance and Federal Disability Insurance Trust Funds," http://www.socialsecurity.gov/OACT/TR/TR08/I_intro.html#1000302 (accessed August 15, 2008).

9. Paulson, "Statement on the Social Security and Medicare Trust Fund Reports."

10. "Falling Short."

CHAPTER 29

1. Germaine L. Odenheimer, "Driving Safety in Older Adults," *Geriatrics* 61, no. 10 (October 2006): 14–21.
2. Ibid.
3. Ibid.
4. Richard M. Dubinsky, Anthony C. Stein, and Kelly Lyons, "Practice Parameter: Risk of Driving and Alzheimer's Disease (an Evidence-Based Review): Report of the Quality Standards Subcommittee of the American Academy of Neurology," *Neurology* 54 (2000): 2205–11.
5. Hartford/MIT AgeLab, "We Need to Talk ... Family Conversations with Older Drivers," http://www.thehartford.com/talkwitholderdrivers/brochure/brochure.htm (accessed February 8, 2008).

CHAPTER 30

1. S. Kuipers et al., "Travel and Venous Thrombosis: A Systematic Review," *Journal of Internal Medicine* 262, no. 6 (December 2007): 615–34.
2. Jim Waterhouse et al., "Jet Lag: Trends and Coping Strategies," *Lancet* 369 (March 31, 2007): 1117–29.

CHAPTER 31

1. Michael A. Silverman et al., "Lessons Learned from Hurricane Andrew: Recommendations for Care of the Elderly in Long-Term Care Facilities," *Southern Medical Journal* 88, no. 6 (June 1995): 603–608.
2. Ibid.
3. Ibid.

CHAPTER 32

1. David I. Shalowitz, Elizabeth Garrett-Mayer, and David Wendler, "The Accuracy of Surrogate Decision Makers," *Archives of Internal Medicine* 166, no. 5 (March 13, 2006): 493–97.
2. Howard B. Degenholtz et al., "Persistence of Racial Disparities in Advance Care Plan Documents among Nursing Home Residents," *Journal of the American Geriatric Society* 50, no. 2 (February 2002): 378–81.
3. American Medical Association's Council on Ethical and Judicial Affairs, "Policy

E-2.22 Do-Not-Resuscitate Orders," www.ama-assn.org/apps/pf_news_online?f_n =resultLink&doc=policyfiles?HnE/E-2.22.htm (accessed August 20, 2008).

4. Robert S. Kane and Edith A. Burns, "Cardiopulmonary Resuscitation Policies in Long-Term Care Facilities," *Journal of the American Geriatric Society* 45, no. 2 (February 1997): 154–57.

CHAPTER 33

1. Christopher Hogan et al., "Medicare Beneficiaries' Costs of Care in the Last Year of Life," *Health Affairs* 20, no. 4 (July/August 2001): 188–95.

2. Michelle T. Weckmann, "The Role of the Family Physician in the Referral and Management of Hospice Patients," *American Family Physician* 77, no. 6 (March 15, 2008): 807–12, 817–18.

3. Susan L. Mitchell, "A 93-Year-Old Man with Advanced Dementia and Eating Problems," *Journal of the American Medical Association* 298, no. 21 (December 5, 2007): 2527–36.

4. Weckmann, "The Role of the Family Physician in the Referral and Management of Hospice Patients."

5. Centers for Medicare and Medicaid, "Medicare Hospice Data—1998–2005," http://www.cms.hhs.gov/ProspMedicareFeeSvcPmtGen/downloads/HospiceData19 98-2005.pdf (accessed February 25, 2009).

6. H. Roeline et al., "Discomfort in Nursing Home Patients with Severe Dementia in Whom Artificial Nutrition and Hydration Is Forgone," *Archives of Internal Medicine* 165, no. 15 (August 8, 2005): 1729–35.

7. R. M. McCann et al., "Comfort Care for Terminally Ill Patients," *Journal of the American Medical Association* 272, no. 16 (October 16, 1994): 1263–66.

INDEX

ABOUT THE AUTHORS

Neil Shulman, MD, is a graduate of Emory University School of Medicine. Among his many responsibilities, he was a former medical director of Pine Knolls nursing home in Carollton, Georgia, for over twenty-three years. He is an associate professor at Emory University School of Medicine. He has authored or coauthored more than twenty-five scientific papers. He has also authored twenty-one books, including *Doc Hollywood*, which was made into a major motion picture starring Michael J. Fox. He speaks and performs comedy around the world and is "Doc Neil" in a series of television spots that have been distributed to public television stations across the United States and Canada. See www. neilshulman.com for more on Neil Shulman's books and projects.

Michael A. Silverman, MD, MPH, is a graduate of the University of Maryland School of Medicine. He is board certified in internal medicine, medical oncology, geriatric medicine, and palliative medicine. He has authored or coauthored more than fifty scientific papers and is a voluntary professor of clinical medicine at the University of Miami Miller School of Medicine. He is also a retired colonel in the US Army Reserve since 1972. He is the current president of the Florida Geriatrics Society and the medical director of the Miami Jewish Home and Hospital (one of the largest nursing homes in the Southeast and the site of Florida's Teaching Nursing Home Program).

Adam Golden, MD, MBA, is a graduate of the University of Miami School of Medicine and is board certified in internal medicine and geriatric medicine.

He was a former medical director at Medco Health Solutions and a former assistant director of the internal medicine residency program at Orlando Regional Medical Center. He is currently on staff at the Miami VA Healthcare System and is an investigator in the Miami Geriatric Research, Education, and Clinical Center (GRECC). He is an assistant professor of clinical medicine at the University of Miami Miller School of Medicine. He is a favorite among the medical students who want to learn about the special medical issues of the frail older adult patient.

MORE PRAISE FOR *THE REAL TRUTH ABOUT AGING*

"I was getting frustrated searching on the Internet for information about a particular type of hip fracture.... I gave up and went to open *The Real Truth about Aging* and it opened right to the page where there were a series of drawings of the location of different types of hip fractures that can be such an important source of disability for older people. This book is chock-full of useful information, like taking a look at nursing homes from all angles: What do the patients think? Or the staff? Are nursing homes REALLY understaffed? Why are older people on too many prescription medications? This book goes beyond the usual fluff of 'aging gracefully' books and provides real information that you can use."
    —J. Douglas Bremner, MD, author of
        Before You Take That Pill: Why the Drug Industry May Be Bad for Your Health and professor of psychiatry and radiology,
        Emory University School of Medicine

"Clearly communicating often-complex health information is more vital today than ever. *The Real Truth about Aging* empowers patients and their families to make good decisions and ask good questions about their care."
    —Cindy W. Hamilton, PharmD, ELS,
        president of the American Medical Writers Association,
        2008–2009, and Melanie Fridl Ross, MSJ, ELS,
        member of American Medical Writers Association
        Executive Committee, 2008–2009

"A well-organized, easy-to-read summary of the problems faced by all older individuals. Practical suggestions regarding drugs, home environment, nursing homes, and hospitals are presented with emphasis on the frail elderly, dementia, and chronic pain. This information should prove valuable to any elderly person wishing to understand aging and to all caregivers who need to be familiar with end-of-life issues."
    —Charles R. Hatcher Jr., MD, vice president for
        Health Affairs and director emeritus, the Robert W. Woodruff Health
        Sciences Center, Emory University, and former chair and CEO of
        Emory Healthcare, Atlanta, Georgia